Injury & Trauma Sourcebook

Learning Disabilities Sourcebook,
2nd Edition

Leukemia Sourcebook

Liver Disorders Sourcebook

Lung Disorders Sourcebook

Medical Tests Sourcebook, 2nd Edition

Men's Health Concerns Sourcebook,
2nd Edition

Mental Health Disorders Sourcebook,
3rd Edition

Mental Retardation Sourcebook

Movement Disorders Sourcebook

Muscular Dystrophy Sourcebook

Obesity Sourcebook

Osteoporosis Sourcebook

Pain Sourcebook, 2nd Edition

Pediatric Cancer Sourcebook

Physical & Mental Issues in Aging
Sourcebook

Podiatry Sourcebook, 2nd Edition

Pregnancy & Birth Sourcebook,
2nd Edition

Prostate Cancer Sourcebook

Prostate & Urological Disorders
Sourcebook

Rehabilitation Sourcebook

Respiratory Diseases & Disorders
Sourcebook

Sexually Transmitted Diseases
Sourcebook, 3rd Edition

Sleep Disorders Sourcebook,
2nd Edition

Smoking Concerns Sourcebook

Sports Injuries Sourcebook, 3rd Edition

Stress-Related Disorders Sourcebook

Stroke Sourcebook

Substance Abuse Sourcebook

Surgery Sourcebook

Thyroid Disorders Sourcebook

Transplantation Sourcebook

Traveler's Health Sourcebook

Urinary Tract & Kidney Diseases &
Disorders Sourcebook, 2nd Edition

Vegeta  **S0-AKH-394**

Women's Health Concerns Sourcebook,
2nd Edition

Workplace Health & Safety Sourcebook

Worldwide Health Sourcebook

## Teen Health Series

Abuse & Violence Information
for Teens

Alcohol Information for Teens

Allergy Information for Teens

Asthma Information for Teens

Body Information for Teens

Cancer Information for Teens

Complementary & Alternative
Medicine Information for
Teens

Diabetes Information for Teens

Diet Information for Teens,
2nd Edition

Drug Information for Teens,
2nd Edition

Eating Disorders Information
for Teens

Fitness Information for Teens

Learning Disabilities Information
for Teens

Mental Health Information for
Teens, 2nd Edition

Pegnancy Information for Teens

Sexual Health Information for
Teens

Skin Health Information for
Teens

Sports Injuries Information
for Teens

Suicide Information for Teens

Tobacco Information for Teens

# Autism
## and Pervasive
## Developmental Disorders
### SOURCEBOOK

*First Edition*

## Health Reference Series

*First Edition*

# Autism
## and Pervasive
## Developmental Disorders
## SOURCEBOOK

*Basic Consumer Health Information about Autism
Spectrum and Pervasive Developmental Disorders, Such as
Classical Autism, Asperger Syndrome, Rett Syndrome, and
Childhood Disintegrative Disorder, Including Information
about Related Genetic Disorders and Medical Problems
and Facts about Causes, Screening Methods, Diagnostic
Criteria, Treatments and Interventions, and Family and
Education Issues*

*Along with a Glossary of Related Terms, Tips for Evaluating
the Validity of Health Claims, and a Directory of Resources
for Additional Help and Information*

*Edited by*
**Sandra J. Judd**

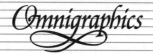

*Omnigraphics*

P.O. Box 31-1640 • Detroit, MI 48231

Bibliographic Note

Because this page cannot legibly accommodate all the copyright notices, the Bibliographic Note portion of the Preface constitutes an extension of the copyright notice.

Edited by Sandra J. Judd

*Health Reference Series*

Karen Bellenir, *Managing Editor*
David A. Cooke, M.D., *Medical Consultant*
Elizabeth Collins, *Research and Permissions Coordinator*
Cherry Stockdale, *Permissions Assistant*
EdIndex, Services for Publishers, *Indexers*

\* \* \*

Omnigraphics, Inc.

Matthew P. Barbour, *Senior Vice President*
Kay Gill, *Vice President—Directories*
Kevin Hayes, *Operations Manager*
David P. Bianco, *Marketing Director*

\* \* \*

Peter E. Ruffner, *Publisher*

Frederick G. Ruffner, Jr., *Chairman*

Copyright © 2007 Omnigraphics, Inc.

ISBN 978-0-7808-0953-6

Library of Congress Cataloging-in-Publication Data

Autism and pervasive developmental disorders sourcebook : basic consumer health information about autism spectrum and pervasive developmental disorders, such as classical autism, Asperger syndrome, Rett syndrome, and childhood disintegrative disorder, including information about related genetic disorders and medical problems and facts about causes, screening methods, diagnostic criteria, treatments and interventions, and family and education issues; along with a glossary of related terms, tips for evaluating the validity of health claims, and a directory of resources for additional help and information / edited by Sandra J. Judd. -- 1st ed.
      p. cm. -- (Health reference series)
      Summary: "Provides basic consumer health information about the causes, symptoms, and diagnosis of autism spectrum disorders, available therapies and interventions, and related conditions. Includes index, glossary, and other resources"--Provided by publisher.
      Includes bibliographical references and index.
      ISBN 978-0-7808-0953-6 (hardcover : alk. paper)  1. Autism in children--Popular works. 2. Developmental disabilities--Popular works. I. Judd, Sandra J.
      RJ506.A9A8929 2007
      618.92'85882--dc22
                                                                    2007028714

# Table of Contents

Visit www.healthreferenceseries.com to view *A Contents Guide to the Health Reference Series*, a listing of more than 13,000 topics and the volumes in which they are covered.

Preface ...................................................................................... xiii

## Part I: Understanding Autism Spectrum and Pervasive Developmental Disorders

Chapter 1—Autism and Pervasive Developmental
Disorders: What We Know ...................................... 3

Chapter 2—Who Develops Autism? ........................................... 19

Section 2.1—Is Autism on the Rise? ................ 20

Section 2.2—Why Do More Boys than
Girls Develop Autism? ................ 23

Chapter 3—Autism Spectrum Disorders: An Overview ......... 27

Chapter 4—Types of Autism Spectrum Disorders .................. 45

Section 4.1—Classical Autism ......................... 46

Section 4.2—Asperger Syndrome .................... 51

Section 4.3—Rett Syndrome ............................ 58

Section 4.4—Childhood Disintegrative
Disorder ...................................... 68

Section 4.5—Pervasive Developmental
Disorder-Not Otherwise
Specified (PDD-NOS) .................. 70

## Part II: Causes of Autism Spectrum Disorders

Chapter 5—What Causes Autism?............................................. 75

Chapter 6—Genes: One of the Suspected Causes of
Autism ................................................................. 77

Chapter 7—Autism and the Measles, Mumps, and
Rubella Vaccine: Current Evidence Does Not
Support a Link ......................................................... 89

Chapter 8—Autism and Other Environmental Exposures...... 99

Chapter 9—Immune System Problems Could Be the
Cause of Autism ...................................................... 103

Chapter 10—Abnormal Brain Development and Function
Linked to Autism .................................................... 109

  Section 10.1—Research on the Biological
Basis of Autism ........................ 110

  Section 10.2—Brain Areas Fail to Work
Together in Autism.................. 113

  Section 10.3—Autism Affects Functioning
of Entire Brain ........................ 116

  Section 10.4—Brain Regions Involving
Memory and Emotion Are
Larger in Children with
Autism ...................................... 119

  Section 10.5—Researchers Find Fewer
Neurons in the Amygdala
of Males with Autism .............. 121

  Section 10.6—Nicotine Receptors in the
Brain May Play Role in
Development of Autism ........... 123

Chapter 11—Parent, Pregnancy, and Birth Factors
Associated with Risk of Autism ........................... 127

## Part III: Conditions That May Accompany Autism Spectrum Disorders

Chapter 12—Understanding Genetic Disorders That
Occur More Frequently in People with
Autism ................................................................. 133

  Section 12.1—Tuberous Sclerosis................... 134

Section 12.2—Fragile X Syndrome ................. 146

Section 12.3—Angelman Syndrome .............. 153

Section 12.4—Landau-Kleffner Syndrome .... 155

Section 12.5—Prader-Willi Syndrome .......... 157

Section 12.6—Williams Syndrome ................ 160

Section 12.7—Tourette Syndrome ................. 163

Chapter 13—Epilepsy Often Accompanies Autism ................. 171

Chapter 14—Auditory Processing Disorder in People
with Autism .......................................................... 187

Chapter 15—Attention Deficit Hyperactivity Disorder
and Autism .......................................................... 193

Chapter 16—Exceptional Abilities in People with Autism ...... 201

Section 16.1—Hyperlexia: Exceptional
Reading Abilities in Young
Children .................................... 202

Section 16.2—Savant Syndrome: An
Extraordinary Condition ......... 205

## Part IV: Diagnosing and Evaluating Autism Spectrum Disorders

Chapter 17—Signs of Autism Spectrum Disorders ................. 213

Chapter 18—The Importance of Early Autism Diagnosis ....... 221

Chapter 19—Screening and Diagnosing Autism Spectrum
Disorders .............................................................. 225

Section 19.1—Guidelines for the Screening
and Diagnosis of Autism ......... 226

Section 19.2—Common Autism Screening
Tools and Tests ....................... 232

Section 19.3—Other Assessments Used in
the Diagnosis of Autism .......... 236

Section 19.4—Medical Tests Used in
Diagnosing and Evaluating
Autism ..................................... 248

Chapter 20—After the Diagnosis: What Comes Next? ........... 253

Section 20.1—Ten Things Parents Need
to Do after a Diagnosis of
Autism ..................................... 254

Section 20.2—Moving Forward with
        Confidence after Your Child
        Is Diagnosed with an Autistic
        Spectrum Disorder .................. 257

Section 20.3—Should You Explain the
        Diagnosis to Your Child
        with Autism or Asperger
        Syndrome? .............................. 260

## Part V: Treatments, Therapies, and Interventions for Autism Spectrum Disorders

Chapter 21—Your Child's Autism Treatment Team ................ 267

Chapter 22—Evaluating Autism Treatments: Rules of
        Thumb and Questions to Ask ............................. 271

Chapter 23—Autism Treatment Options: An Overview ......... 275

Chapter 24—Behavioral Interventions ..................................... 293

Section 24.1—Improving Behavior in
        Children with Autism
        Spectrum Disorders ................ 294

Section 24.2—Applied Behavioral Analysis
        (ABA) ...................................... 297

Section 24.3—Social Stories: Helping
        People with Autism
        Interpret Social Situations ...... 300

Chapter 25—Communication Therapies ................................... 303

Section 25.1—Communication and
        Interaction in Children with
        Autism Spectrum Disorders ... 304

Section 25.2—Picture Exchange
        Communication System .......... 314

Section 25.3—Facilitated Communication:
        A Largely Discredited
        Therapy ................................... 317

Chapter 26—Sensory Interventions ......................................... 323

Section 26.1—Sensory Integration and
        Motor Therapies ..................... 324

Section 26.2—Auditory Integration
        Training ................................... 326

Chapter 27—Dietary Interventions .............................................. 331

    Section 27.1—Diet and Vitamins in the
                Treatment of Autism ............... 332

    Section 27.2—Secretin for Autism: Hope
                and Disappointment ................. 345

    Section 27.3—Is Eliminating Casein
                and Gluten from a Child's
                Diet a Viable Treatment for
                Autism? ..................................... 348

Chapter 28—Pharmacological Interventions ............................ 355

    Section 28.1—Medications Used in the
                Treatment of Autism ............... 356

    Section 28.2—Risperdal Approved to Treat
                Irritability Associated with
                Autism ...................................... 359

    Section 28.3—Oxytocin in the Treatment
                of Repetitive Behaviors and
                Social Cognition Difficulties
                in Adults with Autistic
                Disorders ................................. 360

Chapter 29—Social Intervention Strategies ............................ 363

    Section 29.1—Son-Rise Program:
                Encouraging Love and
                Acceptance of Children ............ 364

    Section 29.2—Daily Life Therapy (Higashi):
                Educating Children with
                Autism through Physical
                Activity, Academic Activity,
                and Vocational Training ......... 376

Chapter 30—Occupational Therapy in the Treatment of
    Autism .................................................................................. 379

Chapter 31—Music Therapy and Individuals with Autism
    Spectrum Disorders ............................................................. 383

## Part VI: Family and Lifestyle Issues for People with Autism

Chapter 32—Autism's Effect on Family Relationships ............ 391

    Section 32.1—Stress on Families of
                Autistic Children .................... 392

Section 32.2—Helping Siblings Understand
Autism and Encouraging
Positive Relationships ............. 397

Chapter 33—Ensuring Safety at Home for People with
Autism ..................................................................... 405

Chapter 34—Understanding Self-Injurious Behavior in
People with Autism ............................................... 409

Chapter 35—Personal Care and Grooming Issues ................... 415

Section 35.1—Handling Dressing and
Bathing Issues with the
Autistic Child ........................... 416

Section 35.2—Tips for Toilet Training the
Autistic Child ........................... 418

Section 35.3—Tips for Dealing with
Sleeping Difficulties in
Autistic Children ..................... 420

Section 35.4—Tips for Dealing with
Eating Difficulties in
Autistic Children ..................... 422

Section 35.5—Dental Care for Children
with Autism .............................. 424

Chapter 36—Encouraging Successful Play Dates for
Autistic Children .................................................. 429

Chapter 37—Integrating the Autistic Child into the World
outside the Home ................................................. 433

Section 37.1—Taking an Autistic Child to
the Grocery Store ..................... 434

Section 37.2—Making Medical Appointments Less Challenging for
Children with Autism .............. 436

Section 37.3—Autism and Airport
Travel Safety Trips .................. 438

Chapter 38—Handling Puberty in Children with Autism
Spectrum Disorders ............................................. 441

## Part VII: Education and Independence Issues for People with Autism

Chapter 39—A Guide to the Individualized Education
Program ................................................................. 449

Chapter 40—Treatment and Education of Autistic
and Related Communication Handicapped
Children (TEACCH) and Structured
Teaching ................................................................. 473

    Section 40.1—Autism Teaching Methods:
                 TEACCH ................................. 474

    Section 40.2—Structured Teaching ................ 475

Chapter 41—School Transitions and the Autistic Child:
Planning for Successful Transitions across
Grade Levels ......................................................... 487

Chapter 42—Transition Planning for Life after High
School: A Team Effort ............................................ 491

Chapter 43—Postsecondary Education for People with
Autism ..................................................................... 523

    Section 43.1—Preparing for Post-
                 secondary Education
                 If You Have Disabilities:
                 Know Your Rights and
                 Responsibilities ........................ 524

    Section 43.2—Lessons Learned: A
                 Parent's Report Regarding
                 Her Son's First Year at
                 College ...................................... 530

Chapter 44—Adults with Autism Spectrum Disorders:
Living and Working Arrangements ..................... 537

    Section 44.1—Living Arrangements
                 for Adults with Autism
                 Spectrum Disorders ................. 538

    Section 44.2—Accommodating Employees
                 with Asperger Syndrome ......... 540

Chapter 45—Estate Planning for Parents of Autistic
Children ................................................................. 549

## Part VIII: Additional Help and Information

Chapter 46—Glossary of Terms Related to Autism
Spectrum Disorders ............................................. 557

Chapter 47—How to Evaluate Health Information on the
Internet ................................................................. 563

Chapter 48—Resources for Information about Autism
        Spectrum Disorders ............................................... 569

**Index** ......................................................................... **581**

# *Preface*

## About This Book

According to the Centers for Disease Control and Prevention, the number of children diagnosed with an autism spectrum disorder who were in public special education programs increased from just over 20,000 to nearly 200,000 between the years of 1994 and 2004. Little is known, however, about the causes of these debilitating disorders, which are characterized by difficulties in social interactions, impairment in verbal or nonverbal communication, and the development of repetitive, unusual, or highly specialized interests. Additionally, there is much disagreement among medical authorities regarding the diagnostic methods and interventions used to care for people with these disorders. Although a wide variety of regimens are available, their effectiveness varies widely, and no cure exists.

*Autism and Pervasive Developmental Disorders Sourcebook* describes the criteria used to differentiate the various types of autism and pervasive developmental disorders. It explains what is known and what is under investigation about their causes. Facts are presented about screening methods, diagnostic indicators, and currently used therapies, including guidelines for evaluating their safety and effectiveness. Information is also provided about coping with common family and lifestyle issues, navigating the educational system, and preparing affected individuals for independence. The book concludes with a glossary of related terms and a directory of resources for further help and information.

## How to Use This Book

This book is divided into parts and chapters. Parts focus on broad areas of interest. Chapters are devoted to single topics within a part.

*Part I: Understanding Autism Spectrum and Pervasive Developmental Disorders* describes the different types of autism spectrum disorders and how they are related to one another. It also provides insight into the current rise in the prevalence of autism, which at one time was believed to occur in four or five out of every 10,000 children and now seems to occur in as many six or seven out of every 1,000.

*Part II: Causes of Autism Spectrum Disorders* discusses theories regarding elements that may contribute to the development of autism and pervasive developmental disorders. Possible genetic links to autism are described, as are the possible links between autism and vaccines, environmental exposures, immune system problems, abnormal brain development, and pregnancy and birth factors.

*Part III: Conditions That May Accompany Autism Spectrum Disorders* describes the many different conditions that occur more frequently in people with autism, including Fragile X syndrome, Tourette syndrome, epilepsy, auditory processing disorder, and attention deficit hyperactivity disorder. It also discusses exceptional abilities—including hyperlexia and savant syndrome—that sometimes accompany autism.

*Part IV: Diagnosing and Evaluating Autism Spectrum Disorders* explains the characteristics of autism spectrum disorders and the types of medical tools used for screening, diagnosis, and assessment. It also discusses strategies parents can use as they cope with the diagnosis, and it offers tips for talking to an autistic child about the diagnosis.

*Part V: Treatments, Therapies, and Interventions for Autism Spectrum Disorders* provides a look at the different methods used to treat autism spectrum disorders. The part begins by defining the members of the treatment team, and it provides guidelines for evaluating autism treatments. It offers a detailed explanation of various behavioral, social, sensory, dietary, and pharmacological interventions, and it discusses the use of communication, occupational, and music therapies.

*Part VI: Family and Lifestyle Issues for People with Autism* provides tips to help families deal with the challenges of daily life with an autistic child. Topics covered include stress, sibling issues, safety, and self-injurious behavior. Personal care and grooming issues are also discussed, and suggestions are provided for integrating the autistic child into the world outside the home.

*Part VII: Education and Independence Issues for People with Autism* explains education laws that apply to people with autism spectrum disorders. It also discusses such issues as instructional approaches, transition between grade levels, postsecondary education, and living and working arrangements for people with autism spectrum disorders. The part concludes with a discussion of estate planning for parents of autistic children.

*Part VIII: Additional Help and Information* provides a glossary of terms related to autism spectrum disorders and a directory of organizations able to provide additional help and support. A guide to evaluating health information on the internet is also included.

## Bibliographic Note

This volume contains documents and excerpts from publications issued by the following U.S. government agencies: Centers for Disease Control and Prevention; Job Accommodation Network; National Guideline Clearinghouse; National Institute of Child Health and Human Development (NICHD); National Institute of Mental Health (NIMH); National Institute of Neurological Disorders and Stroke (NINDS); National Institute on Deafness and Other Communication Disorders (NIDCD); National Institutes of Health (NIH); and the U.S. Department of Education.

In addition, this volume contains copyrighted documents from the following organizations and individuals: American College of Neuropsychopharmacology; American Music Therapy Association; American Occupational Therapy Association; American Psychiatric Association; ASPEN-Asperger Syndrome Education Network; Tony Attwood; Autism National Committee; Autism Outreach; Autism Society Canada; Autism Society of America; Autism Treatment Services of Canada; Autism Web; Cambridge Center for Behavioral Studies; Center for Autism and Related Disabilities–Gainesville; Center for Autism and Related Disorders; Center for Children's Health and the Environment; Center for the Study of Autism; Julie Coulter/Coulter Video; Dennis Debbaudt; EP Global Communications; First Signs; HealthDay/ScoutNews LLC; Help Group; Indiana Resource Center for Autism;

Intermountain Healthcare (IHC); Illinois Autism/PDD Training and Technical Assistance Project; Jessica Kingsley Publishers; Massachusetts General Hospital-School Psychiatry Program; May Institute; Medical University of South Carolina Children's Hospital; National Autistic Society; National Fragile X Foundation; Prader-Willi Syndrome Association; Rady Children's Hospital-San Diego; Society for Treatment of Autism; Susan Stokes; Darold A. Treffert, M.D.; Tuberous Sclerosis Alliance; Ulysses Press; University of California-Davis–M.I.N.D. Institute; University of Kansas-Merrill Advanced Studies Center; University of Michigan Health System; U.S. Food and Drug Administration; *Washington Post*; Williams Syndrome Association; Wrightslaw.com; and the Yale Developmental Disabilities Clinic.

Full citation information is provided on the first page of each chapter. Every effort has been made to secure all necessary rights to reprint the copyrighted material. If any omissions have been made, please contact Omnigraphics to make corrections for future editions.

## *Acknowledgements*

Thanks go to the many organizations, agencies, and individuals who have contributed materials for this *Sourcebook* and to medical consultant Dr. David Cooke and document engineer Bruce Bellenir. Special thanks go to managing editor Karen Bellenir and permissions coordinator Liz Collins for their help and support.

## *About the* Health Reference Series

The *Health Reference Series* is designed to provide basic medical information for patients, families, caregivers, and the general public. Each volume takes a particular topic and provides comprehensive coverage. This is especially important for people who may be dealing with a newly diagnosed disease or a chronic disorder in themselves or in a family member. People looking for preventive guidance, information about disease warning signs, medical statistics, and risk factors for health problems will also find answers to their questions in the *Health Reference Series*. The *Series*, however, is not intended to serve as a tool for diagnosing illness, in prescribing treatments, or as a substitute for the physician/patient relationship. All people concerned about medical symptoms or the possibility of disease are encouraged to seek professional care from an appropriate health care provider.

## A Note about Spelling and Style

*Health Reference Series* editors use *Stedman's Medical Dictionary* as an authority for questions related to the spelling of medical terms and the *Chicago Manual of Style* for questions related to grammatical structures, punctuation, and other editorial concerns. Consistent adherence is not always possible, however, because the individual volumes within the *Series* include many documents from a wide variety of different producers and copyright holders, and the editor's primary goal is to present material from each source as accurately as is possible following the terms specified by each document's producer. This sometimes means that information in different chapters or sections may follow other guidelines and alternate spelling authorities. For example, occasionally a copyright holder may require that eponymous terms be shown in possessive forms (Crohn's disease *vs.* Crohn disease) or that British spelling norms be retained (leukaemia *vs.* leukemia).

## Locating Information within the Health Reference Series

The *Health Reference Series* contains a wealth of information about a wide variety of medical topics. Ensuring easy access to all the fact sheets, research reports, in-depth discussions, and other material contained within the individual books of the series remains one of our highest priorities. As the *Series* continues to grow in size and scope, however, locating the precise information needed by a reader may become more challenging.

*A Contents Guide to the Health Reference Series* was developed to direct readers to the specific volumes that address their concerns. It presents an extensive list of diseases, treatments, and other topics of general interest compiled from the Tables of Contents and major index headings. To access *A Contents Guide to the Health Reference Series*, visit www.healthreferenceseries.com.

## Medical Consultant

Medical consultation services are provided to the *Health Reference Series* editors by David A. Cooke, M.D. Dr. Cooke is a graduate of Brandeis University, and he received his M.D. degree from the University of Michigan. He completed residency training at the University of Wisconsin Hospital and Clinics. He is board-certified in Internal Medicine. Dr. Cooke currently works as part of the University of Michigan Health System and practices in Ann Arbor, MI. In his free time, he enjoys writing, science fiction, and spending time with his family.

## Our Advisory Board

We would like to thank the following board members for providing guidance to the development of this series:

## Health Reference Series *Update Policy*

The inaugural book in the *Health Reference Series* was the first edition of *Cancer Sourcebook* published in 1989. Since then, the *Series* has been enthusiastically received by librarians and in the medical community. In order to maintain the standard of providing high-quality health information for the layperson the editorial staff at Omnigraphics felt it was necessary to implement a policy of updating volumes when warranted.

Medical researchers have been making tremendous strides, and it is the purpose of the *Health Reference Series* to stay current with the most recent advances. Each decision to update a volume is made on an individual basis. Some of the considerations include how much new information is available and the feedback we receive from people who use the books. If there is a topic you would like to see added to the update list, or an area of medical concern you feel has not been adequately addressed, please write to:

Editor
*Health Reference Series*
Omnigraphics, Inc.
P.O. Box 31-1640
Detroit, MI 48231-1640
E-mail: editorial@omnigraphics.com

# Part One

# Understanding Autism Spectrum and Pervasive Developmental Disorders

# Chapter 1

# *Autism and Pervasive Developmental Disorders: What We Know*

Even though autism was first described in the 1940s, little was really known about the disorder until the 1990s. Even today, there is a great deal that researchers, scientists, and health care providers don't know about autism.

But there are things that we do know about autism. This chapter offers broad information about autism and answers some of the more common questions that parents and families often have about the disorder.

## *What is autism?*

Autism is a complex neurobiological disorder of development that lasts throughout a person's life. It is sometimes called a developmental disability because it usually starts before age three, in the developmental period, and because it causes delays or problems in many different skills that arise from infancy to adulthood.

The main signs and symptoms of autism involve[1] language, social behavior, and behaviors concerning objects and routines:

- **Communication:** Both verbal (spoken) and nonverbal (unspoken, such as pointing, eye contact, or smiling)

---

Reprinted from "Autism Overview: What We Know," National Institute of Child Health and Human Development, National Institutes of Health, NIH Publication No. 05-5592, May 2005.

- **Social interactions:** Such as sharing emotions, understanding how others think and feel (sometimes called empathy), and holding a conversation, as well as the amount of time a person spends interacting with others

- **Routines or repetitive behaviors:** Often called stereotyped behaviors, such as repeating words or actions, obsessively following routines or schedules, playing with toys or objects in repetitive and sometimes inappropriate ways, or having very specific and inflexible ways of arranging items

People with autism might have problems talking with you, or they might not look you in the eye when you talk to them. They may have to line up their pencils before they can pay attention, or they may say the same sentence again and again to calm themselves down. They may flap their arms to tell you they are happy, or they might hurt themselves to tell you they are not. Some people with autism never learn how to talk. These behaviors not only make life challenging for people who have autism, but also take a toll on their families, their health care providers, their teachers, and anyone who comes in contact with them.

Because different people with autism can have very different features or symptoms, health care providers think of autism as a "spectrum" disorder—a group of disorders with a range of similar features. Based on their specific strengths and weaknesses, people with autism spectrum disorders (ASDs) may have mild symptoms or more serious symptoms, but they all have an ASD. This chapter uses the terms "ASD" and "autism" to mean the same thing.

## What conditions are in the ASD category?

Currently, the ASD category includes the following:

- Autistic disorder (also called "classic" autism)
- Asperger syndrome
- Pervasive developmental disorder not otherwise specified (or atypical autism)[2]

In some cases, health care providers use a broader term—pervasive developmental disorders (PDD)—to describe autism. The PDD category includes the ASDs mentioned above, plus childhood disintegrative disorder and Rett syndrome.

4

Depending on specific symptoms, a person with autism may fall into the ASD or the PDD category. Sometimes, the terms "ASD" and "PDD" are used to mean the same thing because autism is in both categories.

## What causes autism?

Scientists don't know exactly what causes autism at this time.

Much evidence supports the idea that genetic factors—that is, genes, their function, and their interactions—are one of the main underlying causes of ASDs. But, researchers aren't looking for just one gene. Current evidence suggests that as many as ten or more genes on different chromosomes may be involved in autism, to different degrees.

Some genes may place a person at greater risk for autism, called susceptibility. Other genes may cause specific symptoms or determine how severe those symptoms are. Or, genes with changes or mutations might add to the symptoms of autism because the genes or gene products aren't working properly.

Research has also shown that environmental factors, such as viruses, may also play a role in causing autism.

While some researchers are examining genes and environmental factors, other researchers are looking at possible neurological, infectious, metabolic, and immunologic factors that may be involved in autism.

Because the disorder is so complex, and because no two people with autism are exactly alike, autism is probably the result of many causes.

## Is there a link between autism and vaccines?

To date, there is no conclusive scientific evidence that any part of a vaccine or any combination of vaccines causes autism, even though researchers have carried out many studies to answer this important question. There is also no proof that any material used to make or preserve vaccines plays a role in causing autism.

Although there have been reports of studies that relate vaccines to autism, the findings have not held up under further investigation. Researchers have been unable to replicate the studies that reportedly found a link between autism and vaccines.

There is a great deal of research and discussion on the topic of vaccines and autism—too much to cover here. The U.S. Centers for Disease Control and Prevention (CDC) conducts and supports most of the federal epidemiological studies that seek to answer questions about vaccines and autism.

Currently, the CDC provides the most accurate and up-to-date information about research on autism and vaccine research, both supported by the federal government and funded independently.

### How many people have autism?

Currently, researchers don't know the exact number of people with an ASD in the United States.

Researchers use different ways to determine prevalence that often give different results.

Some estimates of prevalence rely on previously published studies. Researchers review all the published data on a topic and take the averages of these calculations to determine prevalence. Independent researchers[3] recently conducted two such reviews. Based on these studies, the best conservative estimate[4] of the prevalence of ASDs in the United States is that one child in one thousand children has an ASD.

### Is autism more common now than it was in the past?

Researchers are not certain whether autism is more prevalent now than in the past for a number of reasons. Although more cases of autism are being identified, it is not clear why. Some of the increase may result from better education about the symptoms of autism or from more accurate diagnoses of autism.

The new definition of autism as a spectrum disorder means that even people with mild symptoms can be classified as having an ASD, which could also account for the increase in identified cases. As research moves forward using the current definition of ASDs, more definite numbers may be available to answer this question.

### Is autism more common in certain groups of people?

Current figures show that autism occurs in all racial, ethnic, and social groups equally, with individuals in one group no more or less likely to have ASDs than those in other groups. Three groups are at higher-than-normal risk for ASDs:

- **Boys:** Statistics show that boys are three to four times more likely[5] to be affected by autism than are girls.

- **Siblings of those with ASDs:** Among families that have one child with an ASD, recurrence of ASD in another sibling is between[6] 2 percent and 8 percent, a figure much higher than in the general population.

- **People with certain other developmental disorders:** For certain disorders, including Fragile X syndrome, mental retardation, and tuberous sclerosis, autism is common in addition to the primary symptoms of the disorder.

## When do people usually show signs of autism?

A number of the behavioral symptoms[7] of autism are observable by eighteen months of age, including: problems with eye contact, not responding to one's name, joint attention problems, underdeveloped skills in pretend play and imitation, and problems with nonverbal communication and language.

Some studies also note that, although more subtle, some signs of autism are detectable at eight months[8] of age.

In general, the average age of autism diagnosis is currently three years old. In many cases, a delay in the child's starting to speak around age two brings problems to parents' attention, even though other, less noticeable signs may be present at an earlier age.[9]

Studies[10] also show that a subgroup of children with ASDs experiences a "regression," meaning they stop using the language, play, or social skills they had already learned. This regression usually happens between the first and second birthdays.

Researchers are still learning about the features of regression in ASDs, and whether the features differ from those shown by individuals who show signs of autism in early life.

## What are some of the possible signs of autism?

Parents, caregivers, family members, teachers, and others who spend a lot of time with children can look for "red flags." Some may mean a delay in one or more areas of development, while others are more typical of ASDs. Possible red flags for autism are as follows:

- The child does not respond to his or her name.
- The child cannot explain what he or she wants.
- The child's language skills are slow to develop or speech is delayed.
- The child doesn't follow directions.
- At times, the child seems to be deaf.
- The child seems to hear sometimes, but not other times.
- The child doesn't point or wave "bye-bye."

- The child used to say a few words or babble, but now he or she doesn't.

- The child throws intense or violent tantrums.

- The child has odd movement patterns.

- The child is overly active, uncooperative, or resistant.

- The child doesn't know how to play with toys.

- The child doesn't smile when smiled at.

- The child has poor eye contact.

- The child gets "stuck" doing the same things over and over and can't move on to other things.

- The child seems to prefer to play alone.

- The child gets things for him- or herself only.

- The child is very independent for his or her age.

- The child does things "early" compared to other children.

- The child seems to be in his or her "own world."

- The child seems to tune people out.

- The child is not interested in other children.

- The child walks on his or her toes.

- The child shows unusual attachments to toys, objects, or schedules (i.e., always holding a string or having to put socks on before pants).

- The child spends a lot of time lining things up or putting things in a certain order.

In addition, your child's health care provider will send your child for an evaluation if you report any of the following behaviors; such an evaluation would consider ASDs, among other possible causes.[12]
Your child may need further evaluation if he or she:

- Does not babble or coo by twelve months of age;

- Does not gesture (point, wave, grasp, etc.) by twelve months of age;

- Does not say single words by sixteen months of age;

8

- Does not say two-word phrases on his or her own (rather than just repeating what someone says to him or her) by twenty-four months of age;

- Has *any* loss of *any* language or social skill at *any* age.

## What should I do if I think my child has a developmental problem or autism?

Tell your child's health care provider immediately if you think something is wrong. According to the American Academy of Pediatrics (AAP)[13], "Pediatricians should listen carefully to parents discussing their child's development. [Parents] are reliable sources of information and their concerns should be valued and addressed immediately."

Your child's health care provider will note your comments and concerns, will ask some other questions, and will determine the best plan of action. In some cases, the health care provider will ask you to complete a questionnaire about your child to get more specific information about symptoms. To rule out certain conditions, the health care provider will also test your child's hearing and check your child's lead level before deciding on a course of action.

If red flags are present, and if the lead and hearing tests show no problems, your child's health care provider may refer you to a specialist in child development or another specialized health care provider. The specialist will conduct a number of tests to determine whether or not your child has autism or an ASD.

## What if I don't notice any symptoms?

If you don't report any of these signs, your child's health care provider will continue to check for problems at every well-baby and well-child visit.[14] If your child's health care provider does not routinely check your child with such tests, you should ask that he or she do so.

In this developmental screening, the provider asks questions related to normal development that can help measure your child's specific progress. Typically, these questions are similar to the red flags listed earlier. Based on your answers, the health care provider may send your child for further evaluation.

The AAP recommends[15] that health care providers ask questions about different aspects of development. These questions include (but are not limited to) those listed here.

Does your child:

- Not speak as well as other children his or her age?
- Have poor eye contact?
- Act as if he or she is in his or her own world?
- Seem to "tune out" others?
- Not smile when smiled at?
- Seem unable to tell you what he or she wants, and so takes your hand and leads you to what he or she wants, or gets it him- or herself?
- Have trouble following simple directions?
- Not play with toys in a usual way?
- Not bring things to you to "show" you something?
- Not point to interesting things or direct your attention to items of interest?
- Have unusually long or severe temper tantrums?
- Show an unusual attachment to objects, especially "hard" ones, such as a flashlight or key chain, instead of "soft" ones, such as a blanket or stuffed animal?
- Prefer to play alone?
- Not pretend or play "make believe" (if the child is older than age two)?

### Is there a cure for autism?

To date, there is no cure for autism, but sometimes, children with ASDs make so much progress that they no longer show the full syndrome of autism when they are older.

Research[16] shows that early diagnosis and interventions delivered early in life, such as in the preschool period, are more likely to result in major positive effects on later skills and symptoms. The sooner a child begins to get help, the more opportunity for learning. Because a young child's brain is still forming, early intervention gives children the best start possible and the best chance of developing their full potential. Even so, no matter when a person is diagnosed with autism, it's never too late to benefit from treatment. People of all ages with ASDs at all levels of ability generally respond positively to well-designed interventions.

Public Law 108-77: *Individuals with Disabilities Education Improvement Act*[17](2004) and Public Law 105-17: *Individuals with Disabilities Act, or IDEA*[18] (1997) require your child's primary care provider to refer you and your family to an early intervention service. Every state operates an early intervention program for children from birth to age three; children with autism should qualify for these services. Early intervention programs typically include behavioral methods, early developmental education, communication skills, occupational and physical therapy, and structured social play.

### What are the treatments for autism?

Currently there is no definitive, single treatment for ASDs. However, there are a variety of ways to help minimize the symptoms and maximize learning. Persons with an ASD have the best chance of using all of their individual capabilities and skills if they receive appropriate behavioral and other therapies, education, and medication. In some cases, these treatments can help people with autism function at near-normal levels.

Some possible treatments for autism are explained in the following. If you have a question about treatment, you should talk to a health care provider who specializes in caring for people with autism.

**Behavioral therapy and other therapeutic options:** In general, behavior management therapy works to reinforce wanted behaviors and reduce unwanted behaviors. At the same time, these methods also suggest what caregivers should do before or between episodes of problem behaviors, and what to do during or after these episodes. Behavioral therapy is often based on applied behavior analysis (ABA). Different applications of ABA commonly used for people with autism include: positive behavioral interventions and support (PBS), pivotal response training (PRT), incidental teaching, milieu therapy, verbal behavior, and discrete trial teaching (DTT), among others.

Keep in mind that other therapies, beyond ABA, may also be effective for persons with autism. Talk to your health care provider about the best options for your child.

A variety of health care providers can also help individuals with ASDs and their families to work through different situations:

- Speech-language therapists can help people with autism improve their general ability to communicate and interact with others effectively, as well as develop their speech and language skills. These therapists may teach nonverbal ways of communicating and may improve social skills that involve communicating with others. They may also help people to better use words and sentences, and to improve rate and rhythm of speech and conversation.

• Occupational therapists can help people with autism find ways to adjust tasks and conditions that match their needs and abilities. Such help may include finding a specially designed computer mouse and keyboard to ease communication, or identifying skills that build on a person's interests and individual capabilities. Occupational therapists may also do many of the same types of activities as physical therapists do (see following).

• Physical therapists design activities and exercises to build motor control and to improve posture and balance. For example, they can help a child who avoids body contact to participate in activities and games with other children.

Special services are often available to preschool and school-aged children, as well as to teens, through the local public school system. In many cases, services provided by specialists in the school setting are free. More intense and individualized help is available through private clinics, but the family usually has to pay for private services, although some health insurance plans may help cover the cost.

**Educational and school-based options:** Children with ASDs are guaranteed free, appropriate public education under federal laws. *Public Law 108-77: Individuals with Disabilities Education Improvement Act*[17] (2004) and *Public Law 105-17: The Individuals with Disabilities Education Act—IDEA*[18] (1997) make it possible for children with disabilities to get free educational services and educational devices to help them learn as much as they can. Each child is entitled to these services from age three through high school, or until age twenty-one, whichever comes first.

The laws state that children must be taught in the least restrictive environment appropriate for that individual child. This statement does not mean that each child must be placed in a regular classroom. Instead, the laws mean that the teaching environment should be designed to meet a child's learning needs, while minimizing restrictions on the child's access to typical learning experiences and interactions. Educating persons with ASDs often includes a combination of one-to-one, small group, and regular classroom instruction.

To qualify for special education services, the child must meet specific criteria as outlined by federal and state guidelines. You can contact a local school principal or special education coordinator to learn how to have your child assessed to see if he or she qualifies for services under these laws.

If your child qualifies for special services, a team of people, including you and your family, caregivers, teachers, school psychologists, and other child development specialists, will work together to design an Individualized Educational Plan (IEP)[19] for your child. An IEP includes specific academic, communication, motor, learning, functional, and socialization goals for a child based on his or her educational needs. The team also decides how best to carry out the IEP, such as determining any devices or special assistance the child needs, and identifying the developmental specialists who will work with the child.

The special services team should evaluate and re-evaluate your child on a regular basis to see how your child is doing and whether any changes are needed in his or her plan.

A number of parents' organizations, both national and local, provide information on therapeutic and educational services and how to get these services for a child. Check the local phone book for more information.

**Medication options:** Currently, there is no medication that can cure ASDs or all of the associated symptoms. Further, the Food and Drug Administration (FDA) has not approved any drugs specifically for the treatment of autism or its causes. But, in many cases, medication can treat some of the symptoms associated with ASDs. (Please note that the National Institute of Child Health and Human Development [NICHD] does not endorse or support the use of any of these medications for treating symptoms of ASDs, or for other conditions for which the medications are not FDA approved.)

Medication can improve the behavior of a person with autism. Health care providers often use medications to deal with a specific behavior, such as reducing self-injurious behavior. With the symptom minimized, the person with autism can focus on other things, including learning and communication. Some of these medications have serious risks involved with their use; others may make symptoms worse at first or may take several weeks to become effective.

Not every medication helps every person with symptoms of autism. Health care providers usually prescribe medication on a trial basis, to see if it helps. Your child's health care provider may have to try different dosages or different combinations of medications to find the most effective plan. Families, caregivers, and health care providers need to work together to make sure that medications are working and that the overall medication plan is safe.

Medications used to treat the symptoms of autism[20] may include (but are not limited to) the following:

- **Selective serotonin re-uptake inhibitors (SSRIs):** These are a group of antidepressants that treat problems, such as obsessive-compulsive behaviors and anxiety resulting from an imbalance in one of the body's chemical systems, that are sometimes present in autism. These medications may reduce the frequency and intensity of repetitive behaviors; decrease irritability, tantrums, and aggressive behavior; and improve eye contact.

- **Tricyclics:** These are another type of antidepressant used to treat depression and obsessive compulsive behaviors. Although these drugs tend to cause more side effects than the SSRIs, sometimes they are more effective for certain people.

- **Psychoactive or anti-psychotic medications:** These affect the brain of the person taking them. Use of this group of drugs is the most widely studied treatment for autism. In some people with ASDs, these drugs may decrease hyperactivity, reduce stereotyped behaviors, and minimize withdrawal and aggression.

- **Stimulants:** These may be useful in increasing focus and decreasing hyperactivity in people with autism, particularly in higher-functioning individuals. Because of the risk of side effects, health care providers should monitor those using these drugs carefully and often.

- **Anti-anxiety drugs:** These can help relieve anxiousness and panic disorders associated with autism.

## What is secretin and is it an effective treatment for autism?

Secretin is a hormone produced by the small intestine that helps in digestion. Currently, the FDA approves a single dose of secretin only for use in diagnosing digestive problems.

In the 1990s, news reports described a few persons with autism whose behavior improved after getting secretin during a diagnostic test.

However, a series[21] of clinical trials funded by the NICHD and conducted through the Network on the Neurobiology and Genetics of Autism: Collaborative Programs of Excellence in Autism (CPEAs) found no difference in improvement between those taking secretin and those taking placebo. In fact, of the five case-controlled clinical trials published on secretin, not one showed secretin as any better than placebo, no matter what the dosage or frequency. For this reason, secretin is not recommended as a treatment for ASDs.

### *Are there other disorders associated with ASDs?*

In about 5 percent[22] of autism cases, another disorder is also present. Studying this kind of co-occurrence helps researchers who are trying to pinpoint the genes involved in autism. Similar disorders or disorders with similar symptoms may have similar genetic origins. In cases of one disorder commonly occurring with another, it could be that one is actually a risk factor for the other. This kind of information can provide clues to what actually happens in autism.

Some of these co-occurring disorders include the following:

- **Epilepsy or seizure disorder:** Nearly one-third[23] of those with autism also show signs of epilepsy by adulthood. In most cases, medication can control and treat epilepsy effectively.

- **Tuberous sclerosis:** About 6 percent[24] of those with autism also have tuberous sclerosis, a disorder that shares many symptoms with autism, including seizures that result from lesions (cuts) on the brain.

- **Fragile X syndrome:** Nearly 2.1 percent[25] of those with autism also have Fragile X, the most common inherited form of mental retardation.

- **Mental retardation:** About 25 percent[26] of persons with autism also have some degree of mental retardation.

Many people have treatable conditions in addition to their autism. Sleep disorders, allergies, and digestive problems are commonly seen in those with ASDs, and many of these can be treated with environmental interventions or medication. Treatment for these conditions may not cure autism, but it can improve the quality of life for people who have autism and their families.

## References

1.  Filipek, et al. (2000). Practice Parameter: Screening and Diagnosis of Autism—Report of the Quality Standards Subcommittee of

the American Academy of Neurology and the Child Neurology Society. *Neurology*, 55:468–79.

2. *Diagnostic and Statistics Manual, fourth edition*. (1994). American Psychiatric Association: Washington, DC.

3. Fombonne, 2002; and Gilberg and Wing, 1999. As cited in: Immunization Safety Review Committee, Institute of Medicine, National Academy of Sciences. (2004). *Immunization Safety Review: Vaccines and Autism*. Washington, DC: National Academy Press.

4. Immunization Safety Review Committee, Institute of Medicine, National Academy of Sciences. (2004). *Immunization Safety Review: Vaccines and Autism*. Washington, DC: National Academy Press.

5. Volkmar, 1993; and McLennen, 1993. As cited in: Ashley-Koch, et al. (1999). Genetic Studies of Autistic Disorder and Chromosome 7. *Genomics*, 61:227–36.

6. Gillberg, 2000; Chakrabarti, 2001; and Chudley, 1998. As cited in: Muhle, et al. (2004). The genetics of autism. *Pediatrics*, 113(5):e472–e486.

7. Lord, 1995; Stone, 1999; and Charman, 1997. As cited in: Filipek et al. (2000). Practice Parameter: Screening and Diagnosis of Autism—Report of the Quality Standards Subcommittee of the American Academy of Neurology and the Child Neurology Society. *Neurology*, 55:468–79.

8. Cox, 1999; Mars, 1998; Werner, 2000; and Baranek, 1999. As cited in: Filipek, et al. (2000). Practice Parameter: Screening and Diagnosis of Autism—Report of the Quality Standards Subcommittee of the American Academy of Neurology and the Child Neurology Society. *Neurology*, 55:468–79.

9. Johnson, CP. (2004). New tool helps primary care physicians diagnose autism early. *AAP News*, 24(2):74.

10. Goldberg, 2003; and Rodier, 1998. As cited in: Lord, et al. (2004). Regression and word loss in autistic spectrum disorders. *Journal of Child Psychology and Psychiatry*, 45(5):936–55.

11. Filipek et al. (1999). Screening and diagnosis of autistic spectrum disorders. *Journal of Autism and Developmental Disorders*, 29(6):439–84.

12. Filipek et al. (2000). Practice Parameter: Screening and Diagnosis of Autism—Report of the Quality Standards Subcommittee of the American Academy of Neurology and the Child Neurology Society. *Neurology*, 55:468–79.

13. Media Resource Team, American Academy of Pediatrics (AAP). (2001). Guidelines on Diagnosis and Management of Autism. *E-News*, May 2001 [Electronic Version]. Retrieved November 5, 2004, from http://www.aap.org/mrt/May01.htm.

14. Committee on Children with Disabilities, AAP. (2001). The pediatrician's role in the diagnosis and management of autistic spectrum disorder in children. *Pediatrics*, 107:1221–26.

15. Committee on Children with Disabilities, AAP. (2001). Technical report: The pediatrician's role in the diagnosis and management of autistic spectrum disorder in children. *Pediatrics*, 107:e85. Retrieved November 4, 2004, from http://www.pediatrics.org/cgi/content/full/107/5/385.

16. Dawson, 1997; Hurth, 1999; Rogers, 1989; Hoyson, 1984; Lovaas, 1987; Harris, 1991; McEachin, 1993; Greenspan, 1997; Smith, 1997; and Smith, 1998. As cited in Committee on Children with Disabilities, AAP. (2001). The pediatrician's role in the diagnosis and management of autistic spectrum disorder in children. *Pediatrics*, 107:1221–26.

17. For complete information about the reauthorization of IDEA, visit http://www.ed.gov/policy/speced/guid/idea/ idea2004.html.

18. For complete information about the 1997 authorization of IDEA, visit http://www.ed.gov/offices/OSERS/Policy/ IDEA/ regs.html.

19. Adapted from NICHD, NIH, DHHS. (2003). *Are there treatments for Fragile X syndrome? Families and Fragile X Syndrome* (NIH Pub. No. 03-3402). Washington, DC: U.S. Government Printing Office, 24–31.

20. Adapted from: Potenza and McDougle. (2001). *New Findings on the Causes and Treatment of Autism*. CNS Spectrums, Medical Broadcast Limited. Retrieved November 8, 2004, from http://www.patientcenters.com/autism/news/ med_reference .html.

21. Study confirms secretin no more effective than placebo in treating autistic symptoms, NICHD, November 2001. Retrieved

November 08, 2004, from http://www.nichd.nih.gov/new/releases/newskey.cfm?from=autism.

22. Gillberg. (1998). Chromosomal disorders and autism. *Journal of autism and developmental disorders*, 28:415–25.

23. Tuchman, et al. (2002). Epilepsy in autism. *Lancet Neurology*, 1:352–58.

24. Fombonne, et al. (1997). Autism and associated medical disorders in a French epidemiological survey. *Child and Adolescent Psychiatry*, 36:1561–69.

25. Kielinen, et al. (2004). Associated medical disorders and disabilities in children with autistic disorder. *Autism*, 8(1):49–60.

26. Sigman M, Dissanayake C, Arbelle S, and Ruskin E. (1997). Cognition and emotion in children with autism. In Cohen and Volkmar (Eds.) *Handbook of Autism and Pervasive Developmental Disorders, second edition* (pp. 248–65). New York: Wiley and Sons.

# Chapter 2

# *Who Develops Autism?*

## *Chapter Contents*

Section 2.1—Is Autism on the Rise? ........................................... 20
Section 2.2—Why Do More Boys than Girls Develop Autism? ... 23

## Section 2.1

# *Is Autism on the Rise?*

The release last week (February 16, 2007) of statistics on the prevalence of autism spectrum disorders in American children—one case in every 150 eight-year-olds—confirmed that the condition is more common now than it was just a decade ago, when estimates ranged anywhere from one in 500 youngsters to one in 166.

But the new statistics—from a fourteen-state survey conducted by the U.S. Centers for Disease Control and Prevention (CDC)—failed to clear up the mystery of why autism might be striking more and more children with each passing year.

Alison Singer, senior vice president of the nation's leading autism advocacy group, Autism Speaks, said she didn't need the CDC statistics to know that more families are now struggling with the behavioral disorder.

A decade ago, "we didn't have more than year-long waiting lists for places within schools for children with autism," said Singer, whose nine-year-old daughter is autistic. "In fact, we had far fewer schools then for children with autism, because we had far less need. And if you go into any elementary school in the country, you'll see more children with special needs and with autism than you did when I was in elementary school."

Autism spectrum disorders include autism as well as less disabling conditions such as Asperger syndrome and pervasive developmental disorder (PDD). All of these conditions involve some level of difficulty in communication and socialization, according to the CDC. Some children may also engage in repetitive behaviors, have trouble dealing with changes in routine, and be prone to emotional outbursts. As many as four in ten children with autism may not speak at all, the CDC says.

The exact causes of autism remain a mystery. "We know that genes are important," said Dr. Bradley Peterson, professor of child psychiatry at Columbia University Medical Center and the New York State Psychiatric Institute in New York City.

On the other hand, he said, "we know that genes aren't the whole story. Unfortunately, in terms of nongenetic or environmental factors, we just don't have very good leads yet."

Theories as to possible environmental culprits are widespread and hotly debated. They have included a variety of infections (including maternal German measles during pregnancy); drugs such as thalidomide and a labor-inducing agent, Pitocin; synthetic compounds such as PCBs and plastics; and food additives.

Two agents—the mercury-based vaccine preservative thimerosal, and the measles-mumps-rubella (MMR) vaccine—gained widespread public attention after a 1998 study by British researcher Dr. Andrew Wakefield linked vaccination to a spike in childhood autism cases.

Debate still rages on that front, although two more recent and much larger studies—one by the U.S. Institute of Medicine and another British/Japanese effort involving more than thirty thousand Japanese youngsters—have turned up no such link.

So, the question remains: Why are more and more parents discovering their child has autism?

Peterson said the CDC statistics may not be as straightforward as they seem.

"Actually, I think the numbers are comparable to what they were twenty years ago," he said. "Twenty years ago, the estimate [of prevalence] was 5.5 to 6 per 1,000 children, and now it's estimated at 6.6 per 1,000."

While the gap between those numbers is substantial, "it is probably not outside of the margin of error," Peterson said. So, it's still possible that the supposed "rise" is merely a statistical artifact.

Singer discounted that notion, however. "It's not really reflective of the reality of the situation," she said, pointing again to the long waiting lines of parents desperate to get their child treatment or proper schooling, problems Singer said didn't exist ten years ago.

Peterson also pointed to possible changes in "diagnostic trends" to account for rising numbers. For example, "clinically, in the past, people actually thought it was less stigmatizing, and would bring a child greater social services, if they were diagnosed with mental retardation versus autism," he said. That situation has changed with time, however, so more children may be diagnosed with autism now than they were in the past.

Again, Singer challenged that view. "That's a very easy theory to test," she said. In California, she said, "data showed that there was no drop-off in the number of children that were being diagnosed with mental retardation"—even as reported diagnoses for autism disorders were climbing.

Then there's the theory that parents and physicians have simply gotten better at spotting autistic spectrum disorders—even in their milder forms.

"Perhaps, for children that we used to call 'odd' or 'quirky,' the radar is now much more sensitive to detecting them and providing a syndromic label, one that they might not otherwise have had in the past," Peterson said.

But while it is true that the early detection of autism has improved in recent years, Singer said no parent is in any rush to get his or her youngster labeled autistic. "Look, no one would want to send their child to a school for children with autism if they didn't have to," she said. "The demand for those schools, the demand out there for therapists—all of it points to a true increase."

And yet neither expert was ready to point the finger at any one cause for the increase, environmental or otherwise.

Asked about the MMR/thimerosal debate, Singer said only that, "we continue to focus on the need to cast a very wide net when it comes to autism research. We are not ready say that it's 100 percent genetic or environmental. We simply don't know enough to say what it is or is not."

She remains optimistic that dedicated research will bring real answers.

In December 2006, groups like Autism Speaks helped push the Combating Autism Act through to final approval in Congress. The act authorizes that $945 million be spent over the next five years to unravel the root causes of the disorder.

"Now we need to get that money appropriated," Singer said.

She and Peterson agreed that research is the only way to understand what's driving any rise in autism cases—and how to turn that trend around.

"We are only going to find real answers in the laboratory," Singer said. "We have to fund scientists who are looking at the biology, looking at what causes autism, who are looking at environmental exposures, looking at the genetics. That's where we are going to find the answers."

Sources: Alison Singer, senior vice president, Autism Speaks, New York City; Bradley Peterson, M.D., Murphy professor of child psychiatry, Columbia University Medical Center and New York State Psychiatric Institute, New York City; February 9, 2007, *Morbidity and Mortality Weekly Report*.

## Section 2.2

# *Why Do More Boys than Girls Develop Autism?*

Why are boys far more likely to develop autism than girls?

It is not difficult to demonstrate the fact that there are more boys with autistic spectrum disorders than girls. Hans Asperger originally believed that no girls were affected by the syndrome he described in 1944, although clinical evidence later caused him to revise this statement. In Kanner's 1943 study of a small group of children with autistic syndrome there were four times as many boys as girls; and in their much larger study of Asperger syndrome in mainstream schools in Sweden in 1993, Ehlers and Gillberg found the same male to female ratio of 4:1.

In epidemiological research Wing (1981) found that among people with high-functioning autism or Asperger syndrome there were as many as fifteen times as many males as females. On the other hand, when she looked at individuals with learning difficulties as well as autism the ratio of boys to girls was closer to 2:1. This would suggest that, while females are less likely to develop autism, when they do they are more severely impaired.

It is difficult to explain why the sexes should be affected differently by autism.

Attwood (2000), Ehlers and Gillberg (1993), and Wing (1981) have all speculated that many girls with Asperger syndrome are never referred for diagnosis, and so are simply missing from statistics. This might be because the diagnostic criteria for Asperger syndrome are based on the behavioral characteristics of boys, who are often more noticeably "different" or disruptive than girls with the same underlying deficits. Girls with Asperger syndrome may be better at masking

23

their difficulties in order to fit in with their peers, and in general have a more even profile of social skills.

Another hypothesis (Wing 1981) is based on evidence that, in the general population, females have better verbal skills, while males excel in visuospatial tasks. There may be a neurological basis for this, so that autism can be interpreted as exaggeration of "normal" sex differences. Yet environmental and social factors may also play a part in sex differences in ability, which means that no direct analogy can be drawn between the poorer verbal skills of boys and the higher incidence of autism in males.

In 1964 Bernard Rimland pointed out that, overall, males tend to be more susceptible to organic damage than girls, whether through hereditary disease, acquired infection, or other conditions. Since it is now almost universally accepted that there is an organic cause for autism, it should not be surprising that boys are more vulnerable to it than girls.

In recent years researchers have put forward a genetic explanation for the differences. Skuse (2000) has suggested that the gene or genes for autism are located on the X chromosome. Girls inherit X chromosomes from both parents, but boys inherit only one, from their mothers. Skuse's hypothesis is that the X chromosome that girls inherit from their fathers contains an imprinted gene that "protects" the carrier from autism, thus making girls less likely to develop the condition than boys.

This theory has been used to support Asperger's view that autism and Asperger syndrome are at the extreme end of a spectrum of behaviors normally associated with "maleness." Such behaviors can be extremely useful in areas of life such as engineering and science, where attention to detail and single-mindedness may be more valuable than social skills, for example.

Lord and Schopler (1987) have outlined several possible mechanisms for the transmission of autism on the sex-linked X chromosome, and also for autosomal transmission (i.e., involving non-sex chromosomes). However, these are merely theoretical models and in fact researchers are still a long way from identifying a simple genetic cause for autism. It is likely that several genes on different chromosomes will be found to be associated with autism. This means that Skuse's theory, based on the X chromosome alone, may not represent the full picture.

Various theories have been put forward for the excess of males with autism and Asperger syndrome, but the picture is far from complete and until we have a fuller understanding of the causes of autism, it is unlikely that a proper explanation can be reached.

## References

Asperger, H. (1944) Die autistischen Psychopathen im Kindesalter. *Archiv fur Psychiatrie und Nervenkrankheiten,* 117: 76–136.

Attwood, T. (2000) Asperger syndrome: Some common questions: Do girls have a different expression of the syndrome?. Online. Available from: www.asperger.org/asperger/asperger_questions.htm#girls

Ehlers, S. & Gillberg, C. (1993): The Epidemiology of Asperger syndrome. A total population study. *Journal of Child Psychology and Psychiatry,* 34 (8): 1327–50.

Kanner, L. (1943) Autistic disturbances of affective contact. *Nervous Child,* 2: 217–50.

Lord, C. & Schopler, E. (1987) Neurobiological implications of sex differences in autism. In: Schopler, E. & Mesibov, G.M. (Eds.), *Neurobiological issues in autism.* New York: Plenum Press, 191–211.

Rimland, B. (1964) The etiology of infantile autism. In: *Infantile autism: The syndrome and its implications for a neural theory of behaviour.* New York: Appleton-Century-Crofts, 54.

Skuse, D. H. (2000) Imprinting the X-chromosome, and the male brain: Explaining sex differences in the liability to autism. *Pediatric Research,* 47 (1): 9–16.

Wing, L. (1981) Sex ratios in early childhood autism and related conditions. *Psychiatry Research,* 5: 129–37.

# Chapter 3

# *Autism Spectrum Disorders: An Overview*

Great, you figured something out. Congratulations! Now, you may want to share that idea with another human mind. If so, your brain translates the idea into a sequence of words. The words are translated into vibrations that depart from your mouth, sail long distances through the air, and land on my eardrum. These vibrations are turned back into words, and then into meaningful sentences and ideas. My brain also picks up other nonverbal language, such as your facial expression and tone of voice. Meanwhile, I figure out any "hidden agenda" or "subtext" when you said those words. All of these elements mix together to come up with an accurate understanding of what your "self" meant to communicate to my "self."

In this chapter "communication" is used in the broadest possible sense—including spoken speech, nonverbal clues, social skills, and the ability to use imagination and symbolic representations.

With this much involved, it's amazing that humans can communicate fully at all. It is not really amazing that some people have trouble with some aspect of the process. Given all of the ways that communication can go awry, this is a complex topic.

First, we'll start with a discussion of the underlying skills involved in communication, and then move on to the actual disorders. As we pull together a lot of essential information, we'll try to demystify technical terms. Hold on to your hats!

## Skills Involved in Communication

Communication involves two broad areas: literal verbal skills and nonverbal skills. People with an autistic spectrum disorder (ASD) have problems that include (at a minimum) the nonverbal areas—including difficulty with their desire and ability to use language in a social context. Let's examine these categories of communication skills in more detail.

### Literal Verbal/Spoken Communication Skills

Semantic language refers to the ability to use and understand words, phrases, and sentences, including abstract concepts and idioms. These skills involved in the literal use of verbal language may or may not be affected in ASDs. The skills needed for semantic language include the following:

- **Receptive verbal language:** The ability to understand spoken/ written words and ideas. Central auditory processing (CAP) is used to get meaning from sounds and words. Such skills include the ability to distinguish between similar sounds, and to pick out the main voice from the background.

- **Expressive verbal language:** The ability to express our ideas with spoken/written words, including the ability to articulate each word clearly.

### Nonverbal/Nonspoken Communication Skills

By definition, people with ASD have problems in the nonverbal/ nonspoken areas of communication.

Let's explain nonverbal communication by way of analogy. Imagine that a typical three-year-old, English-speaking child is parachuted into Russia. Some Russian women—who don't speak any English— find him on the farm. Even though they would not understand any words from each other, they would be able to have a great deal of communication. The child could let the women know that he was scared and hungry. The women could let him know that he was welcome, and that they'd take care of him. All of this would happen without words. It is just like if you go to a restaurant in a foreign country—everyone would know that you were enjoying the experience, even without your saying it. Such is the power of nonverbal communication.

The communicative skills that are still available to the parachuted child in a foreign country are the areas that are weak in a child with an ASD. These skills include:

- the urge to initiate shared social interaction and two-way communication: theory of mind;
- pragmatic language;
- knowledge of unwritten rules;
- knowing what is and isn't important;
- symbolic play skills;
- the ability to achieve "joint attention";
- nonverbal (nonspoken) transmission of language.

**Urge to initiate shared social interaction and two-way communication—theory of mind:** The ability to socialize/relate/empathize requires a working "theory of mind." Theory of mind refers to the relatively unique ability of humans to understand: that I have a mind; that you have a mind; and most importantly, that our minds may not know or be feeling the same things. Without a theory of mind, there is little point in communicating. There is limited ability to truly recognize that there is another human being in the room. It will be difficult to feel the need to communicate with anyone else. After all, with whom would you be communicating? Eye contact will be poor. It may seem as if there is a pane of glass between the child and others.

With limited ability to "get inside your mind," it will be frequently difficult for the child to demonstrate empathy for what you are feeling. For example, a child with theory of mind problems may assume that since he is happy, then you must be happy; or the child may not understand that someone else is deceptive when he is always bluntly honest.

Thus, the ability to recognize that other people have a mind, the ability to relate to that mind, and the ability to empathize with that mind are all parts of the same skill. Theory of mind problems may underlie many of the difficulties seen in the autistic spectrum disorders.

Closely related to this "interest" in social communication (that arises from a working theory of mind) is the ability to communicate socially. The skills discussed below are required to actually achieve the meaningful interaction. Certainly, if you don't have these required skills, your interest in social interaction may appear blunted.

**Pragmatic language:** Pragmatic language is the practical ability to use language in a social setting, such as knowing what is appropriate to say, where and when to say it, and the give and take nature of conversation. Effective pragmatics requires a working theory of mind: the ability to figure out what the other person does or does not already know—or might or might not be interested in hearing about. Examples of pragmatic language/theory of mind problems would be:

- A new student moves into the school district and enters the classroom for the first time. The teacher asks him where he comes from. The autistic spectrum child responds: "From the hallway."

- As an Asperger child walks into the office, the doctor notices that her pink shirt matches the color of her jacket. He jokes, "If you change into a green shirt, does the color of the jacket change, too?" The child responds: "My wardrobe includes a turquoise shirt, not a green one." This child's spoken language is precise, but she misses the actual meaning of the question; and, more importantly, that the whole purpose of this conversation was just a little fun chitchat to initiate an interaction.

**Knowledge of unwritten rules:** There is an incredible array of essential social norms that most typical children do not need to be explicitly taught. Did your mother have to tell you to look at people when you talk to them? Did your mother have to teach you how close to stand to someone? Did your mother have to teach you how to read facial expressions?

Liane Holliday Willey describes her own frustrating experience with Asperger as follows: "I never got the hang of it. For example, I can never tell how much time should pass before I buy for someone I just met a 'thinking of you gift.' Do I really have to talk on the phone to anyone if I think the conversation is boring or a waste of time? If there is a lapse in the conversation, am I supposed to hang up or tell a joke or just sit there? What if I like the person well enough, but I decide I cannot stand one of their behaviors or habits? The questions are endless, and the concerns are mountain high. This is why human relationships usually take me beyond my limits. They wear me out. (Willey 1999, p. 55)

As a quick rule of thumb, whenever you find yourself saying "I shouldn't have to tell you that . . . ," consider that you might be dealing with an ASD symptom.

**Knowing what is and isn't important:** The skills to know what is—and what is not—important include:

- the ability to see the big picture rather than fixate on details;
- the ability to maintain a full range of interests.

**Symbolic play skills:** Give a child a yellow box on wheels, with thin long black stripes on it. The ability to understand that this object actually represents a school bus is a type of communication. Speech pathologist Elaine Schneider points out that, if a child cannot even recognize that a physical toy bus stands for a real bus, how will he be able to recognize later that the graphic letters "B-U-S" represents a bus, too? Both involve the use of symbols rather than the actual object to communicate (Schneider, verbal communication 2005).

By eighteen months, most toddlers start to use objects as symbols for something else. For example, a cup is for drinking, but it also makes quite a handy telephone. By three years of age, most children are quite good at "let's pretend" activities, such as "You be the cowboy!" The toy school bus is not fascinating because the cold metal box can move, but because little toy figures chat while getting on it as they go to school. Stuffed animals are not just warm rags of cloth to drag around, but appear to be living creatures that have feelings and needs such as to be fed, dressed, and loved.

So, by eighteen to thirty-six months of age, typical children make continuous progress in the skill of appreciating the representational meaning of a toy, rather than focusing on its straightforward physical attributes. Failure to develop representational/symbolic/pretend play is a strong marker of the autistic spectrum disorders.

**Ability to achieve "joint attention":** A really cool limousine passes by. The child excitedly points to it, so that you can share in the experience with him. This important form of social communication is called "joint attention"—you are jointly sharing the same experience. Note that he isn't pointing simply to use you as a mechanical tool, such as pointing to the refrigerator so that you will satisfy his thirst for milk. Delayed ability to point for joint attention may be a marker for an ASD, even before delayed speech is noticed.

31

**Nonverbal (nonspoken) transmission of language:** The simple sounds are not the only thing my body sends through space when it attempts to communicate with you. It also transmits:

- facial expressions;
- body language;
- toned and prosody (rhythm) of speech.

### Secondary Problems Resulting from Failure to Understand

If the child does not understand what is going on around her—especially if pragmatic/socialization cues are difficult—secondary problems usually occur in the autistic spectrum disorders. The child will frequently appear:

- *anxious,* since she doesn't know what she is supposed to do, or where the next blunder will come from;

- *insistent on sameness* and showing ritualistic behavior. Change means that previously hard-learned strategies will not help in this situation. These kids are barely hanging on. One new wrinkle can throw them over the edge. For example, Jill may know that her fist task each day is to take her lunch out of the backpack. What happens, though, if today there is only half a day of school, and the lunch is missing? Now what does she do? The child may be unraveled for the rest of the day.

- *inattentive,* since it's hard to pay attention to something she does not understand;

- *rude,* since she doesn't understand rules of conversation such as waiting your turn;

- *interested in objects rather than people,* after all, objects are more predictable;

- *"hanging back"* from peers, for all of the above reasons, and from simply not knowing how to make conversation and relate;

- *"out of it"* and "odd" looking;

- *socially unwelcome,* which can become quite painful, especially as the child gets older. Says Holliday Willey, "To choose to be left out is one thing, but to be locked out is quite another . . . I was crippled when I found out that it took more than I had to give to make new friends." (Willey 1999, p. 72)

## Categories of Communication Disorders: Sorting Them Out

When a child has difficulties in these areas out of proportion to his or her general cognitive abilities, he or she can be considered to have a communication disorder.

Difficulties in the above skills can group together in varying combinations and severities, allowing for the naming of several communication disorder syndromes. As we shall see, these disorders overlap greatly. Some may even be duplicates of the same condition but approached by different specialties. Additionally, as children develop, their diagnostic classification might change. The human brain is not so simple that its disorders fit into neat, static categories. Nonetheless, we still attempt to find certain patterns. Unless we know about the range of syndromes, we will fail to look for important symptoms that need to be addressed.

Disorders of the communication skills are grouped into two major types of disorders. Let's give an overview of the organizational scheme first, then come back to each condition in detail later:

- **Typical language-based learning disorders** are due to problems in the purely spoken/written language communication skills. These include expressive, receptive, processing, and articulation language disorders. Most routine speech and language evaluations examine these areas. Note that routine psychological testing (such as the WISC "IQ"—Wechsler Intelligence Scale for Children) examines areas of cognition (thinking), rather than language per se.

- **Autistic spectrum disorders (ASD)** are those that include nonspoken communication problems—in particular, problems with socialization/empathy. In other words, the autistic spectrum disorders all share trouble with theory of mind, socialization, the pragmatics of language, and representational play. They may occur with or without additional verbal speech problems.

In turn, the autistic spectrum disorders are written about in two groupings:

- pervasive developmental disorders
- other autistic spectrum disorders

The pervasive developmental disorders (PDDs) defined medically in the *Diagnostic and Statistical Manual of Mental Disorders, Fourth*

*Edition* (*DSM-IV*) by the American Psychiatric Association, are a series of five diagnoses, of which autistic disorder is the most commonly discussed. "Pervasive" means that the problem cuts across multiple types of communication. Note that "PDD" is technically an overlying category for a group of actual individual specific diagnoses. So, it is better to talk of "the PDDs." These five PDDs are as follows

- **Autistic disorder:** Severely disordered verbal and nonverbal language; unusual behaviors; commonly referred to as "autism"

- **Asperger syndrome:** Relatively good verbal language, with "milder" nonverbal language problems; restricted range of interests and relatedness

- **PDD-NOS (pervasive developmental disorder-not otherwise specified):** Nonverbal language problems not meeting strict criteria for other PDD disorders

- **Rett disorder:** Rare neurodegenerative disorder of girls

- **Childhood disintegrative disorder:** A rare disorder that needs to be carefully distinguished from a neurodegenerative condition

Meanwhile, the rest of the world has extended the spectrum beyond those conditions discussed in *DSM-IV* to include other autistic spectrum disorders. To date, these terms have not been formally integrated into *DSM-IV* vocabulary. Presumably, they are subsumed under the category of PDD-NOS. In summary, these include the following:

- **High-functioning autism:** For some authors, synonymous with Asperger; for others, implies milder autism without retardation

- **Nonverbal learning disabilities:** Trouble integrating information in three areas: nonverbal difficulties causing the child to miss the major gestalt in language; spatial perception problems; and motor coordination problems

- **Semantic-pragmatic language disorder:** Delay and trouble with the use of language (both semantic and pragmatic), but socialization relatively spared

- **Hyperlexia:** Most notable for incredible rote reading skills starting at an early age

- **Some aspects of attention deficit hyperactivity disorder (ADHD):** The impulsivity and self-control difficulties in ADHD may cause kids to have trouble showing their empathy.

## DSM-IV *Pervasive Developmental Disorders*

We start our more detailed review of each autistic spectrum disorder by presenting a summary of the key diagnostic criteria for each of the five PDD disorders as defined in *DSM-IV* (APA 1994).

**Autistic disorder:** By *DSM-IV* criteria, children with autistic disorder must have problems in each of the following three areas:

1. *Social interaction problems:* There are significant problems with nonverbal communication like body language, eye contact, and facial expressions. Peer relationships are inadequate, and the child has trouble returning emotions during interactions. The person does not seek to share achievements or interests via pointing or bringing things for praise.

2. *Communication problems:* There are significant spoken language problems (which are not compensated by signing). The person has trouble keeping up or starting a conversation (in those children who can speak). The speech tends to be stereotyped and/or repetitive. There is also a lack of communication via imaginative or imitative play.

3. *Narrow and/or repetitive range of interests or behaviors:* The autistic person has an inappropriately intense fascination with a particular subject, or may be overly preoccupied with the parts of an object. Typically, the child is inflexible and has ritualistic behaviors, including repetitive body movements such as rocking or arm flapping.

Other qualifying criteria include early onset (before three years old) of problems in at least one of the areas of pretend/imaginary play, social interactions, or the pragmatic use of language.

**Asperger syndrome:** Symptoms of Asperger syndrome include the following:

- Impaired ability to utilize social cues such as body language or tone of voice

- Impaired ability to understand irony or other "subtext" of communication
- "Concrete" thinking
- Restricted eye contact and socialization
- Appearance as distant or a loner
- Limited range of encyclopedic interests
- Didactic, verbose, monotone, droning voice
- Perseverative, odd behaviors
- Oversensitivity to certain stimuli
- Unusual movements

The official *DSM-IV* criteria for Asperger syndrome (APA 1994) are similar to those for autistic disorder, except do not include the "communication" problem areas above. In other words, Asperger people are autistic people who talk well. Although verbal speech is preserved in Asperger, other communication problems certainly exist.

You can hear a soundtrack of two children with Asperger at the author's website at www.pediatricneuroligy.com/aspergers_sound.htm Once you hear their typical droning voice, you'll never forget it.

**PDD-NOS (not otherwise specified):** The diagnosis of PDD-NOS is invoked for children in the autistic spectrum who do not completely fit into one of the other categories.

**Rett syndrome:** This is a neurodegenerative disorder of girls who have normal initial development, but then show marked loss of developmental milestones and social interactions, slowing of head growth, and wringing hand movements.

**Childhood disintegrative disorder:** Children with this disorder develop normally for at least the first two years, and then have a deterioration sufficient to meet criteria for autistic disorder, but also show deterioration of language, muscle control, social, play, and toilet training skills. These children need to be carefully evaluated for an underlying neurodegenerative process.

### *Expanded Autistic Spectrum Disorders*

Next, we turn our attention to those autistic spectrum disorders that are not included in *DSM-IV*.

**High-functioning autism:** For some authors, this term is synonymous with Asperger syndrome. For others, it implies milder autism without retardation, or PDD-NOS. Given the lack of consensus for the meaning of this term, it is probably best not to use it.

**Nonverbal learning disabilities:** Nonverbal learning disabilities (NVLDs) are a cluster of symptoms presumably related to poor ability to integrate information. These children have trouble with the ability to integrate it all together, i.e., to see the big gestalt picture rather than the details. In short, they "can't see the forest for the trees." These tasks are usually carried out by the brain's nondominant hemisphere (typically the right hemisphere). Even though rote verbal language is spared, nonverbal areas of difficulty may be debilitating.

Although verbal communication is highly prized in school (good talkers, readers, and writers), up to two-thirds of communication actually occurs nonverbally (Thompson 1996). Thus, in the long run, the maladaptive learning of NVLD may be more destructive than typical LD. Estimates are that 0.1 to 1 percent of the population has an NVLD, compared with as much as 10 percent of the population with an LD (Thompson 1996), although these numbers may be an artifact of who and how we test.

Difficulty integrating nonverbal information occurs in three main areas:

- Motor skills:

  - *Gross motor:* Clumsy, unbalanced walking leading to clinging behaviors, bumping into things, fear of climbing, hesitant to explore physically, difficulty bike-riding, and uncoordinated at sports.

  - *Fine motor:* Difficulty using scissors, shoe tying (which she'll talk herself through), and poor handwriting using awkward and tight grip.

- Visual/spatial orientation skills, with an inability to form visual images:

  - Resultant focus on detail rather than the important gestalt.

  - Labels everything verbally, since that is the only—albeit not always accurate—way she can process the visual/spatial information. For example, she may find her way home by counting houses and labeling landmarks verbally.

- The elaborate "naming" strategies break down with changes in routine, leading to an inability to cope with change.
- Unaware where she is in space, unaware of where to place answers on the homework sheet, or how to navigate the school.

- Social/communication skills:
  - Trouble integrating nonverbal communication with verbal communication in order to achieve full social interaction.
  - Clearly appears to want social acceptance (vs. Asperger, where the children usually do not appear interested socially).
  - Very literal interpretation of others; concrete thinking; seeing the world in black and white; trouble understanding.
  - Dishonesty; trouble seeing hidden meanings, prompting others to say "You know what I meant!"—when they didn't.
  - Don't read the social cues of give-and-take conversation, thus appearing self-centered, weird, or impolite.
  - Typically labeled as "annoying" because of their dependence on others, their constant speech, and their misinterpretation of social cues.

NVLD symptoms change through the lifespan.

- Toddlers:
  - Uncoordinated (gross motor and fine motor).
  - Trouble with social interactions, nonverbal cues (such as a peer's facial expression of "Enough is enough!"), and adjustments to change. They may appear "confused."
  - Warning signal: You always have to tell the child, "I shouldn't have to tell you that." Obviously, with these kids, you *do* have to tell them. That's how you know there is a problem.
  - Trouble with spatial orientation.
- Young children:
  - Often exceptional rote speech, memory, and reading skill, which the children use to compensate for lack of intuitive social interaction. The child tries to "remember" how to interact, rather than the skill coming automatically in each different situation.

- The pedantic speech patterns and the exceptional reading abilities may be interpreted as precociousness.
- Clumsy monologues replace typical give-and-take conversations.
- Older children:
  - Academic problems in the later elementary years with organization, inferential reading, and written output.
  - Math facts better than concepts.
  - Typically performance IQ is lower than verbal IQ.
  - Sustains focus on details, does not attend to big picture.
  - A life of social blunders, without ever figuring out why.
  - May have secondary depression or anxiety.

NVLD is determined by neuropsychological testing, whereas Asperger syndrome is determined by detailed history and observation. There is great overlap in these two conditions—perhaps due to comorbidity; or perhaps, as some authors feel, they are essentially the same condition but labeled by different specialties. However, people with Asperger are primarily notable for *not appearing* interested in forming human bonds. (The degree to which Asperger kids actually are painfully aware of their trouble making bonds is debated in the literature. Nevertheless, they typically appear uninterested.) NVLD kids, though, do typically appear interested in human bonds—even though they may be clueless how to actually achieve them successfully. Additionally, children with Asperger syndrome typically have more diminished "symbolic play" than in NVLD.

So, how about this for a gross oversimplification? NVLD kids recognize that you exist while they miss the subtext of what you are saying. Asperger kids appear as if outside a window as they miss the subtext of what you are saying.

**Semantic-pragmatic language disorder:** "Semantics refers to the ability to use and understand words, phrases, and sentences, including abstract concepts and idioms. "Pragmatics" refers to the practical ability to use language in a social setting, such as knowing what is appropriate to say, where and when to say it, the give-and-take nature of a conversation, and the ability to know what the other person does or does not already know. Thus, semantic-pragmatic language disorder (SPLD) kids have:

- Difficulty understanding the literal meaning of words and sentences (semantics);
- Difficulty with abstract words, words about emotions, idioms, and words about status such as "expert" (semantics);
- Difficulty extracting the central idea (pragmatics);
- Trouble with the appropriate rules of conversation, such as talking "at" you or using monologues (pragmatics).

This inability to understand verbal language and the purpose of language leads to the typical secondary problems we have discussed above.

Here is what we might expect in the life of a child with SPLD through the years:

- Often very easy infants
- Delayed development of speech with few words even by two years old
- Trouble with creative or symbolic play
- Simple speech improves with therapy, but in school child is "odd"
- Good rote skills in math and computers, perhaps, but poor writing and socialization skills
- Parrot back more than they understand, leading to an aura of intellectual maturity out of synch with their social skills
- Trouble understanding what others are really thinking or feeling, i.e., trouble with theory of mind
- Many have fine motor problems; some have gross motor difficulties as well
- May have trouble knowing what is socially acceptable, but are not usually conduct disorder teens
- May be "eccentric" adults

SPLD can be differentiated from Asperger syndrome as follows:

- SPLD kids tend to have more early speech delays than Asperger kids.
- SPLD kids tend to have somewhat better socialization skills than Asperger kids.

- The appropriate label may change over time as the child matures.

**Hyperlexia:** Hyperlexia is a condition, occurring almost always in boys, where autistic spectrum symptoms are accompanied by a striking capacity for rote reading. By eighteen to twenty-four months of age, these kids have taught themselves the ability to name letters and numbers. By three years old, they may read printed words, exceeding even their ability to talk. By five years old, all have a fascination with the printed word. Some of the children seemed to have a mild regression at eighteen to twenty-four months (less severe than as in autism).

In addition to this unusual reading skill, there are the other typical common autistic spectrum disorder symptoms we have seen, such as the following:

- Language problems:
  - Good rote or echoed language
  - Trouble translating words into larger gestalt ideas
  - Repetitive, idiosyncratic speech
  - Pragmatic language problems
  - Unusual prosody (rhythm) of speech
- Socialization problems:
  - See "Secondary problems resulting from failure to understand" (above)
  - Stereotyped, ritualistic behaviors
  - Anxiety
  - Trouble making friends

The above description is based on an article by Phyllis Kupperman and others from the Center for Speech and Language Disorders (Kupperman et al. n.d.)

**Attention deficit hyperactivity disorder (ADHD):** ADHDers typically have adequate capacity for empathy—but may have trouble inhibiting their behavior long enough to show it. Conversely, many children on the autistic spectrum may appear to have a short attention span, but this may actually be due to an inability to stay focused

41

on situations they don't understand. Of course, ADHD and ASD can—and do—frequently co-occur as parts of the syndrome mix.

It is probably best to consider ADHD not as part of, but as sometimes sharing the following symptoms with autistic spectrum disorders:

- *Poor reading of social cues:* "Johnny, you're such a social klutz. Can't you see that the other children think that's weird?"

- *Poor ability to utilize "self-talk" to work through a problem:* "Johnny, what were you thinking? Did you ever think this through?"

- *Poor sense of self-awareness:* Johnny's true answer to the above question is probably "I don't have a clue. I guess I wasn't actually thinking."

- *Better performance with predictable routine.*

- *Poor generalization of rules:* "Johnny, I told you to shake hands with your teachers. Why didn't you shake hands with the *principal?*"

## Conclusion (Finally!)

The classification of the autistic spectrum disorders is in a state of flux. The problems can overlap, cause each other, occur simultaneously in different combinations and severities, change over time, and don't even have one "official" group attempting the classification of the whole spectrum.

However, unless we know all of the possible syndromes, we will continue to squeeze everyone into the same category or two. Most importantly, unless we know the full range of the autistic spectrum disorders, we will not identify all of the individual symptoms that require treatment.

With trepidation, I offer the following gross oversimplifications. I am reminded of my professor's comment on the first day of medical school: "One-third of what I am going to tell you this year is wrong. Unfortunately, I don't know which third":

- Autistic spectrum disorders are marked by difficulty in communication/socialization in areas other than the literal meaning of words.

- Once a child has trouble with getting the big picture of communication and socialization, there will often be secondary symptoms, such as anxiety, holding back from peers, a rigid adherence to sameness, a relative preference for things (which are predictable) rather than people, and an appearance of "oddness."

- Asperger and autism share primarily the difficulty of recognizing the existence of others—trouble with theory of mind. People with Asperger can talk; autism usually has limited speech.

- Asperger children *appear* less interested in forming bonds and have more trouble with "theory of mind" than NVLD and semantic-pragmatic disorder.

- NVLDs are marked by integration problems of pragmatic language gestalt; spatial orientation; and motor coordination.

- Hyperlexia is marked by fascination with the printed word starting at an early age.

- "High-functioning autism" is used by different authors to mean either autistic disorder with relatively spared speech and cognition, Asperger syndrome, or PDD-NOS.

Autistic spectrum disorders such as Asperger syndrome tend to be highly "comorbid"—occur in conjunction with other conditions of the syndrome mix. ADHD, anxiety, obsessive-compulsive disorder (OCD), and sensory integration problems are particularly common.

## References

American Psychiatric Association (APA) (1994) *Diagnostic and Statistical Manual of Mental Disorders* (4th edition). Washington, DC: American Psychiatric Association.

Kupperman, P., Bligh, S., and Barouski, K. (n.d.) *Hyperlexia.* www.hyperlexia.org/hyperlexia.html

Thompson, S. (1996) "Non verbal learning disabilities." http://www.nldontheweb.org/thompson-1.htm

Willey, L. H. (1999) *Pretending to Be Normal: Living with Asperger's Syndrome.* London: Jessica Kingsley Publishers.

# Chapter 4

# *Types of Autism Spectrum Disorders*

## Chapter Contents

Section 4.1—Classical Autism ........................................................ 46

Section 4.2—Asperger Syndrome ................................................. 51

Section 4.3—Rett Syndrome .......................................................... 58

Section 4.4—Childhood Disintegrative Disorder ....................... 68

Section 4.5—Pervasive Developmental Disorder-Not
Otherwise Specified (PDD-NOS)............................ 70

Section 4.1

# *Classical Autism*

Reprinted from "Autism Fact Sheet," National Institute of
Neurological Disorders and Stroke, National Institutes of Health,
NIH Publication No. 06-1877, July 17, 2006.

### *What is autism?*

Autism (sometimes called "classical autism") is the most common
condition in a group of developmental disorders known as the autism
spectrum disorders (ASDs). Autism is characterized by impaired social interaction, problems with verbal and nonverbal communication,
and unusual, repetitive, or severely limited activities and interests.
Other ASDs include Asperger syndrome, Rett syndrome, childhood disintegrative disorder, and pervasive developmental disorder not otherwise specified (usually referred to as PDD-NOS). Experts estimate
that three to six children out of every one thousand will have autism.
Males are four times more likely to have autism than females.

### *What are some common signs of autism?*

There are three distinctive behaviors that characterize autism.
Autistic children have difficulties with social interaction, problems
with verbal and nonverbal communication, and repetitive behaviors
or narrow, obsessive interests. These behaviors can range in impact
from mild to disabling.

The hallmark feature of autism is impaired social interaction.
Parents are usually the first to notice symptoms of autism in their
child. As early as infancy, a baby with autism may be unresponsive
to people or focus intently on one item to the exclusion of others for
long periods of time. A child with autism may appear to develop
normally and then withdraw and become indifferent to social engagement.

Children with autism may fail to respond to their name and often
avoid eye contact with other people. They have difficulty interpreting what others are thinking or feeling because they can't understand
social cues, such as tone of voice or facial expressions, and don't watch

other people's faces for clues about appropriate behavior. They lack empathy.

Many children with autism engage in repetitive movements such as rocking and twirling, or in self-abusive behavior such as biting or head banging. They also tend to start speaking later than other children and may refer to themselves by name instead of using "I" or "me." Children with autism don't know how to play interactively with other children. Some speak in a singsong voice about a narrow range of favorite topics, with little regard for the interests of the person to whom they are speaking.

Many children with autism have a reduced sensitivity to pain, but are abnormally sensitive to sound, touch, or other sensory stimulation. These unusual reactions may contribute to behavioral symptoms such as a resistance to being cuddled or hugged.

Children with autism appear to have a higher than normal risk for certain coexisting conditions, including fragile X syndrome (which causes mental retardation), tuberous sclerosis (in which tumors grow on the brain), epileptic seizures, Tourette syndrome, learning disabilities, and attention deficit disorder. For reasons that are still unclear, about 20 to 30 percent of children with autism develop epilepsy by the time they reach adulthood. While people with schizophrenia may show some autistic-like behavior, their symptoms usually do not appear until the late teens or early adulthood. Most people with schizophrenia also have hallucinations and delusions, which are not found in autism.

### How is autism diagnosed?

Autism varies widely in its severity and symptoms and may go unrecognized, especially in mildly affected children or when it is masked by more debilitating handicaps. Doctors rely on a core group of behaviors to alert them to the possibility of a diagnosis of autism. These behaviors are as follows:

- Impaired ability to make friends with peers
- Impaired ability to initiate or sustain a conversation with others
- Absence or impairment of imaginative and social play
- Stereotyped, repetitive, or unusual use of language
- Restricted patterns of interest that are abnormal in intensity or focus
- Preoccupation with certain objects or subjects
- Inflexible adherence to specific routines or rituals

Doctors will often use a questionnaire or other screening instrument to gather information about a child's development and behavior. Some screening instruments rely solely on parent observations; others rely on a combination of parent and doctor observations. If screening instruments indicate the possibility of autism, doctors will ask for a more comprehensive evaluation.

Autism is a complex disorder. A comprehensive evaluation requires a multidisciplinary team including a psychologist, a neurologist, a psychiatrist, a speech therapist, and other professionals who diagnose children with ASDs. The team members will conduct a thorough neurological assessment and in-depth cognitive and language testing. Because hearing problems can cause behaviors that could be mistaken for autism, children with delayed speech development should also have their hearing tested. After a thorough evaluation, the team usually meets with parents to explain the results of the evaluation and present the diagnosis.

Children with some symptoms of autism, but not enough to be diagnosed with classical autism, are often diagnosed with PDD-NOS. Children with autistic behaviors but well-developed language skills are often diagnosed with Asperger syndrome. Children who develop normally and then suddenly deteriorate between the ages of three to ten years and show marked autistic behaviors may be diagnosed with childhood disintegrative disorder. Girls with autistic symptoms may be suffering from Rett syndrome, a sex-linked genetic disorder characterized by social withdrawal, regressed language skills, and hand wringing.

### What causes autism?

Scientists aren't certain what causes autism, but it's likely that both genetics and environment play a role. Researchers have identified a number of genes associated with the disorder. Studies of people with autism have found irregularities in several regions of the brain. Other studies suggest that people with autism have abnormal levels of serotonin or other neurotransmitters in the brain. These abnormalities suggest that autism could result from the disruption of normal brain development early in fetal development caused by defects in genes that control brain growth and that regulate how neurons communicate with each other. While these findings are intriguing, they are preliminary and require further study. The theory that parental practices are responsible for autism has now been disproved.

## What role does inheritance play?

Recent studies strongly suggest that some people have a genetic predisposition to autism. In families with one autistic child, the risk of having a second child with the disorder is approximately 5 percent, or one in twenty. This is greater than the risk for the general population. Researchers are looking for clues about which genes contribute to this increased susceptibility. In some cases, parents and other relatives of an autistic child show mild impairments in social and communicative skills or engage in repetitive behaviors. Evidence also suggests that some emotional disorders, such as manic depression, occur more frequently than average in the families of people with autism.

## Do symptoms of autism change over time?

For many children, autism symptoms improve with treatment and with age. Some children with autism grow up to lead normal or near-normal lives. Children whose language skills regress early in life, usually before the age of three, appear to be at risk of developing epilepsy or seizure-like brain activity. During adolescence, some children with autism may become depressed or experience behavioral problems. Parents of these children should be ready to adjust treatment for their child as needed.

## How is autism treated?

There is no cure for autism. Therapies and behavioral interventions are designed to remedy specific symptoms and can bring about substantial improvement. The ideal treatment plan coordinates therapies and interventions that target the core symptoms of autism: impaired social interaction, problems with verbal and nonverbal communication, and obsessive or repetitive routines and interests. Most professionals agree that the earlier the intervention, the better.

**Educational/behavioral interventions:** Therapists use highly structured and intensive skill-oriented training sessions to help children develop social and language skills. Family counseling for the parents and siblings of children with autism often helps families cope with the particular challenges of living with an autistic child.

**Medications:** Doctors often prescribe an antidepressant medication to handle symptoms of anxiety, depression, or obsessive-compulsive disorder. Anti-psychotic medications are used to treat severe behavioral problems. Seizures can be treated with one or more of the anticonvulsant drugs. Stimulant drugs, such as those used for children with attention deficit disorder (ADD), are sometimes used effectively to help decrease impulsivity and hyperactivity.

**Other therapies:** There are a number of controversial therapies or interventions available for autistic children, but few, if any, are supported by scientific studies. Parents should use caution before adopting any of these treatments.

## What research is being done?

The National Institute of Neurological Disorders and Stroke (NINDS) is one of the federal government's leading supporters of biomedical research on brain and nervous system disorders. The NINDS conducts research in its laboratories at the National Institutes of Health in Bethesda, Maryland, and also awards grants to support research at universities and other facilities.

As part of the Children's Health Act of 2000, the NINDS and three sister institutes have formed the National Institutes of Health (NIH) Autism Coordinating Committee to expand, intensify, and coordinate NIH's autism research. Eight dedicated research centers across the country have been established as "Centers of Excellence in Autism Research" to bring together researchers and the resources they need. The centers are conducting basic and clinical research, including investigations into causes, diagnosis, early detection, prevention, and treatment, such as the studies highlighted below:

- Investigators are using animal models to study how the neurotransmitter serotonin establishes connections between neurons in hopes of discovering why these connections are impaired in autism.

- Researchers are testing a computer-assisted program that would help autistic children interpret facial expressions.

- A brain imaging study is investigating areas of the brain that are active during obsessive/repetitive behaviors in adults and very young children with autism.

- Other imaging studies are searching for brain abnormalities that could cause impaired social communication in children with autism.

50

- Clinical studies are testing the effectiveness of a program that combines parent training and medication to reduce the disruptive behavior of children with autism and other ASDs.

## Section 4.2

# *Asperger Syndrome*

Reprinted from "Asperger Syndrome Fact Sheet," National Institute of Neurological Disorders and Stroke, National Institutes of Health, NIH Publication No. 05-5624, July 17, 2006.

### *What is Asperger syndrome?*

Asperger syndrome (AS) is a developmental disorder that is characterized by the following traits:[1]

- Limited interests or an unusual preoccupation with a particular subject to the exclusion of other activities

- Repetitive routines or rituals

- Peculiarities in speech and language, such as speaking in an overly formal manner or in a monotone, or taking figures of speech literally

- Socially and emotionally inappropriate behavior and the inability to interact successfully with peers

- Problems with nonverbal communication, including the restricted use of gestures, limited or inappropriate facial expressions, or a peculiar, stiff gaze

- Clumsy and uncoordinated motor movements

AS is an autism spectrum disorder (ASD), one of a distinct group of neurological conditions characterized by a greater or lesser degree of impairment in language and communication skills, as well as repetitive or restrictive patterns of thought and behavior. Other ASDs include: classic autism, Rett syndrome, childhood disintegrative disorder, and

51

pervasive developmental disorder not otherwise specified (usually referred to as PDD-NOS).

Parents usually sense there is something unusual about a child with AS by the time of his or her third birthday, and some children may exhibit symptoms as early as infancy. Unlike children with autism, children with AS retain their early language skills. Motor development delays—crawling or walking late, clumsiness—are sometimes the first indicator of the disorder.

The incidence of AS is not well established, but experts in population studies conservatively estimate that two out of every ten thousand children have the disorder. Boys are three to four times more likely than girls to have AS.

Studies of children with AS suggest that their problems with socialization and communication continue into adulthood. Some of these children develop additional psychiatric symptoms and disorders in adolescence and adulthood.

Although diagnosed mainly in children, AS is being increasingly diagnosed in adults who seek medical help for mental health conditions such as depression, obsessive-compulsive disorder (OCD), and attention deficit hyperactivity disorder (ADHD). No studies have yet been conducted to determine the incidence of AS in adult populations.

### Why is it called Asperger syndrome?

In 1944, an Austrian pediatrician named Hans Asperger observed four children in his practice who had difficulty integrating socially. Although their intelligence appeared normal, the children lacked nonverbal communication skills, failed to demonstrate empathy with their peers, and were physically clumsy. Their way of speaking was either disjointed or overly formal, and their all-absorbing interest in a single topic dominated their conversations. Dr. Asperger called the condition "autistic psychopathy" and described it as a personality disorder primarily marked by social isolation.

Asperger's observations, published in German, were not widely known until 1981, when an English doctor named Lorna Wing published a series of case studies of children showing similar symptoms, which she called "Asperger's" syndrome. Wing's writings were widely published and popularized. AS became a distinct disease and diagnosis in 1992, when it was included in the tenth published edition of the World Health Organization's diagnostic manual, *International Classification of Diseases (ICD-10)*, and in 1995 it was added to the

*Diagnostic and Statistical Manual of Mental Disorders* (*DSM-IV*), the American Psychiatric Association's diagnostic reference book.

### What are some common signs or symptoms?

The most distinguishing symptom of AS is a child's obsessive interest in a single object or topic to the exclusion of any other. Some children with AS have become experts on vacuum cleaners, makes and models of cars, even objects as odd as deep fat fryers. Children with AS want to know everything about their topic of interest, and their conversations with others will be about little else. Their expertise, high level of vocabulary, and formal speech patterns make them seem like little professors.

Children with AS will gather enormous amounts of factual information about their favorite subject and will talk incessantly about it, but the conversation may seem like a random collection of facts or statistics, with no point or conclusion.

Their speech may be marked by a lack of rhythm, an odd inflection, or a monotone pitch. Children with AS often lack the ability to modulate the volume of their voice to match their surroundings. For example, they will have to be reminded to talk softly every time they enter a library or a movie theatre.

Unlike the severe withdrawal from the rest of the world that is characteristic of autism, children with AS are isolated because of their poor social skills and narrow interests. In fact, they may approach other people, but make normal conversation impossible by inappropriate or eccentric behavior, or by wanting to talk about only their singular interest.

Children with AS usually have a history of developmental delays in motor skills such as pedaling a bike, catching a ball, or climbing outdoor play equipment. They are often awkward and poorly coordinated with a walk that can appear either stilted or bouncy.

Many children with AS are highly active in early childhood, and then develop anxiety or depression in young adulthood. Other conditions that often coexist with AS are ADHD, tic disorders (such as Tourette syndrome), depression, anxiety disorders, and OCD.

### What causes AS? Is it genetic?

Twin and family studies suggest there is a genetic vulnerability to AS and the other ASDs, but a specific gene for AS hasn't been identified. It is likely that multiple genes cause AS, since the symptoms and the severity of symptoms vary so widely among individuals.

Researchers recently identified an association between certain behavioral traits (the insistence on strict routines and repetitive behavior) in a group of children with autism and a specific gene—GABRB3. Another study discovered a strong association between autism and the mutation of a gene the researchers call ENGRAILED 2. Additional evidence for the link between inheritable genetic mutations and AS is seen in the higher incidence of family members of children with an ASD who have similar behavioral symptoms, but in a more limited form. For example they may have mild social, language, or reading problems.

Current research points to structural abnormalities in the brain as a cause of AS. These abnormalities impact neural circuits that control thought and behavior. Researchers think that gene/environment interactions cause some genes to turn on or turn off, or turn on too much or too little in the wrong places, and this interferes with the normal migration and wiring of embryonic brain cells during early development.

Researchers at the University of California, supported in part by the National Institutes of Health, have proposed the disorder stems from abnormal changes that happen during critical stages of fetal development. Defects in the genes that control and regulate normal brain growth create abnormal growth patterns, which cause overgrowth in some brain structures and reduced growth, or excessive cell loss, in others.

Using advanced brain imaging techniques, scientists have revealed structural and functional differences in specific brain regions between the brains of normal versus AS children. One study found a lack of activity in the frontal lobe of AS children when asked to respond to tasks that required them to use their judgment. Another found differences in brain activity when children were asked to respond to facial expressions. Other methods of investigating brain function have revealed abnormal levels of particular proteins in the brains of adults with AS, which correlate with obsessive and repetitive behaviors.

### How is it diagnosed?

The diagnosis of AS is complicated by the lack of a standardized diagnostic screen or schedule. In fact, because there are several screening instruments in current use, each with different criteria, the same child could receive different diagnoses, depending on the screening tool the doctor uses.

To further complicate the issue, some doctors believe that AS is not a separate and distinct disorder. Instead, they call it high-functioning autism (HFA), and view it as being on the mild end of the ASD spectrum with symptoms that differ—only in degree—from classic autism. Some clinicians use the two diagnoses, AS or HFA, interchangeably. This makes gathering data about the incidence of AS difficult, since some children will be diagnosed with HFA instead of AS, and vice versa.

Most doctors rely on the presence of a core group of behaviors to alert them to the possibility of a diagnosis of AS:

- Abnormal eye contact

- Aloofness

- The failure to turn when called by name

- The failure to use gestures to point or show

- A lack of interactive play

- A lack of interest in peers

Some of these behaviors may be apparent in the first few months of a child's life, or they may appear later. Problems in at least one of the areas of communication and socialization or repetitive, restricted behavior must be present before the age of three.

The diagnosis of AS is a two-stage process. The first stage begins with developmental screening during a "well-child" check-up with a family doctor or pediatrician. The second stage is a comprehensive team evaluation to either rule in or rule out AS. This team generally includes a psychologist, a neurologist, a psychiatrist, a speech therapist, and additional professionals who have expertise in diagnosing children with AS.

The comprehensive evaluation includes neurologic and genetic assessment, with in-depth cognitive and language testing to establish IQ and evaluate psychomotor function, verbal and nonverbal strengths and weaknesses, style of learning, and independent living skills. An assessment of communication strengths and weaknesses includes evaluating nonverbal forms of communication (gaze and gestures); the use of nonliteral language (metaphor, irony, absurdities, and humor); patterns of inflection, stress, and volume modulation; pragmatics (turn-taking and sensitivity to verbal cues); and the content, clarity, and coherence of conversation. The physician will look at the testing results and combine them with the child's developmental history and current symptoms to make a diagnosis.

### Are there treatments available?

The ideal treatment for AS coordinates therapies that address the three core symptoms of the disorder: poor communication skills, obsessive or repetitive routines, and physical clumsiness. There is no single best treatment package for all children with AS, but most professionals agree that the earlier the intervention, the better.

An effective treatment program builds on the child's interests, offers a predictable schedule, teaches tasks as a series of simple steps, actively engages the child's attention in highly structured activities, and provides regular reinforcement of behavior. This kind of program generally includes the following elements:

- **Social skills training:** A form of group therapy that teaches children with AS the skills they need to interact more successfully with other children

- **Cognitive behavioral therapy:** A type of "talk" therapy that can help the more explosive or anxious children to manage their emotions better and cut back on obsessive interests and repetitive routines

- **Medication:** For coexisting conditions such as depression and anxiety

- **Occupational or physical therapy:** For children with sensory integration problems or poor motor coordination

- **Specialized speech/language therapy:** To help children who have trouble with the pragmatics of speech—the give and take of normal conversation

- **Parent training and support:** To teach parents behavioral techniques to use at home

### Do children with AS get better? What happens when they become adults?

With effective treatment, children with AS can learn to cope with their disabilities, but they may still find social situations and personal relationships challenging. Many adults with AS are able to work successfully in mainstream jobs, although they may continue to need encouragement and moral support to maintain an independent life.

## *What research is being done?*

The National Institute of Neurological Disorders and Stroke (NINDS) is one of the federal government's leading supporters of biomedical research on brain and nervous system disorders. The NINDS conducts research in its laboratories at the National Institutes of Health in Bethesda, Maryland, and also awards grants to support research at universities and other facilities.

Many of the Institutes at the NIH, including the NINDS, are sponsoring research to understand what causes AS and how it can be effectively treated. One study is using functional magnetic resonance imaging (fMRI) to show how abnormalities in particular areas of the brain cause changes in brain function that result in the symptoms of AS and other ASDs. A large-scale study is comparing neuropsychological and psychiatric assessments of children with possible diagnoses of AS or HFA to those of their parents and siblings to see if there are patterns of symptoms that link AS and HFA to specific neuropsychological profiles. A clinical trial is testing the effectiveness of an anti-depressant in individuals with AS and HFA who exhibit high levels of obsessive/ritualistic behavior. Other investigators are conducting a long-range study to collect and analyze DNA samples from a large group of children with AS and HFA and their families to identify genes and genetic interactions that are linked to AS and HFA.

## *Notes*

1.  Adapted from the *Diagnostic and Statistical Manual of Mental Disorders IV* and the *International Classification of Diseases - 10.*

Section 4.3

# *Rett Syndrome*

Reprinted from National Institute of Child Health and
Human Development, National Institutes of Health, NIH
Publication No. 06-5590, April 2006.

## *What is Rett syndrome?*

Rett syndrome[1] is a complex neurobiological disorder of development in which an infant seems to grow and develop normally at first, but then stops developing and even loses skills and abilities.

For instance, they stop talking, even though they used to say certain words. They lose their ability to walk properly, even though they used to walk normally. They stop using their hands to do things, even though they had already started to grab and point. They often develop stereotyped hand movements, such as wringing, clapping, or patting their hands. They stop responding to and interacting with others normally, even though they used to smile at others and follow them with their eyes.

Until recently, researchers thought that Rett syndrome affected only females, but they now know that Rett syndrome affects a few males as well.[2] Because the number of males with Rett syndrome is very small, most of the statistics and research on Rett syndrome are specific to females. You will notice that this section refers mostly to females when talking about Rett syndrome.

Although many people with Rett syndrome live into their forties and fifties, their lives are not easy. Many of them can't walk or talk, but can communicate with their eyes. Most need special education, diets, and treatments for their various problems.

Most people with Rett syndrome can't care for themselves and need someone to care for them throughout their lives.

## *What causes Rett syndrome?*

For most females with Rett syndrome, the disorder results from a change in a single gene.

## What are genes?

Genes are pieces of DNA, material that contains all the information needed to "build" a person. Genes are hereditary, meaning parents pass genes on to their children.

Most of this material is found in the nucleus of the cell, a storage area that keeps these materials together in one place. The nucleus stores the material in packages called chromosomes.

Most people have forty-six chromosomes in most of their cells—twenty-three from their mother and twenty-three from their father. Each chromosome is made up of different numbers of individual genes.

Genes contain the information your body uses to make proteins, the body's building blocks. Proteins make up the structure of your organs and tissues; your body needs them for chemical functions and interacting chemical pathways. Each protein performs a specific job in the body's different types of cells, and a single gene usually contains the information for making at least one protein.

The pattern, or sequence, of your genes is like a blueprint that tells your body how to build its different parts. For example, your genes control how tall you are, what color your hair and eyes are, and other features of your body and mind. Changes, or mutations, in that blueprint can cause changes in how your body or mind grows and develops.

## How do genes cause Rett syndrome?

In 1999, scientists supported by the National Institute of Child Health and Human Development (NICHD)[3] discovered that most girls with Rett syndrome have a change in the pattern of a single gene—the Methyl-CpG-binding Protein 2 (*MECP2*) gene on the X chromosome. Between 90 and 95 percent of girls with Rett syndrome have a mutation in this gene.[4,5]

This gene makes methyl-CpG-binding protein 2 (MeCP2), which is necessary for the development of the nervous system—especially the brain. The mutation causes the gene to make less than the needed amounts of the protein, or to make a damaged protein that the body can't use. As a result, there may not be enough usable amount of the protein for the brain to develop normally.

Researchers are still trying to understand exactly how the brain uses MeCP2 and how problems with the protein cause the typical features of Rett syndrome. Normally, MeCP2 helps to "turn off" certain genes that make different proteins in nerve cells and other cells. Without MeCP2, the body keeps making these materials, even when it no longer needs them. After a while, having high amounts of these materials in the body may actually start to hurt the nervous system and cause the problems of Rett syndrome.

But not all people with Rett syndrome have a genetic mutation. In 5 percent[4,6] of people with Rett syndrome an *MECP2* mutation is not present or is not detectable. Furthermore, some people who have mutations on the *MECP2* gene don't show the typical features of Rett syndrome. Researchers are looking at different genes to see if they, too, can cause the symptoms of Rett syndrome.

### If Rett syndrome is a genetic disorder, does that mean it is inherited?

In more than 99.9 percent[2] of cases of Rett syndrome, the genetic mutation is spontaneous, meaning that it occurs randomly. Random mutations are usually not inherited or passed from one generation to the next. In a very small percentage of families—about 1 percent[5]—Rett mutations are inherited and passed on by female carriers. Scientists are working to learn more about these families to understand how this inherited mutation arises.

### How many people have Rett syndrome?

To date, researchers don't know exactly how many people have Rett syndrome. However, current estimates of the prevalence of Rett syndrome are that about one female out of ten thousand[7] has the disorder.

### What are the typical features of Rett syndrome?

Beginning between three months and three years of age, most children with Rett syndrome start to show some of the following symptoms:

- **Loss of purposeful hand movements:** They lose the ability to do things with their hands, such as grasping with fingers, reaching for things, or touching things on purpose.

- **Loss of speech:** Initially, they may stop saying words or phrases that they once said; later, they may make sounds, but do not say any purposeful words.

- **Balance and coordination problems:** These problems may start out as clumsiness and trouble walking. About 60 percent[8] of those with Rett syndrome are still able to walk later in life; others may become unable to sit up or walk or may become immobile.

- **Stereotypic movements:** One of the unique features of Rett syndrome is stereotypic hand movements—such as hand wringing—that can intensify and become almost continuous.

- **Breathing problems:** These problems may include hyperventilation and breath holding or apnea. These problems occur only while the person with Rett syndrome is awake, not during sleep.

- **Anxiety and social-behavioral problems:** These issues can range from not being comfortable in new places or situations, such as a mall, to autistic-like features, such as lack of eye contact.

- **Intellectual disability/mental retardation:** Intellectual disability is often significant. In fact, Rett syndrome is one of the leading causes of intellectual disability and autism in females.

During the last several years, researchers have described a broader set of features for Rett syndrome. Some people may be more or less affected by symptoms of Rett syndrome than others. Some people with Rett syndrome may still be able to say single words, while others are never able to talk. Some people with Rett syndrome are not able to sit up on their own and stay upright, while others have no problems with sitting.

### Are there other problems associated with Rett syndrome?

A number of problems are common among those who have Rett syndrome. Yet having these other problems is not necessary to get a diagnosis of Rett syndrome. These problems can include the following:

- Approximately 80 percent[8] of girls with Rett syndrome have scoliosis. In some cases, the curving of the spine is so severe that the girls require surgery. For some, bracing relieves the problem, prevents it from getting worse, or delays or eliminates the need for surgery.

- Seizures are also a common problem[9] for those with Rett syndrome. Seizures may involve the whole body, or they may be staring spells with no movement.

- Many persons with Rett syndrome also have constipation and gastroesophageal reflux. Gallbladder problems[10] may also occur and can range from gallstones to pain or discomfort in the abdomen.

- Some persons[11,12] with Rett syndrome have cardiac or heart problems, specifically problems with the rhythm of their hearts. For example, they may have abnormally long pauses between heartbeats (as measured by an electrocardiogram or ECG), or they may experience other types of arrhythmia.

- Many girls[2] with Rett syndrome cannot feed themselves. Some have trouble swallowing, and others never develop the ability to chew food properly. In some cases, too, in spite of healthy appetites, girls with Rett syndrome do not gain weight or have trouble maintaining a healthy weight. As a result, some girls with Rett syndrome rely on feeding tubes.

- Problems with sleep, specifically disrupted sleep patterns at night (during childhood) and an increase in total and daytime sleep (after age five years) are also common[13] among those with Rett syndrome. Some researchers[14] suggest that problems with sleep are among the earliest symptoms of Rett syndrome and can appear between one and two months of age.

### What is the usual course of Rett syndrome?

As mentioned earlier, children with Rett syndrome seem to develop normally as infants, then regress or lose skills. Many persons with Rett syndrome also experience a period of stability.

Health care providers, relying on consensus criteria,[15] view the onset of symptoms in four stages:

- **Early onset phase:** Development stalls or stops. Sometimes, the slowing or stopping is so subtle that parents and health care providers don't notice it at first.

- **Rapid destructive phase:** The child loses skills (regresses) quickly. Purposeful hand movements and speech are usually the first skills lost. Breathing problems and stereotypic hand movements usually also start during this stage.

- **Plateau phase:** Regression slows, and other problems may seem to lessen or improve. Seizures and movement problems are common in this stage. Most people with Rett syndrome spend most of their lives in this stage.

- **Late motor deterioration phase:** Individuals with Rett syndrome may become stiff or lose muscle tone; some become immobile. Scoliosis may be severe and require bracing or surgery. Stereotypic hand movements and breathing problems seem to lessen.

Researchers once thought that stage one began around six months of age. But after analyzing videotapes of Rett individuals taken from birth, they now know[16] that some infants with Rett syndrome only seem to develop normally. In fact, these infants show problems with very early development.

In one study,[17] all of the infants with Rett syndrome showed problems with body movements from birth through age six months. Another 42 percent[17] showed stereotyped hand movements during this time period.

In light of these new findings, some health care providers feel that genetic screening for Rett syndrome is critical to ensure that these infants get help as early in life as possible. Yet, because genetic testing would miss 5 percent of infants with the disorder, clinical followup[18] is also critical to establish a diagnosis.

### Is there a cure for Rett syndrome?

To date, there is no cure for Rett syndrome. However, research[19] shows that early diagnosis of developmental disorders, such as Rett syndrome, is important for improving outcomes.

Interventions delivered early in life are more likely to result in positive effects on later skills and symptoms. The sooner treatment begins, the greater the opportunity for learning. Most people with Rett syndrome, no matter what their age, benefit from well-designed interventions.

### Are there treatments for Rett syndrome?

There are a variety of ways to help minimize the effects of Rett syndrome. Rather than addressing the syndrome as a whole, most treatments[20] try to reduce specific symptoms of Rett syndrome. These treatments generally aim to slow the loss of abilities, improve or preserve movement, and encourage communication and social contact.

People with Rett syndrome often benefit from a team approach to care, in which many different kinds of health care providers play a role along with family members. Members of this care team may include (but are not limited to) the following:

- Physical therapists, who can help patients improve or maintain mobility and balance and reduce misshapen back and limbs

- Occupational therapists, who can help patients improve or maintain use of their hands and reduce stereotypic hand movements

- Speech-language therapists, who can help patients use nonverbal ways of communication and improve social interaction

Other members of the team may also include developmental specialists, developmental pediatricians, orthopedic surgeons, gastroenterologists, pulmonologists, cardiologists, neurologists, special education providers, and nurses. The involvement of family members is also critical to ensuring the well-being of those with Rett syndrome.

Other options, such as medication or surgery, are also effective. For instance, surgery can correct scoliosis for some persons with Rett syndrome. Similarly, anti-seizure medications can effectively control seizures for many affected by Rett syndrome. Other medications can reduce breathing problems and can eliminate problems with heartbeat rhythm.

Over-the-counter aids for indigestion and constipation can help to reduce these problems. Calcium and mineral supplements may also help to strengthen bones, which slows the progress of the scoliosis.

If you have a question about treatments, talk to your health care provider.

### *What are researchers doing to learn more about Rett syndrome?*

The NICHD and other organizations continue their efforts to support research to understand Rett syndrome, in hopes of learning to slow, stop, and reverse its effects.

The 1999 finding of the *MECP2* gene was a big step forward and has provided many new avenues for research.

Some researchers[21] suggest that the specific type of mutation in the *MECP2* gene affects how mild or severe symptoms of Rett syndrome are. Studies are now underway to understand each mutation that may cause the features of Rett syndrome, and how these mutations might change the features of the syndrome. One study (funded by the National Institutes of Health [NIH]) of the natural history of Rett syndrome should also provide new information about these topics.

Researchers are also trying to find other genes that may be involved in Rett syndrome. Some studies have helped to narrow the search for these genes, but much is still unknown about how these genes may cause or contribute to Rett syndrome.

Current findings[1] suggest that a congenital type of Rett-like syndrome, in which children have very severe seizures in early infancy, may involve the cyclin-dependent kinase-like 5 gene, *CDKL5*. But researchers still don't know how this gene might be involved, or what its protein product, cyclin-dependent kinase-like 5, specifically does in the brain. Studies on this and other genes are ongoing.

Other research focuses on understanding how X chromosome inactivation (XCI) affects people with Rett syndrome. Cells randomly choose which X chromosome to use and which one not to use—called XCI. Because females have two X chromosomes, those with Rett syndrome usually have one mutated *MECP2* gene and one normal *MECP2* gene in most of their cells. Yet, only one X chromosome is active in each cell, and only the active chromosome makes proteins.

For some girls, then, XCI may mean that many cells use the normal chromosome, so they have higher levels of MeCP2 protein and milder features of Rett syndrome. In some females, only the normal chromosome is active, so these individuals are normal, even though they have a mutated gene.

Studies are also looking into XCI in males with Rett syndrome. For some males, the features of Rett syndrome occur with another genetic condition called Klinefelter syndrome. Most males have one X and one Y chromosome in most of their cells. But, males with Klinefelter syndrome have two X chromosomes and one Y chromosome, which means they may have one mutated *MECP2* gene and one normal *MECP2* gene.

In these cases, the normal gene may be able to make MeCP2, making the features of Rett syndrome less severe; or the mutated gene may cause the characteristic features of Rett syndrome.

In other males with Rett syndrome, not all the cells in the body have the mutated *MECP2* gene. In these cases, the cells are mosaic, meaning that they are different because some have the mutation and some do not. Efforts are ongoing to try and understand mosaicism and how it impacts the features of Rett syndrome.

With an understanding of how Rett syndrome affects the entire body, health care providers can better treat the problems associated with the syndrome. This knowledge is important not just for those affected by Rett syndrome, but also for any person touched by a developmental disorder.

## References

1.  Weaving, L.S., Ellaway, C.J, Gécz, J., and Christodoulou, J. (2005). Rett syndrome: Clinical review and genetic update. *Journal of Medical Genetics*, 42:1–7.

2.  Percy, A.K., Dragich, J., and Schanen, C. (2003). Rett Syndrome: Clinical-Molecular Correlates. In G. Fisch (Ed.), *Genetics and Neurobehavioral Disorders* (pp. 391–418). Totowa, NJ: Humana Press.

3.  Amir, R.E., Van den Veyver, I.B., Wan, M., Tran, C.Q., Francke, U., and Zoghbi, H.Y. (1999). Rett syndrome is caused by mutations in X-linked *MECP2*. *Nature Genetics*, Oct; 23(2): 185–88.

4.  Schollen, E., Smeets, E., Deflem, E., Fryns, J.P., and Mathis, G. (2003). Gross rearrangements in the *MECP2* gene in three patients with Rett syndrome: Implications for routine diagnosis of Rett syndrome. *Human Mutations*, 22:116–20.

5.  Zoghbi, H.Y. (2005). MeCP2 dysfunction in humans and mice. *Journal of Child Neurology*, 20:736–40.

6.  Fang, P., Ward, P.A., Berry, S.A., Irons, M., Chong, B., Van den Veyver, I.B., Neul, J., Glaze, D.G., Zoghbi, H.Y., and Roa, B.B. (2005 October). *MECP2* gene rearrangements in female and male patients with features of Rett syndrome. Poster session presented at the American Society of Human Genetics 2005 Annual Meeting, Salt Lake City, Utah. Retrieved November 28, 2005, from http://www.ashg.org/genetics/ashg/ashgmenu.htm.

7.  Hagberg, B. (1993). Rett Syndrome: Clinical and Biological Aspects. In G. Hberg, J. Wahlstrom, and M. Anvret (Eds.), *Clinics in Developmental Medicine No. 127* (pp. 4–20). London: McKeith Press.

8.  Kerr, A.M., Webb, P., Prescott, R.J., and Milne, Y. (2003). Results of surgery for scoliosis in Rett syndrome. *Journal of Child Neurology*, 18:703–8.

9.  Glaze, D., Schultz, R., and Frost, J. (1998). Rett syndrome: Characterization of seizures and nonseizures. Electroencephalography and Clinical Neurophysiology, 106:79–83.

10. Percy, A.K., and Lane, J.B. (2004). Rett syndrome: Clinical and molecular update. *Current Opinions in Pediatrics*, 16:660–77.

11. Ellaway, C.J., Sholler, G., Leonard, H., and Christodoulou, J. (1999). Prolonged QT interval in Rett syndrome. *Archives of Disease in Childhood*, 80:470–72.

12. Guideri, F., Acampa, M., DiPerri, T., Zapella, M., and Hayek, Y. (2004). Progressive cardiac dysautonomia observed in patients affected by classic Rett syndrome and not in the preserved speech variant. *Journal of Child Neurology*, 16:370–73.

13. Ellaway, C., Peat, J., Leonard, H., and Christodoulou, J. (2001). Sleep dysfunction in Rett syndrome: Lack of age-related decrease in sleep duration. *Brain Development*, Dec; 23(Suppl 1): S101–S103.

14. Nomura, Y. (2005). Early behavior characteristics and sleep disturbance in Rett syndrome. *Brain and Development*, Nov; 27(Suppl 1): S35–S42.

15. Hagberg, B., Hanefiled, F., Percy, A., and Skjeldal, O. (2002). An update on clinically applicable diagnostic criteria in Rett syndrome. Comments to Rett Syndrome Clinical Criteria Consensus Panel Satellite to European Pediatric Neurology Society Meeting, Germany 2001. *European Journal of Pediatric Neurology*, 6:293–97.

16. Nomura, Y., and Segawa, M. (1990). Clinical features of the early stage of the Rett syndrome. *Brain Development*, 12(1): 16–19.

17. Einspieler, C., Kerr, A.M., and Prechtl, H.F.R. (2005). Is the early development of girls with Rett disorder really normal? *Pediatric Research*, 57:696–700.

18. Zoghbi, H.Y. (Updated 11 February 2004). Rett syndrome. In: GeneReviews at GeneTests: Medical Genetics Information Resource (database online). Copyright University of Washington, Seattle. 1997–2005. Available at http://www.genetests.org. Accessed October 7, 2005.

19. Committee on Children with Disabilities, American Academy of Pediatrics. (2001). The pediatrician's role in the diagnosis and management of autistic spectrum disorder in children. *Pediatrics*, 107:1221–26.

20.  Segawa, M., and Nomura, Y. (2005). Rett syndrome. *Current Opinions in Neurology*, 18:97–104.

21.  Schanen, C., Houwink-Manville, I., Dorrani, N., Lane, J., Everett, R., Feng, A., Cantor, R.M., and Percy, A. (2004). Phenotypic manifestations of *MECP2* mutations in classical and atypical Rett syndrome.

# Section 4.4

# *Childhood Disintegrative Disorder*

This rather rare condition was described many years before autism (Heller, 1908) but has only recently been "officially" recognized. With childhood disintegrative disorder (CDD) children develop a condition that resembles autism but only after a relatively prolonged period (usually two to four years) of clearly normal development (Volkmar, 1994). This condition apparently differs from autism in the pattern of onset, course, and outcome (Volkmar, 1994). Although apparently rare the condition probably has frequently been incorrectly diagnosed.

## *Criteria and Clinical Features*

Both the *DSM-IV* and *ICD-10* provide criteria for this condition. The criteria are rather similar in both, although some differences between the two systems are apparent. The condition develops in children who have previously seemed perfectly normal. Typically language, interest in the social environment, and often toileting and self-care abilities are lost, and there may be a general loss of interest in the environment. The child usually comes to look very "autistic," that is, the clinical presentation (but not the history) is then typical of a child with autism.

## History

A special educator in Vienna, Theodore Heller, proposed the term *dementia infantilis* to account for the condition. Few papers on the topic appeared and these were mostly case reports. The presumption until recently was that this condition was *always* associated with some specific neuropathological process. However, current data do not support this, and in most cases after even very extensive testing no specific medical cause for the condition is found. As with autism, children who suffer from this condition are at increased risk for seizures.

## Course and Prognosis

Several different patterns of onset and course have been identified. Patterns of onset include gradual versus insidious, while patterns of course or development include progressive deterioration, developmental plateau with little subsequent improvement, and (much less frequently) marked improvement. The available data suggest that generally the prognosis for this condition is worse than that for autism.

## Etiology/Cause

The etiology is unknown but several lines of evidence suggest that it arises as a result of some form of central nervous system pathology.

## Epidemiology

More boys than girls appear to be affected. Childhood disintegrative disorder is perhaps ten times less common than more strictly defined autism (Volkmar, 1994).

## Case Illustration

John's early history was within normal limits. By age two he was speaking in sentences, and his development appeared to be proceeding appropriately. At age thirty months he was noted to abruptly exhibit a period of marked behavioral regression shortly after the birth of a sibling. He lost previously acquired skills in communication and was no longer toilet trained. He became uninterested in social interaction, and various unusual self-stimulatory behaviors became evident.

Comprehensive medical examination failed to reveal any conditions that might account for this development regression. Behaviorally he exhibited features of autism. At follow-up at age twelve he still was not speaking, apart from an occasional single word, and had been placed in a school for the severely disabled.

## Section 4.5

# *Pervasive Developmental Disorder-Not Otherwise Specified (PDD-NOS)*

Pervasive developmental disorder-not otherwise specified (PDD-NOS) is a "subthreshold" condition in which some—but not all—features of autism or another explicitly identified pervasive developmental disorder are identified. PDD-NOS is often incorrectly referred to as simply "PDD." The term PDD refers to the class of conditions to which autism belongs. PDD is *not* itself a diagnosis, while PDD-NOS *is* a diagnosis. The term pervasive developmental disorder-not otherwise specified (PDD-NOS; also referred to as "atypical personality development," "atypical PDD," or "atypical autism") is included in *DSM-IV* to encompass cases where there is marked impairment of social interaction, communication, and/or stereotyped behavior patterns or interest, but when full features for autism or another explicitly defined PDD are not met.

It should be emphasized that this "subthreshold" category is thus defined implicitly, that is, no specific guidelines for diagnosis are provided. While deficits in peer relations and unusual sensitivities are typically noted, social skills are less impaired than in classical autism. The lack of definition(s) for this relatively heterogeneous group of children presents problems for research on this condition. The limited available evidence suggest that children with PDD-NOS probably come to professional attention rather later than is the case with autistic children, and that intellectual deficits are less common.

## Case Illustration

Leslie was the oldest of two children. She was noted to be a difficult baby who was not easy to console but whose motor and communicative development seemed appropriate. She was socially related and sometimes enjoyed social interaction but was easily overstimulated. She was noted to exhibit some unusual sensitivities to aspects of the environment and at times of excitement exhibited some hand flapping. Her parents sought evaluation when she was four years of age because of difficulties in nursery school. Leslie was noted to have problems with peer interaction. She was often preoccupied with possible adverse events. At evaluation she was noted to have both communicative and cognitive functions within the normal range. Although differential social relatedness was present, Leslie had difficulty using her parents as sources of support and comfort. Behavioral rigidity was noted, as was a tendency to impose routines on social interaction. Subsequently Leslie was enrolled in a therapeutic nursery school where she made significant gains in social skills. Subsequently she was placed in a transitional kindergarten and did well academically, although problems in peer interaction and unusual affective responses persisted. As an adolescent she describes herself as a "loner" who has difficulties with social interaction and who tends to enjoy solitary activities.

# Part Two

# Causes of Autism Spectrum Disorders

# Chapter 5

# *What Causes Autism?*

There is no known single cause for autism, but it is generally accepted that it is caused by abnormalities in brain structure or function. Brain scans show differences in the shape and structure of the brain in children with autism versus children without autism. Researchers are investigating a number of theories, including the link between heredity, genetics, and medical problems. In many families, there appears to be a pattern of autism or related conditions, further supporting a genetic basis to the disorder. While no one gene has been identified as causing autism, researchers are searching for irregular segments of genetic code that may have been inherited. It also appears that some children are born with a susceptibility to autism, but researchers have not yet identified a single "trigger" that causes autism to develop.

Other researchers are investigating the possibility that under certain conditions, a cluster of unstable genes may interfere with brain development, resulting in autism. Still other researchers are investigating problems during pregnancy or delivery as well as environmental factors such as viral infections, metabolic imbalances, and exposure to environmental chemicals.

Autism tends to occur more frequently than expected among individuals who have certain medical conditions, including fragile X syndrome, tuberous sclerosis, congenital rubella syndrome, and untreated phenylketonuria (PKU). Some harmful substances ingested during pregnancy also have been associated with an increased risk of autism.

The question of a relationship between vaccines and autism continues to be debated. In a 2001 investigation by the Institute of Medicine, a committee concluded that the "evidence favors rejection of a causal relationship . . . between MMR [measles, mumps, and rubella] vaccines and autistic spectrum disorders (ASD)." The committee acknowledged, however, that "they could not rule out" the possibility that the MMR vaccine could contribute to ASD in a small number of children. While other researchers agree the data does not support a link between the MMR and autism, more research is clearly needed.

Whatever the cause, it is clear that children with ASD are born with the disorder or born with the potential to develop it. It is not caused by bad parenting. Autism is not a mental illness. Children on the autism spectrum are not unruly kids who choose not to behave. Furthermore, no known psychological factors in the development of the child have been shown to cause autism.

Chapter 6

# *Genes: One of the Suspected Causes of Autism*

### *What are genes?*

Genes are pieces of DNA, material that contains all the information needed to "build" a person. Genes are hereditary, meaning parents pass genes on to their children.

Most genetic material is found in the nucleus of a cell, a storage area that keeps these materials together in one place. The nucleus stores genetic materials in packages called chromosomes. Most people have forty-six chromosomes in most of their cells: twenty-three from their mother and twenty-three from their father. Each chromosome is made up of genes.

Genes contain the information your body uses to make proteins, the body's building blocks. Proteins make up the structure of your organs and tissues; they are also needed for the body's chemical functions and pathways. Each protein performs a specific job in the body's different types of cells, and the information for making at least one protein is contained in a single gene.

The pattern or sequence of your genes is like a blueprint that tells your body how to build its different parts. For example, your genes control how tall you are, what color your eyes and hair are, and other features of your body and mind. Changes, or mutations, in the blueprint can change how the body or mind grows and develops.

Excerpted from "Autism and Genes," National Institute of Child Health and Human Development, National Institutes of Health, NIH Publication No. 05-5590, May 2005.

## What is autism?

Autism is a complex neurobiological disorder of development that lasts throughout a person's life. It is sometimes called a developmental disability because it usually starts before age three, in the developmental period, and because it causes delays or problems in many different skills that arise from infancy to adulthood.

The main signs and symptoms of autism involve[1] language, social behavior, and behaviors concerning objects and routines:

- **Communication:** Both verbal (spoken) and nonverbal (unspoken, such as pointing, eye contact, or smiling)

- **Social interactions:** Such actions as sharing emotions, understanding how others think and feel (sometimes called empathy), and holding a conversation, as well as the amount of time a person spends interacting with others

- **Routines or repetitive behaviors:** Often called stereotyped behaviors, such as repeating words or actions over and over, obsessively following routines or schedules, playing with toys or objects in repetitive and sometimes inappropriate ways, or having very specific and inflexible ways of arranging items

People with autism might have problems talking with you, or they might not want to look you in the eye when you talk to them. They may have to line up their pencils before they can pay attention, or they may say the same sentence again and again to calm themselves down. They may flap their arms to tell you they are happy, or they might hurt themselves to tell you they are not. Some people with autism never learn how to talk.

These behaviors not only make life difficult for people who have autism, but also take a toll on their families, their health care providers, their teachers, and anyone who comes in contact with them.

Because different people with autism can have very different features or symptoms, health care providers think of autism as a "spectrum" disorder—a group of disorders with a range of similar features. Based on their specific strengths and weaknesses, people with autism spectrum disorders (ASDs) may have mild symptoms or more serious symptoms, but they all have an ASD. This chapter uses the terms "ASD" and "autism" to mean the same thing.

## What causes autism?

Scientists don't know exactly what causes autism.

Much evidence supports the idea that genetic factors—that is, genes, their function, and their interactions—are one of the main underlying causes of ASDs. But, researchers aren't looking for just one gene. Current evidence suggests that as many as twelve or more genes on different chromosomes may be involved in autism to different degrees.

Some genes may place a person at greater risk for autism, called susceptibility. Other genes may cause specific symptoms or determine how severe those symptoms are. Or, genes with mutations might add to the symptoms of autism because the genes or gene products aren't working properly.

Research has also shown that environmental factors, such as viruses, may also play a role in autism.

While some researchers are examining genes and environmental factors, other researchers are looking at possible neurological, infectious, metabolic, and immunologic factors that may be involved in autism.

Because the disorder is so complex, and because no two people with autism are exactly alike, autism is probably the result of many causes.

### Why study genes to learn about autism?

Past research links autism and genes:

- **Studies of twins with autism:** Scientists have studied autism in both identical twins—who are genetically the same—and fraternal twins—who are genetically similar, but not the same. When identical twins have autism, both have autism more than 60 percent[1] of the time, depending on the criteria used. When fraternal twins have autism, both have autism between 0 percent[2] and 6 percent of the time. If genes were not involved in autism, the rate of autism would be the same for both types of twins.

- **Family studies of autism:** Studies of family histories show that the chances a brother or sister of someone who has autism will also have autism is between 2 percent and 8 percent,[3] which is much higher than in the general population. Also, some of the autism-like symptoms, such as delays in language development, occur more often[4] in parents and adult brothers and sisters of people with autism than in families who have no members or relatives with ASDs. Because members of the same family are more likely to share genes, something about these genes' sequences appears to be related to autism.

- **Diagnosable disorders and autism:** In about 5 percent[5] of autism cases, another single-gene disorder, chromosome disorder, or developmental disorder is also present. This type of co-occurrence helps researchers who are trying to pinpoint the genes involved in autism. Similar disorders or conditions with similar symptoms may have similar genetic beginnings. In cases of one disorder commonly occurring with another, it could be that one is actually a risk factor for the other. This kind of information can provide clues to what actually happens in autism. For example, many people with ASDs also have epilepsy, a condition marked by seizures. If scientists can understand what happens in epilepsy, they may also find clues to what happens in autism.

Based on these and other findings, scientists have long felt that there was a likely link between genes and autism, but how symptoms of ASDs affect family members and the wide variety of symptoms in ASDs tell researchers that they aren't looking for just one gene. So, even when scientists find the genes involved in autism, their work will be just beginning. They will still have to uncover what roles the genes play in the condition.

### How do researchers look for the genes involved in autism?

Scientists generally use a combination of methods to find candidate genes—genes likely to be involved in autism.

**Screen the whole genome:** A genome is all the genetic material in a person's cells—their DNA, their genes, and their chromosomes. Usually, researchers screen the genome of a family or a set of families that has more than one member with an ASD, to look for common features and differences. They look for so-called links between those diagnosed with ASDs and the genes within these families. Using "marker" locations—genes whose position in the genome is known—researchers can narrow down the location of genes involved in ASD. If a gene involved with autism is close to a particular marker, scientists can identify this gene by mapping it in relation to the known markers.

**Conduct cytogenetic studies:** In a cytogenetic study, researchers stain chromosomes with a dye and then look at them under a microscope. The dye creates light and dark bands that are unique to each chromosome. Researchers compare the resulting bands of two people with autism, of one person with autism and one relative, or of one person with autism and one person not affected by ASD. These comparisons can point out similarities and differences between regions on the chromosome, which researchers can then study further based on the traits of that specific region.

**Examine linkage ratios:** Researchers use this approach to find hot spots—areas on chromosomes that may contain genes involved in autism. Hot spots are like neighborhoods on the chromosome where the genes involved in autism might "reside." In many cases, genes in the same area of a chromosome are tightly connected to one another, and this connection is hard to break. If the connection is present in more people than you might expect by chance, the situation is called linkage disequilibrium. Linkage disequilibrium helps researchers narrow their genetic search to find the spot in the chromosomal neighborhood where the gene might be.

**Evaluate genes based on their known functions:** In some cases, researchers already know what the normal function of a specific gene or genes is. If that specific function is abnormal or incomplete in autism, researchers can look at the genes controlling that function in a person with autism to see what is different or missing. Or, they can look at what kinds of medications are useful in correcting or controlling that function to reduce the symptoms of autism. They can then study the chemical pathways that these medications affect to see what step might be changed or missing in autism. Once they've found the pathway or the change, they can look at the genes that control these features for more information about autism. This approach is known as genetic association analysis.

## What have researchers found by studying genes and autism?

Researchers in the Network on the Neurobiology and Genetics of Autism: Collaborative Programs of Excellence (CPEA) and their colleagues around the world have learned a lot about autism through genetic studies, but they still have a great deal to learn. To date, some of their findings include the following.

**Chromosomes where important genes are likely to be found:** Using genome-wide screens, scientists have identified a number of genes that might be involved in autism. Although some analyses suggest that as many as twelve genes[6] might be involved in ASDs, the strongest evidence[7,13] points to areas on the following chromosomes:

- *Chromosome 2:* Scientists know[7,10,11,12] that areas of chromosome 2 are the neighborhoods for "homeobox" or HOX genes, the group of genes that control growth and development very early in life. You have thirty-eight different HOX genes in your chromosomal neighborhoods, and each one directs the action of other genes in building your body and body systems. Expression of these HOX genes is critical to building the brain stem and the cerebellum, two areas of the brain where functions are disrupted in ASDs.

- *Chromosome 7:* Researchers have found[6,7,8,9] a very strong link between this chromosome and autism. Their investigations now focus on a region called *AUTS1*, which is very likely associated with autism. Most of the genome studies completed to date have found that *AUTS1* plays some role in autism. There is evidence that a region of chromosome 7 is also related to speech and language disorders. Because ASDs affect these functions, autism may involve this chromosome.

- *Chromosome 13:* In one study, 35 percent[7,9] of families tested showed linkage for chromosome 13. Researchers are now trying to replicate these findings with other populations of families affected by autism.

- *Chromosome 15:* Genome-wide screens and cytogenetic studies show that a part of this chromosome may play a role in autism. Genetic errors on this chromosome cause Angelman syndrome and Prader-Willi syndrome, both of which share behavioral symptoms with autism. Cytogenetic errors on chromosome 15 occur[9] in up to 4 percent of patients with autism.

- *Chromosome 16:* Genes found on this chromosome control a wide variety of functions[7] that, if disrupted, cause problems that are similar or related to symptoms of autism. For example, a genetic error on this chromosome causes tuberous sclerosis, a disorder that shares many symptoms with autism, including seizures. So, regions on this chromosome may be responsible for certain similar behavioral aspects of the two disorders.

- *Chromosome 17:* A recent study found the strongest evidence[13] of linkage on this chromosome among a set of more than five hundred families whose male members were diagnosed with autism.

Missing or disrupted genes on this chromosome can cause problems, such as galactosemia, a metabolic disorder that, if left untreated, can result in mental retardation. Chromosome 17 also contains the gene for the serotonin transporter, which allows nerve cells to collect serotonin. Serotonin is involved in emotions and helps nerve cells communicate. Problems with the serotonin transporter can cause obsessive-compulsive disorder (OCD), which is marked by recurrent, unwanted thoughts (obsessions) and/or repetitive behaviors (compulsions).

- *The X chromosome:* Two disorders that share symptoms with autism—fragile X syndrome and Rett syndrome—are typically caused by genes on the X chromosome, which suggests that genes on the X chromosome may also play a role in ASDs. People generally have forty-six chromosomes in most of their cells—twenty-three from their mother and twenty-three from their father. After fertilization, the two sets match up to form twenty-three pairs of chromosomes. The chromosomes in the twenty-third pair are called the "sex chromosomes," X and Y. This combination determines a person's sex—males usually have one X and one Y chromosome, and females usually have two X chromosomes. The fact that more males than females have autism supports[5,9] the idea that the disorder involves genes on the X chromosome. Females may be able to use their other X chromosome to function normally, while males, without such a "back up," show symptoms of the condition.

**Potential candidate genes:** By focusing their studies on hot spots, researchers have narrowed their search for candidate genes. They need to do more work to understand how many genes are involved, and how these genes interact with each other and with the environment to cause autism. Researchers do have some promising leads—more leads than can be mentioned in this chapter, but these are a few.

Researchers have found evidence that autism may involve the *HOXA1* gene. *HOXA1*, a homeobox gene, plays a critical role in the development of important brain structures, cranial nerves, the ear, and the skeleton of the head and neck. Researchers know that the *HOXA1* gene is active very early in life—between the twentieth and twenty-fourth days after conception—and that any problem with the gene's function causes problems with the development of these structures. Such problems may contribute to the features of autism.

In one study,[10] nearly 40 percent of the persons with autism carried a specific mutation in the *HOXA1* gene sequence—nearly twice as many as those who had the same change, but who did not have autism and were not related to anyone with autism. In addition, 33 percent of those who did not have autism but were related to someone with autism also had the mutation in their *HOXA1* gene. These findings mean that autism does not result from genetics alone, but that some other factors are also involved in causing the condition. If researchers can confirm an association between this mutation and ASDs, they may be able to detect the mutation as an early test for autism, allowing important interventions to start as early in life as possible.

Another study[11] found that increased head size in ASD patients was associated with a different mutation in the *HOXA1* gene. About 20 percent of persons with autism have large head size. It is one of the most consistently reported physical features of persons with autism. Now researchers want to know whether the mutation affects head size in persons with autism only, or if it affects head size in general, regardless of ASD status.

Several other genes have come forward as potential candidates, including the following:

- *The Reelin (RELN) gene on chromosome 7:* This gene plays a crucial role in the development of connections between cells of the nervous system. Researchers think that abnormal brain connectivity plays a role in autism, which makes Reelin a good candidate. In addition, persons with autism and their parents and siblings have lower levels of certain types of the Reelin protein, which may mean that gene is not functioning normally.

- *The HOXD1 gene:* This homeobox gene is critical to the formation of certain brain structures. This gene is involved in Duane syndrome, a disorder that causes eye- movement problems and sometimes occurs with autism. In one study[12] of persons with autism, nearly 94 percent of participants had mutations in the same regions of *HOXD1*, which could mean that the region contributes to ASDs.

- *Gamma-amino-butyric acid (GABA) pathway genes:* GABA compounds are neurotransmitters, which means they help parts of the nervous system communicate with each other. GABA receptor genes are involved in early development of parts of the nervous system and help with communication between these parts throughout life. A problem in the GABA pathway can cause some of the symptoms of ASDs. For instance, epilepsy may result, in part, from low levels of GABA compounds. Many persons with autism also have epilepsy and also show low levels of GABA. Current research focuses on genes that, when their structure or function is incorrect, cause autism-like problems in mice.

- *Serotonin transporter gene on chromosome 17:* The serotonin transporter allows nerve cells to collect serotonin so that they can communicate. Serotonin is a neurotransmitter involved in depression, alcoholism/problem drinking, OCD, and other disorders. Research shows that persons with autism have higher-than-normal levels of serotonin—ranging between 25 percent and 50 percent[9,13] higher than persons without autism. This higher serotonin level may result from problems with the serotonin transporter that arise from errors in the gene.

**Body chemicals that may play a role in autism:** The body makes many chemicals that help it function correctly. When these chemicals are missing or incorrect, the body may have problems functioning properly, which may result in symptoms of autism or other disorders. Researchers are now trying to uncover how body chemicals might be involved in autism, so they can learn how the genes that make these chemicals might also play a role. Researchers are also studying whether medications might regulate or control these chemicals to create normal chemical levels. Normalizing the chemicals in a person with ASDs might reduce symptoms.

As mentioned earlier, GABA may play a role in autism and definitely plays a role in epilepsy. Levels of different types of GABA compounds are abnormally low in persons with autism. Researchers believe that these low levels may contribute to autism. In studies of mice, disrupting the GABA pathway causes seizures, extreme reactions to touch and sound, and stereotyped actions—symptoms also common in autism. Research now focuses on whether medications used to treat these problems can also reduce some of the symptoms of autism.

Another brain chemical mentioned earlier—serotonin—is also out of balance in many persons with autism. High serotonin levels may explain why persons with autism have problems showing emotion and handling sensory information, such as sounds, touch, and smells. Researchers now focus on whether medications that regulate serotonin levels may improve behavior in persons with autism. They also examine the genes that make and regulate serotonin and its pathway components to see if they can find any changes or patterns.

## What does the future hold for studies of genes and autism?

Scientists in the CPEA Network and their colleagues who study the genetic mechanisms of autism hope that these studies will reveal the main cause or causes of autism. Doctors could then test for the gene or genes to detect autism early in life so that intervention can begin when it is most effective. Or, researchers could develop drugs that change or regulate the gene or genes to help normalize body chemicals and body functions.

Researchers share their information and their methods to see if other researchers can replicate their findings. Having several scientists get the same results "confirms" that discovery. Once confirmed, a discovery becomes the stepping-stone to other discoveries. To date, however, not all genetic studies have gotten the same results. Therefore, additional work is still important.

Scientists also look beyond genes to find factors that may play a role in autism, including things in the environment. Environmental features can affect how genes function, which may contribute to the symptoms of ASDs. By understanding genetic and environmental causes of autism, scientists may better understand how to treat it and maybe even how to prevent it. Doctors and scientists will continue to study genes, the environment, and gene-environment interactions until they solve the mysteries of autism.

### References

1.  Folstein & Rutter, 1977; Bailey, et al, 1995; Smalley, et al, 1988, as cited in Ingram, 2000.

2.  Steffenburg, et al, 1989, as cited in Muhle, 2004.

3.  Gillberg, et al, 2000; Chakrabarti, et al, 2001; Chudley, et al, 1998, as cited in Muhle 2004.

4.  Landa, et al, 1991; Landa, et al, 1992; Volkmar, et al, 1998; MacLean, et al, 1999, as cited in Ingram, 2000.

5.  Gillberg. (1998). Chromosomal disorders and autism. *Journal of Autism and Developmental Disorders*, 28:415–25.

6.  IMGSAC. (1998). A full genome screen for autism with evidence for linkage to a region of chromosome 7q. *Human Molecular Genetics*, 7:571–78.

7.  Collaborative Linkage Study of Autism. (1999). An autosomal genomic screen for autism. *American Journal of Medical Genetics*, 88:609–15; and International Molecular Genetic Study of Autism Consortium. (2001). A genome-wide screen for autism: Strong evidence for linkage to chromosomes 2q, 7q, and 16p. *American Journal of Human Genetics*, 69:570–81.

8.  IMGSAC. (2001). Further characterization of autism susceptibility locus *AUTS1* on chromosome 7q. *Human Molecular Genetics*, 10(9): 973–82.

9.  Muhle, et al. (2004). The Genetics of Autism. *Pediatrics*, 113(5): e472–e486.

10. Ingram JL, Stodgell CJ, Hyman SL, Figlewicz DA, Weitkamp LR, and Rodier PM. (2000). Discovery of allelic variants of *HOXA1* and *HOXB1*: genetic susceptibility to autism spectrum disorders. *Teratology*, 62:393–405.

11. Conciatori, et al. (2004). Association between the *HOXA1* A218G polymorphism and increased head circumference in patients with autism. *Journal of Biological Psychiatry*, 55: 413–19.

12. Stodgell, et al. (2004). Association of *HOXD1* and *GBX2* allelic variants with autism spectrum disorders. Presented at the CPEA/STAART Annual Scientific Meeting.

13. Cantor, et al. (2005). Replication of autism linkage: Fine mapping peak at 17q21. *American Journal of Human Genetics*, 76: 1050–56.

Chapter 7

# Autism and the Measles, Mumps, and Rubella Vaccine: Current Evidence Does Not Support a Link

## What is autism?

Autism is a term that refers to a collection of neurologically based developmental disorders in which individuals have impairments in social interaction and communication skills, along with a tendency to have repetitive behaviors or interests. The severity of autism varies greatly, from individuals with little speech and poor daily living skills, to others who function well in most settings. Autism is typically diagnosed during the toddler or preschool years, although some children are diagnosed at older ages. It has been reported that approximately 20 percent of children with autism experience a "regression"; that is, they have apparently normal development followed by a loss of communication and social skills. Boys are three to four times more likely to have autism than girls. Autism occurs in all racial, ethnic, and social groups. A variety of factors could be associated with some forms of autism, including infectious, metabolic, genetic, neurological, and environmental factors. Genetic factors and brain abnormalities at birth are considered to be some of the most recognized causes of autism.

## Does the measles-mumps-rubella (MMR) vaccine cause autism?

Current scientific evidence does not support the hypothesis that measles-mumps-rubella (MMR) vaccine, or any combination of vaccines,

Reprinted from "FAQs about MMR Vaccine and Autism," National Immunization Program, Centers for Disease Control and Prevention, May 19, 2004.

causes the development of autism, including regressive forms of autism. The question about a possible link between MMR vaccine and autism has been extensively reviewed by independent groups of experts in the United States, including the National Academy of Sciences, Institute of Medicine. These reviews have concluded that the available epidemiologic evidence does not support a causal link between MMR vaccine and autism.

## What have studies found regarding MMR vaccine and autism?

Epidemiologic studies have shown no relationship between MMR vaccination in children and development of autism.

In 1997, the National Childhood Encephalopathy Study (NCES) was examined to see if there was any link between measles vaccine and neurological events. The researchers found no indication that measles vaccine contributes to the development of long-term neurological damage, including educational and behavioral deficits (Miller et al., 1997).

A study by Gillberg and Heijbel (1998) examined the prevalence of autism in children born in Sweden from 1975 to 1984. There was no difference in the prevalence of autism among children born before the introduction of the MMR vaccine in Sweden and those born after the vaccine was introduced.

In 1999, the British Committee on Safety of Medicines convened a "Working Party on MMR Vaccine" to conduct a systematic review of reports of autism, gastrointestinal disease, and similar disorders after receipt of MMR or measles/rubella vaccine. It was concluded that the available information did not support the posited associations between MMR and autism and other disorders.

Taylor and colleagues (1999) studied 498 children with autism in the United Kingdom (U.K.) and found the age at which they were diagnosed was the same regardless of whether they received the MMR vaccine before or after eighteen months of age or whether they were never vaccinated. Importantly, the first signs or diagnoses of autism were not more likely to occur within time periods following MMR vaccination than during other time periods. Also, there was no sudden increase in cases of autism after the introduction of MMR vaccine in the U.K. Such a jump would have been expected if MMR vaccine were causing a substantial increase in autism.

Kaye and colleagues (2001) assessed the relationship between the risk of autism among children in the U.K. and MMR vaccine. Among a subgroup of boys aged two to five years, the risk of autism increased almost fourfold from 1988 to 1993, while MMR vaccination coverage remained constant at approximately 95 percent over these same years. Researchers in the United States found that among children born between 1980 and 1994 and enrolled in California kindergartens, there was a 373 percent relative increase in autism cases, though the relative increase in MMR vaccine coverage by the age of twenty-four months was only 14 percent (Dales et al., 2001).

Researchers in the U.K. (Frombonne and Chakrabarti, 2001) conducted a study to test the idea that a new form, or "new variant," of inflammatory bowel disease (IBD) exists. This new variant IBD has been described as a combination of developmental regression and gastrointestinal symptoms occurring shortly after MMR immunization. Information on ninety-six children (ninety-five immunized with MMR) who were born between 1992 and 1995 and were diagnosed with pervasive developmental disorder was compared with data from two groups of autistic patients (one group of ninety-eight born before MMR was ever used and one group of sixty-eight who were likely to have received MMR vaccine). No evidence was found to support a new syndrome of MMR-induced IBD/autism. For instance, the researchers found that there were no differences between vaccinated and unvaccinated groups with regard to when their parents first became concerned about their child's development. Similarly, the rate of developmental regression reported in the vaccinated and unvaccinated groups was not different; therefore, there was no suggestion that developmental regression had increased in frequency since MMR was introduced. Of the ninety-six children in the first group, no inflammatory bowel disorder was reported. Furthermore, there was no association found between developmental regression and gastrointestinal symptoms.

Another group of researchers in the U.K. (Taylor et al., 2002) also examined whether MMR vaccination is associated with bowel problems and developmental regression in children with autism, looking for evidence of a "new variant" form of IBD/autism. The study included 278 cases of children with autism and 195 with atypical autism (cases with many of the features of childhood autism but not quite meeting the required criteria for that diagnosis, or with atypical features such as onset of symptoms after the age of three years). The cases included in this study were born between 1979 and 1998. The proportion of children with developmental regression or bowel symptoms did not change significantly from 1979 to 1988, a period that included the introduction of MMR vaccination in the U.K. in 1988. No significant difference was found in rates of bowel problems or regression in children who received the MMR vaccine before their parents became concerned about their development, compared with those who received it only after such concern and those who had not received the MMR vaccine. The findings provide no support for an MMR-associated "new variant" form of autism and further evidence against involvement of MMR vaccine in autism.

Madsen et al. (2002) conducted a study of all children born in Denmark from January 1991 through December 1998. There were a total of 537,303 children in the study; 440,655 of the children were vaccinated with MMR and 96,648 were not. The researchers did not find a higher risk of autism in the vaccinated than in the unvaccinated group of children. Furthermore, there was no association between the age at time of vaccination, the amount of time that had passed since vaccination, or the date of vaccination and the development of any autistic disorder. Though there were many more vaccinated than unvaccinated children in the study group, the sample was large enough to contain more statistical power than other MMR and autism studies. Therefore, this study provides strong evidence against the hypothesis that MMR vaccination causes autism.

DeStefano et al. (2004) conducted a study to see if there was a difference in the age at which children with autism and without autism received their first MMR vaccination. The study's findings showed that children with autism received their first MMR vaccination at similar ages as children without autism.

## *Are there studies that suggest there might be a connection between autism and MMR vaccine?*

The existing studies that suggest a causal relationship between MMR vaccine and autism have generated media attention. However, these studies have significant weaknesses and are far outweighed by the epidemiologic studies described previously that have consistently failed to show a causal relationship between MMR vaccine and autism.

The MMR-autism theory is based on the idea that intestinal problems, like Crohn disease, are the result of viral infection and can contribute to the development of autism. The theory has its origins in research by Wakefield and colleagues (1989, 1990) that suggested that inflammatory bowel disease (IBD) is linked to persistent viral infection.

In 1993, Wakefield and colleagues reported isolating measles virus in the intestinal tissue of persons with IBD. However, the validity of this finding was later called into question when it could not be reproduced by other researchers (Afzal, 1998; Iizuka et al., 2000).

Thompson and colleagues (1995) suggested in a retrospective cohort study that MMR vaccine might be a risk factor for Crohn disease. However, the selection and recall biases and the differences in data collection in this study were so substantial as to cast doubt on the validity of the findings.

Two studies out of Sweden linked measles infection in utero to the development of IBD (Ekbom et al., 1994; Ekbom et al., 1996). However, these studies involved a very small number of cases and when researchers identified the persons to be included in the 1996 study, they had prior knowledge that cases of Crohn disease had occurred in the offspring of two women who were infected with measles during pregnancy. This is called "selection bias" and limits the strength of the study.

The MMR-autism theory came to the forefront when, in 1998, Wakefield and colleagues reviewed reports of children with bowel disease and regressive developmental disorders, mostly autism. The researchers suggested that MMR vaccination led to intestinal abnormalities, resulting in impaired intestinal function and developmental regression within twenty-four hours to a few weeks of vaccination. This hypothesis was based on twelve children. In nine of the cases, the child's parents or pediatrician speculated that the MMR vaccine had contributed to the behavioral problems of the children in the study. There are a number of limitations in the Wakefield et al. (1998) study:

- The study used too few cases to make any generalizations about the causes of autism; only twelve children were included in the study. Further, the cases were referred to the researchers and may not be a representative sample of cases of autism.

- There were no healthy control children for comparison. As a result, it is difficult to determine whether the bowel changes seen in the twelve children included in the study were similar to changes in normal children, or to determine if the rate of vaccination in autistic children was higher than in the general population.

- The study did not identify the time period during which the cases were identified.

- In at least four of the twelve cases, behavioral problems appeared before the onset of symptoms of bowel disease; that is, the effect preceded the proposed cause. It is unlikely, therefore, that bowel disease or the MMR vaccine triggered the autism.

In 2004, ten of the thirteen authors of the study retracted the paper's interpretation, stating that the data were insufficient to establish a causal link between MMR vaccine and autism (Murch et al., 2004).

In another study that generated media attention and raised public concern in the U.K. (Uhlmann et al, 2002), researchers found measles virus fragments in the intestines of children with "new variant" IBD (children with both IBD and developmental disorder). Scientists looked for the presence of measles virus in the intestinal tissue of ninety-one children with new variant IBD and seventy "controls" (children without this type of IBD). The researchers found measles virus fragments in seventy-five out of the ninety-one children with "new variant" IBD, and in only five of the seventy controls. While this provides evidence for an association between the presence of measles virus and IBD in children with developmental disorder, it does not mean that the measles component of the MMR vaccine causes IBD or developmental disorder. As a commentary published with the article asserts, the data could just as easily be interpreted as indicating that the IBD or the developmental disorder cause the persistence of measles in the intestines (Morris and Aldulaimi, 2002). In addition, the researchers did not compare the virus found in the intestines of patients with the virus used in the MMR vaccine; nor did they provide information regarding whether or not the children in the study had been previously vaccinated with MMR or had previously contracted measles disease. The limitations of this study are further discussed in a letter written by the director of the Center for Disease Control's National Immunization Program to the United Kingdom's chief medical officer.

### What about the claim that the number of children with autism has been increasing ever since the MMR vaccine has been in use?

Data from California (Department. of Developmental Services, 1999) have been used to illustrate an increase in cases of autism since the introduction of MMR vaccine. However, the data have been presented inaccurately (Fombonne, 2001). Fombonne (2001) lists several reasons why the data are misrepresented:

- The figures presented are based on numbers, not rates, and do not account for population growth and changes in the composition of the population.

- Changes in diagnostic definitions were not controlled in the report.

- As in other areas of the country, children with autism are currently being diagnosed at earlier ages, meaning that there will be an increase in the number of reported cases.

A 2001 study (Dales et al.) used the autism case numbers provided by the California Department of Developmental Services and compared them with early childhood MMR immunization level estimates for California children. Results showed that for children born from 1980 through 1987, there was no major change in MMR immunization levels, with the exception of a small increase in children born in 1988. This small increase was followed again by steady levels in children born through 1994. On the other hand, the cases of autism increased markedly, from 44 cases per 100,000 live births in 1980 to 208 cases per 100,000 live births in 1994. Even if one allows that a true increase in autism has occurred and the increase is not due to changes in diagnostic methods, diagnostic categorization, and improved identification of individuals with autism because of the level of services offered (Fombonne, 2001), this analysis shows that receipt of the MMR vaccine is not a factor. If it were a factor, one would expect the shape of the MMR level of immunization curve to be very similar to that of the autism case numbers. This is not the case, thus the analysis in this study argues against a link between MMR vaccination and autism.

*Would it be safer to separate the MMR vaccine into its individual components—in other words, give children three separate shots, at different times (e.g., six months or one year apart), instead of one combined shot?*

There is no confirmed scientific research or data to indicate that there is any benefit to separating the MMR vaccine into its individual components. A publication by Wakefield and Montgomery (2001) suggests that there is an increased risk of immune-mediated disease when the MMR vaccine is administered as one vaccine versus when the three vaccines are administered separately. The specific issue of the safety of multiple vaccines given as one vaccine was addressed by the Institute of Medicine (IOM) (1994, p. 63). They stated that the number of separate antigens in a vaccine would not likely result in a significant burden on the immune system that would result in immunosuppression.

The issue of multiple vaccines and immune dysfunction was addressed again by the IOM in 2002. An IOM Immunization Safety Review Committee concluded that a review of the available scientific evidence does not support the suggestion that the infant immune system is inherently incapable of handling the number of antigens that children are exposed to during routine immunizations. The IOM committee also did not suggest any need to change the current U.S. vaccination schedule for MMR.

Splitting the MMR vaccine into three separate doses given at three different times would cause more discomfort from additional injections and would leave children exposed to potentially serious diseases. For instance, if rubella vaccine were delayed, four million children would be susceptible to rubella for an additional six to twelve months. This would potentially allow otherwise preventable cases of congenital rubella syndrome (CRS) to occur through transmission of rubella from infected children to pregnant women. Ironically, infection of pregnant woman with "wild" rubella virus is one of the few known causes of autism. Thus, by preventing rubella infection of pregnant women, MMR vaccine also prevents autism.

*Should a younger sibling of an autistic child or a child of someone who has autism be vaccinated with MMR or other vaccines?*

Yes. Current scientific evidence does not show that MMR vaccine, or any combination of vaccines, causes the development of autism, including regressive forms of autism.

A younger sibling or the child of someone who suffered a vaccine side effect usually can, and should, safely receive the same vaccine. This is especially true since the large majority of side effects after vaccination are local reactions and fever, which do not represent a contraindication.

*Should we delay vaccination until we know more about the negative effects of vaccines?*

No. There is no convincing evidence that vaccines such as MMR cause long-term health effects. On the other hand, we do know that people will become ill and some will die from the diseases this vaccine prevents. Measles outbreaks have recently occurred in the U.K. and Germany following an increase in the number of parents who chose not to have their children vaccinated with the MMR vaccine.

Discontinuing a vaccine program based on unproven theories would not be in anyone's best interest. Isolated reports about these vaccines causing long-term health problems may sound alarming at first. However, careful review of the science reveals that these reports are isolated and not confirmed by scientifically sound research. Detailed medical reviews of health effects reported after receipt of vaccines have often proven to be unrelated to vaccines, but rather have been related to other health factors. Because these vaccines are recommended widely to protect the health of the public, research on any serious hypotheses about their safety are important to pursue. Several studies are underway to investigate still unproven theories about vaccinations and severe side effects.

Chapter 8

# Autism and Other Environmental Exposures

### *How common is autism spectrum disorder?*

Autism spectrum disorder, or ASD, is a group of developmental disorders that includes autistic disorder, atypical autism, and Asperger syndrome. It is unknown how many children in the United States have ASD, but recent research indicates that ASD may affect 2 per 1,000 children.[1]

### *How common is autism?*

Autistic disorder, which is commonly known as autism, falls within the larger category of ASD. Autistic children have impaired sociability, language, and communication, often coupled with mental retardation. A recent analysis of data from the 1992–94 National Health Interview Survey showed a national prevalence estimate for autism of 0.38 per 1,000.[2]

### *Is autism on the rise?*

There has been a global increase in prevalence rates for autism in recent years, rising from less than 0.5 per 1000 children in studies of children born before 1970, to a mean rate of about 1 per 1000 in children born in or after 1970.[3] Causes for the rise in prevalence are not known but might include change in diagnostic criteria, a greater awareness of autism, increased exposure to environmental pollutants and exposure to newly synthesized environmental pollutants, and increased survival of premature infants.[4] There are lower prevalence rates of autism in children from the United States (0.33 per 1,000 and 0.36 per 1,000) than in children from other parts of the world (from 0.40 to 3.1 per 1,000). The rise in prevalence was not seen in U.S. data. This geographic variation has not been explained.

Despite lack of evidence for an increase in prevalence in the United States, an increasing number of autistic patients seem to be using public services. California, for example, reported in 1999 that the autistic population receiving public services in the state had increased by 210 percent between 1987 and 1998, while the population served had increased in size by only 60 percent.[5] Moreover, the population with autism grew faster during that decade than the population with other developmental disabilities. The cause of such an increase is not known, but could include an increased recognition of the disorder and/ or an increased willingness to access public services for the disorder.

### What causes autism?

Several studies have found that genes may cause autism.[6,7,8,9,10] But in light of what may be rising rates of autism, genetics does not appear to be the only factor. Genes may interact with the environment to cause the disorder. One potentially important factor is infectious disease. A recent study found that levels of a particular antibody to streptococcus were significantly higher in children with autism than in controls.[11] This raises the possibility that infection during pregnancy may be correlated with the development of autism.

Another important factor may be in utero disturbance of neural tube closure. A 1994 study showed an association between autism and malformations caused by thalidomide.[12] Because thalidomide is known to act on the embryo during a particular developmental window (twenty to thirty-six days after conception), it has been speculated that autism may be caused by a disturbance of brain development during that same developmental window.[13,14]

### Have specific environmental substances been implicated?

Despite the suggestion of gene-environment interactions in the etiology of autism, there have been few efforts to link autism with specific exposures and/or exposure levels.[15] One such project has begun in

Brick Township, New Jersey, where residents are concerned that there are an unusually high number of children with autism. Parents in the township suspect a relationship between these cases and a high level of industrial contamination of the area, particularly in drinking water. As a result of the residents' concerns, the Centers for Disease Control and Prevention(CDC) and the Agency for Toxic Substances and Disease Registry (ATSDR) initiated an investigation that found a high rate of autism in the area but did not examine the role of environmental contaminants.[16]

## References

1.  Centers for Disease Control and Prevention, Developmental Disabilities Branch, Division of Child Development, Disability and Health. *Fact Sheet: Autism among children.*

2.  Halfon N, Newacheck PW. Prevalence and impact of parent-reported disabling mental health conditions among U.S. children. *J Am Acad Child Adolesc Psychiatry.* 1999; 38:600–609.

3.  Gillberg C, Wing L. Autism: not an extremely rare disorder. *Acta Psychiatrica Scand.* 1999; 99:399–406.

4.  Gillberg C, Wing L. Autism: not an extremely rare disorder. *Acta Psychiatrica* Scand. 1999; 99:399–406.

5.  California Department of Developmental Services. *Changes in the population of persons with autism and pervasive developmental disorders in California's developmental services system: 1987 through 1998.* A report to the legislature. March 1, 1999.

6.  Smalley SL, Asarnow RF, Spence MA. Autism and genetics. A decade of research. *Arch Gen Psychiatry* 1988; 45:953–61.

7.  Wahlstrom J, Steffenburg S, Hellgren L, Gillberg C. Chromosome findings in twins with early-onset autistic disorder. *Am J Med Genet* 1989; 32:19–21.

8.  Bailey A, Le Couteur A, Gottesman I, Bolton P, Simonoff E, Yuzda E, Rutter M. Autism as a strongly genetic disorder: evidence from a British twin study. *Psychol Med* 1995; 25:63–77.

9.  Le Couteur A, Bailey A, Goode S, Pickles A, Robertson S, Gottesman I, Rutter M. A broader phenotype of autism: the clinical spectrum in twins. *J Child Psychol Psychiatry* 1996; 37:785–801.

10. Risch N, Spiker D, Lotspeich L, Nouri N, Hinds D, Hallmayer J, Kalaydjieva L, McCague P, Dimiceli S, Pitts T, Nguyen L, Yang J, Harper C, Thorpe D, Vermeer S, Young H, Hebert J, Lin A, Ferguson J, Chiotti C, Wiese-Slater S, Rogers T, Salmon B, Nicholas P, Myers RM. A genomic screen of autism: evidence for a multilocus etiology. *Am J Hum Genet* 1999; 65:493–507.

11. Hollander E, DelGiudice-Asch G, Simon L, Schmeidler J, Cartwright C, DeCaria CM, Kwon J, Cunningham-Rundles C, Chapman F, Zabriskie JB. B lymphocyte antigen D8/17 and repetitive behaviors in autism. *Am J Psychiatry* 1999; 156:317–20.

12. Strömland K, Nordin V, Miller M, Akerström B, Gillberg C. Autism in thalidomide embryopathy: a population study. *Developmental Medicine and Child Neurology* 1994; 36:351–56.

13. Rodier PM, Ingram JL, Tisdale B, Croog VJ. Linking etiologies in humans and animal models: studies of autism. *Reprod Toxicol* 1997; 11:417–22.

14. Rodier PM, Ingram JL, Tisdale B, Nelson S, Romano J. Embryological origin for autism: developmental anomalies of the cranial nerve motor nuclei. *J Comp Neurol* 1996; 370:247–61.

15. Goldman L. *Healthy From the Start*. Pew Environmental Health Commission. 1999.

16. *Prevalence of Autism in Brick Township, New Jersey, 1998: Community Report*. CDC. April 2000.

Chapter 9

# Immune System Problems Could Be the Cause of Autism

## The Link Between the Immune System and Autism

If you think autism is only "a brain disorder," you may be surprised to hear that new research carried out by M.I.N.D. Institute scientists suggests that problems with the immune system may be one of the causes or consequences of the disorder. Some autism patients appear to have abnormalities in immune cell subsets that could result in an inappropriate or ineffective immune response to pathogens, such as bacteria or viruses.

One way to determine the health of the immune system in humans is to analyze the overall levels of antibody produced as well as the antibody response to proteins to which the individual has been exposed. Therefore, to better define the immune status of children with autism, M.I.N.D. Institute scientists Judy Van de Water, associate professor of rheumatology, allergy, and clinical immunology,

This chapter begins with "The Link Between the Immune System and Autism," *M.I.N.D. Matters*, Volume 6, Number 2, Winter 2006, © 2006 Regents of the University of California. It continues with "Children with Autism Have Distinctly Different Immune System Reactions" and "Scientists Report Strong Evidence of Immune and Protein Alterations in Blood Samples of Children with Autism, Raising Hope for an Early Diagnostic Blood Test," May 5, 2005, © 2005 Regents of the University of California. All three documents are reprinted with permission from the University of California-Davis M.I.N.D. Institute. All rights reserved.

103

and Paul Ashwood, assistant professor of medical microbiology and immunology, examined the blood levels of different types of antibodies (IgG, IgM, and IgA), along with the responses of these antibodies when challenged with common vaccine antigens in patients and age-matched typically developing children. These antigens included bacterial proteins from the diphtheria-tetanus-pertussis vaccine and the viral proteins from the measles, mumps, and rubella vaccine (MMR).

The most striking difference was that children with autism had a significantly lower antibody response to *Bordetella*, diphtheria, and tetanus proteins. They also had an overall reduction in blood antibody levels when compared both to typically developing children and to children with mental retardation. Interestingly, the siblings of patients with autism also had reduced antibody levels.

A different result was observed when the antibody response to MMR vaccine was analyzed. Surprisingly, there was an apparent increase in reactivity in the patients with autism and their siblings. However, when the time between vaccination and the analysis was taken into account, this apparent increase disappeared—an example of how carefully one must consider various factors in autism research.

In contrast to these studies, other investigators (V. Singh et al., 2004) have reported an increased response in patients with autism to measles vaccine antigens. However, it is important to note that the controls for these studies were not age-matched. This is critical, since the antibody response to these vaccines can drop dramatically in the year following vaccination.

In addition to the decreased immune response to bacterial vaccine proteins, the M.I.N.D. Institute investigators have also identified the presence of antibodies in some patients with autism that recognize proteins from the human brain. While the impact of these autoantibodies is currently unknown, such autoantibodies have the potential to either inhibit cell function or cause damage to neuronal tissue. Alternatively, they may be a harmless marker of tissue damage, having arisen during a brief, early exposure of the immune system to brain proteins. Current research is attempting to determine the identity of these brain proteins and their relationship to the development of autism.

Research on the role of immune system dysfunction is still in its infancy, but it is already clear that, for at least some forms of autism, immune problems may play a substantial role in the disorder. These M.I.N.D. Institute studies are leading the way to new strategies for prevention and treatment of autism.

## Children with Autism Have Distinctly Different Immune System Reactions Compared to Typical Children

A new study by researchers at the University of California, Davis, M.I.N.D. Institute and the National Institute of Environmental Health Sciences (NIEHS) Center for Children's Environmental Health demonstrate that children with autism have different immune system responses than children who do not have the disorder. This is important evidence that autism, currently defined primarily by distinct behaviors, may potentially be defined by distinct biologic changes as well.

The study was released at the Fourth International Meeting for Autism Research (IMFAR), a meeting of autism scientists started by Cure Autism Now, the University of California (UC) Davis M.I.N.D. Institute, and the National Alliance for Autism Research to accelerate knowledge of this increasingly common and perplexing disorder. It is estimated that autism now affects 1 in every 166 children.

"Understanding the biology of autism is crucial to developing better ways to diagnose and treat it," said Judy Van de Water, associate professor of rheumatology, allergy, and clinical immunology at the UC Davis School of Medicine and the UC Davis M.I.N.D. Institute. "While impaired communication and social skills are the hallmarks of the disorder, there has not yet been strong scientific evidence that the immune system is implicated as well. We now need to design carefully controlled studies that tell us even more about the way in which a dysfunctional immune system may or may not play a role in the disorder itself."

Van de Water, along with co-investigator of the study Paul Ashwood, assistant professor of medical microbiology and immunology at the UC Davis M.I.N.D. Institute, isolated immune cells from blood samples taken from thirty children with autism and twenty-six typically developing children between two and five years of age. The cells from both groups were then exposed to bacterial and viral agents that usually provoke T-cells, B-cells, and macrophages—primary players in the immune system.

Of the agents tested in the study—tetanus toxoid, lipopolysaccharide derived from E. coli cell walls, a plant lectin known as PHA, and a preparation of the measles, mumps, and rubella vaccine antigens—the researchers found clear differences in cellular responses between patients and controls following exposure to the bacterial agents and PHA.

In response to bacteria, the researchers saw lower levels of protein molecules called cytokines in the group with autism. Cytokines function as mediators of the immune response, carrying messages between B, T, and other immune cells. They also are known to be capable of having profound effects on the central nervous system, including sleep and the fever response. Immune system responses to PHA, in contrast, produced more varied cytokine levels: Higher levels of certain cytokines and lower levels of others.

According to Van de Water and Ashwood, these studies illustrate that under similar circumstances, the cytokine responses elicited by the T-cells, B-cells, and macrophage cell populations following their activation differs markedly in children with autism compared to age-matched children in the general population. Cytokines are known to affect mood and behavior, and while their specific role in the development of autism remains unclear, the potential connection is an intriguing area of research that warrants further investigation.

"This study is part of a larger effort to learn how changes in immune system response may make some children more susceptible to the harmful effects of environmental agents," said Kenneth Olden, director of the National Institute of Environmental Health Sciences, the federal agency that provided funding for the study. "A better understanding of the connection between altered immune response and autism may lead to significant advances in the early detection, prevention, and treatment of this complex neurological disorder."

"We would like to take these findings and explore whether, for example, the cytokine differences are specific to certain subsets of patients with autism, such as those with early onset, or those who exhibit signs of autism later during development," Ashwood said. He added that the logical next step is to look directly at specific cell populations that may be responsible for the diverging responses between patients and controls.

This study was supported by grants from the National Institutes of Environmental Health Sciences, the U.S. Environmental Protection Agency, the UC Davis M.I.N.D. Institute, Ted Lindsay Foundation, and Visceral. The UC Davis M.I.N.D. (Medical Investigation of Neurodevelopmental Disorders) Institute is a unique collaborative center for research into the causes and treatments of autism, bringing together parents, scientists, clinicians, and educators.

## Scientists Report Strong Evidence of Immune and Protein Alterations in Blood Samples of Children with Autism

Offering a new and exciting direction in the effort to develop a diagnostic test for autism in infancy, scientists from the UC Davis M.I.N.D. Institute have presented new evidence indicating that components of the immune system and proteins and metabolites found in the blood of children with autism differ substantially from those found in typically developing children.

Investigators at the Institute believe the discovery, announced at the Fourth International Meeting for Autism Research (IMFAR) in Boston, could be a major step toward developing a routine blood test that would allow autism to be detected in newborns and treatment or even prevention to be initiated early in life.

Over the last two decades, parents, educators, scientists, and pediatricians have been alarmed by a dramatic and baffling rise in the prevalence of autism, which now affects as many as 1 in every 166 children. But diagnosing autism, a brain disorder that leaves children in apparent isolation from their families and communities, is currently accomplished through a series of behavioral observations that are not reliable until a child is between two and three years old.

"Finding a sensitive and accurate biological marker for autism that can be revealed by a simple blood test would have enormous implications for diagnosing, treating, and understanding more about the underlying causes of autism," said David G. Amaral, research director at the UC Davis M.I.N.D. Institute and one of the co-authors of the paper presented at IMFAR. "Not being able to detect autism until a child is close to three years old eliminates a valuable window of treatment opportunity during the first few years of life when the brain is undergoing tremendous development."

Amaral, along with pediatric neuropsychologist Blythe Corbett and other M.I.N.D. Institute colleagues, took blood samples from seventy children with autism who were between four and six years old and from thirty-five children of the same age who didn't have the disorder. The samples were then analyzed by a biotech company, SurroMed, LLC, Menlo Park, Calif., which has developed technology that can identify differences in the number and types of immune cells, proteins, peptides, and metabolites in small amounts of blood. SurroMed was recently acquired by PPD, Inc., and its biomarker services have been integrated into PPD's discovery and development services and products provided to biopharmaceutical companies.

The study has generated an enormous amount of data and M.I.N.D. Institute researchers say it will take months before all of the information has been fully evaluated. But initial findings clearly demonstrate differences in the immune system, as well as proteins and other metabolites in children with autism:

- The antibody-producing B-cells are increased by 20 percent in the autism group.

- Natural killer cells are increased by 40 percent.

- More than one hundred proteins demonstrated significant differential expression between the autism and typically developing groups.

- Other small molecules (metabolites) also show many differences.

"This is an important pilot experiment, a proof of principle," said Amaral. "From these results we think it is highly likely that there are differences we can detect in blood samples that will be predictive of the disorder, though we are still some years away from having an actual diagnostic blood test for autism. Scientists have long suspected there were distinct biological components to autism but the technology needed to reveal them has only recently become available."

Future research studies need to be done to confirm the findings in a larger group and with younger children. For example, researchers might take blood samples from newborns and then see if the results predicting autism are later confirmed by a behavioral diagnosis. Other studies would also use bioinformatics approaches to narrow down the number of proteins or metabolites that would need to be assayed to show the strongest link to autism.

"Discovering an early diagnostic test is an important focus of research," said Amaral. "There is a growing view among experts that not all children with autism are 'doomed to autism' at birth. It may be that some children have a vulnerability—such as a genetic abnormality—and that something they encounter after being born, perhaps in their environment, triggers the disorder. Studying the biological signs of autism could lead to new ways to prevent the disorder from ever occurring. And even if it can't be prevented, intervening early in life—ideally shortly after birth—could greatly improve the lifetime outlook for children with autism, particularly those who now respond poorly to therapy initiated when they are three or older."

Chapter 10

# Abnormal Brain Development and Function Linked to Autism

## Chapter Contents

Section 10.1—Research on the Biological Basis of Autism ...... 110

Section 10.2—Brain Areas Fail to Work Together in
Autism ............................................................. 113

Section 10.3—Autism Affects Functioning of Entire Brain ..... 116

Section 10.4—Brain Regions Involving Memory and
Emotion Are Larger in Children with Autism ... 119

Section 10.5—Researchers Find Fewer Neurons in the
Amygdala of Males with Autism ...................... 121

Section 10.6—Nicotine Receptors in the Brain May Play
Role in Development of Autism ........................ 123

Section 10.1

## *Research on the Biological Basis of Autism*

Excerpted from "Autism Spectrum Disorders: Pervasive Developmental Disorders," National Institute of Mental Health, National Institutes of Health, NIH Publication No. 06-5511, July 11, 2006.

Because of its relative inaccessibility, scientists have only recently been able to study the brain systematically. But with the emergence of new brain imaging tools—computerized tomography (CT), positron emission tomography (PET), single photon emission computed tomography (SPECT), and magnetic resonance imaging (MRI), study of the structure and the functioning of the brain can be done. With the aid of modern technology and the new availability of both normal and autism tissue samples to do postmortem studies, researchers will be able to learn much through comparative studies.

Postmortem and MRI studies have shown that many major brain structures are implicated in autism. This includes the cerebellum, cerebral cortex, limbic system, corpus callosum, basal ganglia, and brain stem.[1] Other research is focusing on the role of neurotransmitters such as serotonin, dopamine, and epinephrine.

Research into the causes of autism spectrum disorders is being fueled by other recent developments. Evidence points to genetic factors playing a prominent role in the causes for autism spectrum disorders (ASD). Twin and family studies have suggested an underlying genetic vulnerability to ASD.[2] To further research in this field, the Autism Genetic Resource Exchange, a project initiated by the Cure Autism Now Foundation, and aided by a grant from the National Institute of Mental Health (NIMH), is recruiting genetic samples from several hundred families. Each family with more than one member diagnosed with ASD is given a two-hour, in-home screening. With a large number of DNA samples, it is hoped that the most important genes will be found. This will enable scientists to learn what the culprit genes do and how they can go wrong.

Another exciting development is the Autism Tissue Program (http://www.brainbank.org), supported by the Autism Society of America Foundation, the Medical Investigation of Neurodevelopmental Disorders

(M.I.N.D.) Institute at the University of California, Davis, and the National Alliance for Autism Research. The program is aided by a grant to the Harvard Brain Tissue Resource Center (http://www.brainbank .mclean.org), and funded by the National Institute of Mental Health (NIMH) and the National Institute of Neurological Disorders and

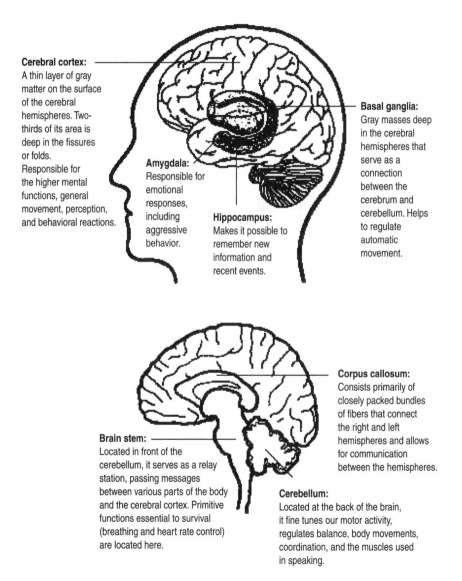

**Cerebral cortex:** A thin layer of gray matter on the surface of the cerebral hemispheres. Two-thirds of its area is deep in the fissures or folds. Responsible for the higher mental functions, general movement, perception, and behavioral reactions.

**Amygdala:** Responsible for emotional responses, including aggressive behavior.

**Hippocampus:** Makes it possible to remember new information and recent events.

**Basal ganglia:** Gray masses deep in the cerebral hemispheres that serve as a connection between the cerebrum and cerebellum. Helps to regulate automatic movement.

**Brain stem:** Located in front of the cerebellum, it serves as a relay station, passing messages between various parts of the body and the cerebral cortex. Primitive functions essential to survival (breathing and heart rate control) are located here.

**Corpus callosum:** Consists primarily of closely packed bundles of fibers that connect the right and left hemispheres and allows for communication between the hemispheres.

**Cerebellum:** Located at the back of the brain, it fine tunes our motor activity, regulates balance, body movements, coordination, and the muscles used in speaking.

*Figure 10.1.* Major Brain Structures Implicated in Autism

111

Stroke (NINDS). Studies of the postmortem brain with imaging methods will help us learn why some brains are large, how the limbic system develops, and how the brain changes as it ages. Tissue samples can be stained and will show which neurotransmitters are being made in the cells and how they are transported and released to other cells. By focusing on specific brain regions and neurotransmitters, it will become easier to identify susceptibility genes.

Recent neuroimaging studies have shown that a contributing cause for autism may be abnormal brain development beginning in the infant's first months. This "growth dysregulation hypothesis" holds that the anatomical abnormalities seen in autism are caused by genetic defects in brain growth factors. It is possible that sudden, rapid head growth in an infant may be an early warning signal that will lead to early diagnosis and effective biological intervention or possible prevention of autism.[3]

## References

1. Akshoomoff N, Pierce K, Courchesne E. The neurobiological basis of autism from a developmental perspective. *Development and Psychopathology*, 2002; 14: 613–34.

2. Korvatska E, Van de Water J, Anders TF, Gershwin ME. Genetic and immunologic considerations in autism. *Neurobiology of Disease*, 2002; 9: 107–25.

3. Courchesne E, Carper R, Akshoomoff N. Evidence of brain overgrowth in the first year of life in autism. *JAMA*, 2003; 290(3): 337–44.

## Section 10.2

# *Brain Areas Fail to Work Together in Autism*

Reprinted from "Researchers Gain Insight into Why Brain Areas Fail to Work Together in Autism," NIH News, National Institutes of Health, July 12, 2006.

Researchers have found in two studies that autism may involve a lack of connections and coordination in separate areas of the brain.

In people with autism, the brain areas that perform complex analysis appear less likely to work together during problem-solving tasks than in people who do not have the disorder, report researchers working in a network funded by the National Institutes of Health (NIH). The researchers found that communications between these higher-order centers in the brains of people with autism appear to be directly related to the thickness of the anatomical connections between them.

In a separate report, the same research team found that, in people with autism, brain areas normally associated with visual tasks also appear to be active during language-related tasks, providing evidence to explain a bias toward visual thinking common in autism.

"These findings provide support to a new theory that views autism as a failure of brain regions to communicate with each other," said Duane Alexander, M.D., director of NIH's National Institute of Child Health and Human Development (NICHD). "The findings may one day provide the basis for improved treatments for autism that stimulate communication between brain areas."

The studies and the theory are the work of Marcel Just, Ph.D., D.O., Hebb Professor of psychology at Carnegie Mellon University in Pittsburgh, Pennsylvania, and Nancy Minshew, M.D., professor of psychiatry and neurology at the University of Pittsburgh School of Medicine, and their colleagues.

The research was conducted by the Collaborative Program of Excellence in Autism, a research network funded by the NICHD and the National Institute on Deafness and Other Communication Disorders.

People with autism often have difficulty communicating and interacting socially with other people. The saying "unable to see the forest for the trees" describes how people with autism frequently excel at

113

details, yet struggle to comprehend the larger picture. For example, some children with autism may become spelling bee champions, but have difficulty understanding the meaning of a sentence or a story.

An earlier finding by these researchers described how a group of people with autism tended to use parts of the brain typically associated with processing shapes to remember letters of the alphabet.

Participants with autism in both current studies had normal I.Q. There were no significant differences between the participants with and without autism in age or I.Q.

The first of the two new studies recently was published online in the journal *Cerebral Cortex*. In that study, the researchers used a brain imaging technique known as functional magnetic resonance imaging, or fMRI, to view the brains of people with autism as well as a comparison group of people who do not have autism. All of the study participants were asked to complete the Tower of London test. The task involves moving three balls into a specified arrangement in an array of three receptacles. The Tower of London is used to gauge the functioning of the prefrontal cortex.

This brain area, located in the front, upper part of the brain, deals with strategic planning and problem solving. The prefrontal cortex is the executive area of the brain, in which decision-making, judgment, and impulse control reside.

A little further back is the parietal cortex, which controls high-level visual thinking and visual imagery, supporting the visual aspects of problem solving. Both the prefrontal and parietal cortex play a critical part in performing the Tower of London test.

In the normal participants, the prefrontal cortex and the parietal cortex tended to function in synchrony (increasing and decreasing their activity at the same time) while solving the Tower of London task. This suggests that the two brain areas were working together to solve the problem.

In the participants with autism, however, the two brain areas, prefrontal and parietal, were less likely to function in synchrony while working on the task.

The researchers made another discovery, for the first time finding a relationship between this lower level of synchrony and the properties of some of the neurological "cables" or white matter fiber tracts that connect brain areas.

White matter consists of fibers that, like cabling, connect brain areas. The largest of the white matter tracts is known as the corpus callosum, which allows communication between the two hemispheres (halves) of the brain.

"The size of the corpus callosum was smaller in the group with autism, suggesting that inter-regional brain cabling is disrupted in autism," Dr. Just said.

In essence, the extent to which the two key brain areas (prefrontal and parietal) of the autistic participants worked in synchrony was correlated with the size of the corpus callosum. The smaller the corpus callosum, the less likely the two areas were to function in synchrony. In the normal participants, however, the size of the corpus callosum did not appear to be correlated with the ability of the two areas to work in synchrony.

"This finding provides strong evidence that autism is a disorder involving the biological connections and the coordination of processing between brain areas," Dr. Just said.

He added, however, that the thickness, or extent, of connections between brain areas may not be the basis for the disorder. Although the neurological connections between the prefrontal cortex appear to be reduced in autism, the brains of people with autism have thicker connections between certain brain regions within each hemisphere.

"At this point, we can say that autism appears to be a disorder of abnormal neurological and informational connections of the brain, but we can't yet explain the nature of that abnormality," Dr. Just said.

In the second study, published online in the journal *Brain*, the researchers examined the extent to which brain areas involved in language interact with brain regions that process images. Dr. Just explained that earlier studies, as well as anecdotal accounts, suggest that people with autism rely more heavily on visual and spatial areas of the brain than do other people.

In this study, the researchers used fMRI to examine brain functioning in participants with autism and in normal participants during a true-false test involving reading sentences with low imagery content and high imagery content. A typical low-imagery sentence consisted of constructions like "Addition, subtraction, and multiplication are all math skills." A high-imagery sentence, "The number eight when rotated ninety degrees looks like a pair of eyeglasses," would first activate left prefrontal brain areas involved with language, and then would involve parietal areas dealing with vision and imagery as the study participant mentally manipulated the number eight.

As the researchers expected, the visual brain areas of the normal participants were active only when evaluating sentences with imagery content. In contrast, the visual centers in the brains of participants with autism were active when evaluating both high-imagery and low-imagery sentences.

"The heavy reliance on visualization in people with autism may be an adaptation to compensate for a diminished ability to call on prefrontal regions of the brain," Dr. Just said.

The second study also confirmed the observations in the first study—that the prefrontal and parietal brain regions of the cortex in people with autism were less likely to work in synchrony than were the brains of normal volunteers. The second study also confirmed that the extent to which the two parts of the cortex could work together was correlated with the size of the corpus callosum that connected them.

Dr. Just and his colleagues are conducting additional studies to ascertain the nature of the abnormality of the connections in the brains of people with autism.

# Section 10.3

# *Autism Affects Functioning of Entire Brain*

Reprinted from "Study Provides Evidence That Autism Affects Functioning of Entire Brain," NIH News, National Institutes of Health, August 16, 2006.

A recent study provides evidence that autism affects the functioning of virtually the entire brain, and is not limited to the brain areas involved with social interactions, communication behaviors, and reasoning abilities, as had been previously thought. The study, conducted by scientists in a research network supported by the National Institutes of Health (NIH), found that autism also affects a broad array of skills and abilities, including those involved with sensory perception, movement, and memory.

The findings, appearing in the August 2006 *Child Neuropsychology*, strongly suggest that autism is a disorder in which the various parts of the brain have difficulty working together to accomplish complex tasks.

The study was conducted by researchers in the Collaborative Program of Excellence in Autism (CPEA), a research network funded by two components of the NIH, the National Institute of Child Health and Human Development and the National Institute on Deafness and Other Communication Disorders.

"These findings suggest that further understanding of autism will likely come not from the study of factors affecting one brain area or system, but from studying factors affecting many systems," said the director of NICHD, Duane Alexander, M.D.

People with autism tend to display three characteristic behaviors, which are the basis of the diagnosis of autism, explained the study's senior author, Nancy Minshew, M.D., professor of psychiatry and neurology at the University of Pittsburgh School of Medicine. These behaviors involve difficulty interacting socially, problems with verbal and nonverbal communications, and repetitive behaviors or narrow, obsessive interests. Traditionally, Dr. Minshew said, researchers studying autism have concentrated on these behavioral areas.

Within the last twenty years, however, researchers began studying other aspects of thinking and brain functioning in autism, discovering that people with autism have difficulty in many other areas, including balance, movement, memory, and visual perception skills.

In the current study, Dr. Minshew and her colleagues administered a comprehensive array of neuropsychological tests to a group of children with autism. The researchers tested fifty-six autistic children, and compared their responses to those of fifty-six children who did not have autism. The children with autism were classified as having higher functioning autism—an I.Q. of 80 or above, and the ability to speak, read, and write. All of the children in the study ranged in age from eight to fifteen years. The purpose of the test array, Dr. Minshew said, was to determine whether there were any patterns in mental functioning unique to autism.

"We set out to find commonalities across a broad range of measures, so that we could make inferences about what's going on in the brain," Dr. Minshew said.

The researchers found that, across the entire series of tests, the children with autism performed as well as—and in some instances even better than—the other children on measures of basic functioning. Uniformly, however, they had trouble with complex tasks.

For example, regarding visual and spatial skills, the children with autism were very good at finding small objects in a cluttered visual field, on tasks like finding Waldo in the "Where's Waldo" picture books series. However, when asked to perform a complex task, like telling the difference between the faces of similar-looking people, they had great difficulty.

Although their memory for the detail in a story was phenomenal, the children with autism had great difficulty comprehending the story. Many were highly proficient at spelling and had a good command of grammar, but had difficulty understanding complex figures of speech, like idioms and metaphors.

"We see this with our patients," Dr. Minshew said. "If you use an expression like 'hop to it,' a child with autism may literally hop."

Other complex tasks were also difficult for them. The children with autism either had poor handwriting or wrote very slowly. Many had difficulty tying their shoes and with using scissors.

"These findings show that you can't compartmentalize autism under three basic areas," Dr. Minshew said. "It's much more complex than that."

Dr. Minshew explained that the major implication of the finding is that when seeking to understand autism, researchers need to look for a cause or causes that affect multiple brain areas, rather than limiting their search to brain areas dealing with the three characteristic behaviors involving social interactions, communication, and repetitive behaviors or obsessive interests.

"Our paper strongly suggests that autism is not primarily a disorder of social interaction, but a global disorder affecting how the brain processes the information it receives—especially when the information becomes complicated."

In previous research with an imaging technology known as functional magnetic resonance imaging, or fMRI, Dr. Minshew and her coworkers determined that adults with autism have abnormalities in the neurological wiring through which brain areas communicate. In those studies, the researchers found that people with autism had difficulty performing certain complex tasks that involved brain areas working together.

Dr. Minshew said that such abnormalities in brain circuitry provide the most likely explanation for why the children with autism in the current study have difficulty with complex tasks that require coordination among brain regions but do well on tasks that require only one region of the brain at a time.

The researchers undertook the current study as a follow-up to an earlier study they did of adults with autism. The researchers studied children to determine if the features of autism were consistent throughout life, or changed as people with autism grow older. For the most part, the current study revealed that both adults and children with autism experience the same kinds of difficulties with complex tasks.

One difference is that adults with autism appear to score higher on tests involving sensory interpretation than do children with autism. Such tests would involve identifying a number traced on a fingertip, or identifying an object placed in one's hand without looking at it. Dr. Minshew said that as people with autism grow older, they may have less sensory difficulty than they did as children.

Still, adults with autism fare much worse on tests of complex language and reasoning than do other adults. This gap in complex language and reasoning ability between the two groups is not as pronounced when children with autism are compared to other children. This is because children's brains have not yet developed these skills, Dr. Minshew said. However, the gap widens with time. As typical children get older, they develop these higher-order language and reasoning skills while adolescents and adults with autism do not.

## Section 10.4

# *Brain Regions Involving Memory and Emotion Are Larger in Children with Autism*

Researchers at the UC Davis M.I.N.D. Institute, in collaboration with scientists in the Department of Psychiatry and Behavioral Sciences at Stanford University, have carried out a comprehensive magnetic resonance imaging (MRI) brain analysis finding that the brain regions responsible for memory and emotion are larger in children with autism. This study appears in the July 14, 2004, issue of the *Journal of Neuroscience.*

David Amaral, the principal investigator on the project, notes, "Our study shows that the amygdala develops abnormally in autism. This brain region grows too quickly in boys with autism and does not seem to have the opportunity to benefit from information derived from the environment for normal development. We also found that the hippocampus is about 10 percent larger in boys with autism at all ages."

The research team studied ninety-eight boys, aged seven to eighteen years, with a diagnosis of autism or Asperger syndrome. One autism group had mental retardation and the second autism group had normal intelligence, and both were compared to a volunteer group of typically developing children.

The study examined two brain regions located in the temporal lobe, using high-resolution MRI and specially designed computer software to measure the volume of the amygdala or hippocampus. The amygdala is involved with emotional processing, especially fear, and the hippocampus is involved in making memories of episodes from our lives.

The amygdala in the typically developing boys underwent a tremendous expansion of approximately 40 percent over the age range studied. The volume of the total brain actually decreased slightly over this age range. For both groups of children with autism, the amygdala was initially larger than in the typically developing children but did not undergo the age-related increase in size seen in the control group. Thus, for younger children (7.5–12.5 years) the amygdala is significantly larger in the boys with autism than the control group, whereas in the older boys (12.5–18.5 years), there is no significant difference between the groups.

These data support the growing view that autism is associated with a precocious growth of the brain or at least of certain brain regions. Additional research is needed to determine: what percentage of children with autism have abnormal development of the amygdala and hippocampus; what symptoms of autism might result from this abnormal development; what causes these brain regions to be too large; and if it is possible that the increased size of the hippocampus could actually reflect better than average ability for certain types of memory in autism. Many of these issues are being addressed in research currently under way at the M.I.N.D. Institute.

Section 10.5

# Researchers Find Fewer Neurons in the Amygdala of Males with Autism

Researchers at the University of California, Davis, M.I.N.D. Institute have discovered that the brains of males with autism have fewer neurons in the amygdala, a part of the brain involved in emotion and memory. The study, published in the July 19, 2006, issue of the *Journal of Neuroscience*, is the first neuroanatomical study to quantify a key difference in the autistic amygdala.

David Amaral, research director of the UC Davis M.I.N.D. Institute, and former graduate student Cynthia Mills Schumann counted and measured representative samples of neurons in the amygdala of nine postmortem brains of males who had autism and ten postmortem brains of males who did not have autism. Both subject groups ranged in age from ten to forty-four years at the time of death. Using a technique known as "unbiased stereological analysis," Schumann and Amaral counted neurons using a computer-aided microscope system. They found significantly fewer neurons—cells responsible for creating and transmitting electrical impulses—in the whole amygdala and its lateral nucleus in the brains of people with autism.

"This is the first quantitative evidence of an abnormal number of neurons in the autistic amygdala and the first study to use modern unbiased sampling techniques for autism research," Amaral said.

"While we have known that autism is a developmental brain disorder, where, how and when the autistic brain develops abnormally has been a mystery," said Thomas R. Insel, a physician and director of the National Institute of Mental Health. "This new finding is important because it demonstrates that the structure of the amygdala is abnormal in autism. Along with other findings on the abnormal function of the amygdala, research is beginning to narrow the search for the brain basis of autism."

121

Now affecting 1 in every 166 children and primarily affecting males, autism is a lifelong neurodevelopmental disorder characterized by social and communication deficits. While autism has clear behavioral indicators, the neural alterations leading to the deficits have been difficult to pinpoint. In studies dating back to the mid-1980s, researchers began focusing on the amygdala because of its importance in generating appropriate emotional responses and assimilating memories that are key to social learning—functions that are impaired by autism.

"Previous magnetic resonance imaging studies from several laboratories, including the M.I.N.D. Institute, have indicated precocious enlargement of the amygdala in young children with autism," said Schumann, who is now a postdoctoral researcher at the UC San Diego School of Medicine. "But these studies were not able to determine whether the number of neurons were different in the autistic amygdala."

Interpreting these earlier qualitative studies was hampered because many postmortem brains available for research were from individuals who had autism as well as epilepsy, a condition known to cause pathology of the amygdala.

"Back when these studies were conducted, it wasn't easy to acquire the brain of a deceased person who just had autism," Amaral explained. "We are fortunate now to have the Autism Tissue Program, funded by the National Alliance for Autism Research and the National Institutes of Health. With their help, we were able to analyze more than double the number of previously examined postmortem brains, none of which had seizure disorders or any major neurological disorder other than autism."

"A better understanding of the neurobiology of the amygdala is crucial to advance autism research, and this study helps answer many important questions about the fundamental basis of autism," said Andy Shih, chief science officer for the National Alliance for Autism Research, which is now merged with Autism Speaks. "Autism Speaks and the Autism Tissue Program were proud to support this project so that these important discoveries could be made."

By counting the actual number of neurons in tissue samples, the researchers also overcame a methodological concern raised by studies that described changes in neuronal density, or neurons per unit volume, in portions of the amygdala.

"Differences in neuron density could just indicate changes in tissue volume rather than changes in total cell number. The only way to determine the actual difference is to systematically count samples of neurons in a defined volume," Amaral said.

With this latest confirmation that the amygdala is pathological in autism, Amaral and colleagues will now determine why there are fewer neurons in the amygdala and if other parts of the brain are similarly affected.

"We need to look at other brain regions to find out if the cell loss is idiosyncratic to the amygdala or a more general phenomenon," he said. "We're in the very early stages of understanding autism and its neurological pathologies. It's clearly a process with many steps, and at least we are now one step further."

Additional research will also help identify the developmental point in time at which the neuron reduction actually occurs, which the current study does not address.

"One possibility is that there are always fewer neurons in the amygdala of people with autism. Another possibility is that a degenerative process occurs later in life and leads to neuron loss. More studies are needed to refine our findings," said Schumann.

## Section 10.6

# Nicotine Receptors in the Brain May Play Role in Development of Autism

"Nicotine Receptors May Play Role in Development of Autism," by Joan Archart-Treidhel, *Psychiatric News*, July 20, 2001. Reprinted with permission from the *Psychiatric News*, © 2001 American Psychiatric Association. Updated by David A. Cooke, M.D., March 2007.

Deep inside the human brain, cholinergic nicotinic receptors are busy plying their trade, and one might view them as triple agents. They release the nerve transmitter acetylcholine from certain nerve ends, they receive it at others, and they can be stimulated by nicotine—yes, from cigarette smoking!

Even more intriguing, these receptors have been implicated of late in a spate of psychiatric and neurological disorders such as Alzheimer disease, Parkinson disease, schizophrenia, and Tourette syndrome (*Psychiatric News*, March 13, 2000).

And now the receptors have been linked to yet another psychiatric-neurological condition—autism.

The finding comes from Elaine Perry, Ph.D., of Newcastle General Hospital in Newcastle-Upon-Tyne, England, and her colleagues. It is reported in the July 2001 *American Journal of Psychiatry*.

"This is an important paper," Peter Whitehouse, M.D., Ph.D., a neurologist-psychologist with Case Western Reserve University in Cleveland, told *Psychiatric News*. "It is probably the first [neurochemical] investigation of cholinergic systems in autism. And the findings regarding the nicotinic receptors do suggest a potential role for them in the mechanisms of autism, particularly related to the ability to focus attention and to interact with other people."

During the past few years, there have been intimations that the nerves and other brain mechanics that concern themselves with acetylcholine—the so-called cholinergic systems—might be implicated in autism. For example, cholinergic neurons in the basal forebrain, an area of the brain known to be involved in attention, have been found to be abnormally plentiful, and abnormally large, in children with autism.

As for a chemical known to influence the development and function of cholinergic neurons in the basal forebrain area—brain-derived neurotrophic factor—abnormally high levels of it have been found in the bloodstreams of newborns with autism. Thus, these and some other discoveries prompted Perry and her team to try to determine whether, and how, various cholinergic players conspire in the autism disease process.

They acquired frozen brain samples from seven deceased adults who had had autism and from ten deceased adults who had no mental disorder. They then examined the activities of specific cholinergic functions in the brain samples and compared the activity of each function in brain samples from the autistic subjects with the activity in brain samples from the control subjects.

If any functions were found to behave abnormally in brain samples from autistic subjects, they reasoned, then those functions might well be culprits in the autism disease process.

For instance, the researchers measured in the brain samples the activity of acetylcholinesterase, the enzyme that makes acetylcholine. They then compared the activity of the enzyme in samples from the autism group with the activity of the enzyme in samples from the control group. They found no difference. So they concluded that this particular enzyme is probably not implicated in autism.

They also measured the activity of the enzyme that breaks down acetylcholine. They then compared the activity of this enzyme in samples from the autism group with the activity of this enzyme in samples from the control group. Again they found no difference. So they concluded that this enzyme, too, is not involved in autism.

However, they did find something interesting regarding the chemical that is known to influence the development and function of cholinergic neurons in the basal forebrain—that is, brain-derived neurotrophic factor.

They found three times more of the factor in the basal forebrain area of brain samples taken from autism subjects than in samples taken from mentally normal subjects. So they think that this factor might indeed be involved in autism.

And they also found considerably less nicotinic receptor activity in the cerebral cortex of brain samples taken from autism subjects than in the cerebral cortex of samples taken from mentally normal subjects. So they believe that faulty nicotinic receptors might also be culprits in autism.

Such findings, they concluded in their paper, suggest that "the role of the cholinergic system in autism should be investigated further. . . ."

Also of interest, they wrote, is that the abnormalities they have detected in brain samples from autism subjects more closely resemble those in brain samples from schizophrenia subjects than those in brain samples from Alzheimer disease or Parkinson disease subjects. Such similarities, they believe, are not surprising since "there is an extensive overlap in clinical symptoms between autism and schizophrenia, both behaviorally and cognitively . . . and the same neural systems are likely to be involved in both, although differing in developmental staging and etiology."

But the findings by Perry and her team are especially provocative because they may point the way to an effective treatment for autism—something that does not currently exist. For instance, might nicotine or another drug that stimulates the nicotinic receptors possibly help autism patients? Perry thinks so. In fact, she told *Psychiatric News*, she would like to explore this possibility. The most recently approved drug for Alzheimer disease—galantamine—might also be able to counter autism, Whitehouse conjectures. The reason, he said, is that the drug is thought to be capable of influencing the nicotinic receptors (*Psychiatric News*, April 20, 2001).

To date, there have been three published reports of treating autistic patients with galantamine. All three of these reports did report some positive change. However, all involved very small numbers of patients, and only one was a placebo-controlled, double-blind study— the most scientifically rigorous kind.

There is a long history of drugs that have been called "promising" for treatment of autism, only to be later shown ineffective in larger and better-designed studies. This is because symptoms of autism can be difficult to measure, and vary greatly over time. In addition, the hopes of caregivers and well-meaning researchers can generate false impressions of medication effectiveness where none exists.

Will galantamine prove to be different? Only large, very carefully designed studies can answer this question, and they have not yet been completed.

Chapter 11

# Parent, Pregnancy, and Birth Factors Associated with Risk of Autism

## Associations of Parent, Pregnancy, and Birth Factors with the Risk of Autism

Pregnancy factors, parental psychiatric history, and preterm delivery may be associated with the risk of autism, according to a recent study supported in part by the Centers for Disease Control and Prevention (CDC). The study, "Risk Factors for Autism: Perinatal Factors, Parental Psychiatric History, and Socioeconomic Status," appears in the May 15, 2005, issue of the *American Journal of Epidemiology*.

The research, which involved a national study of all 698 Danish children with autism born after 1972 and diagnosed before 2000, focused on perinatal risk factors (i.e., delivery and newborn characteristics, pregnancy characteristics, and parental characteristics), parental psychiatric history (i.e., whether a parent had a diagnosed psychiatric illness before the date that autism was diagnosed in the child), and socioeconomic status (i.e., the mother's formal education and parental wealth at the child's birth). Previous research had suggested each category might represent or include risk factors for autism.

"This study is a helpful step forward in identifying possible risk factors for autism," said Dr. José Cordero, director of the Center for

Disease Control and Prevention (CDC)'s National Center on Birth Defects and Developmental Disabilities. "It also indicates there may be some children for whom we need extra vigilance in watching for signs of developmental delay. In recent years, many programs and studies have found that early recognition of autism and other developmental disabilities is important because early treatment can significantly improve a child's development."

Some of the specific factors that the study found to be associated with the risk of autism included: breech presentation at birth, delivery before thirty-five weeks, a parent who had a diagnosis of schizophrenia-like psychosis before the date that autism was diagnosed in the child, and low birth weight at delivery. The study also found that many of these factors were independently associated with autism. For example, there was an association between adverse pregnancy events and autism, regardless of whether one of the parents had a diagnosed psychiatric illness.

"We need to further investigate the role of events during pregnancy, including their possible interaction with genetic factors, to learn more about potential causes of autism," said Diana Schendel, CDC epidemiologist and one of the authors. "We also need additional research to determine if the factors identified here really play a role in causing autism. Right now, we have only identified possible associations. But if we can find a cause-and-effect relationship, it may help our efforts to prevent autism."

Autism spectrum disorders (ASDs) are a group of developmental disabilities that are caused by unusual brain development. People with ASDs tend to have problems with social and communication skills. Many people with ASDs also have unusual ways of learning, paying attention, or reacting to different sensations. ASDs begin during childhood and last throughout a person's life. CDC funds projects on ASDs in several states. These projects track the number of children who have an ASD, conduct studies to find out what factors make it more likely that a child will have an ASD, and offer education and outreach programs for researchers, families, and other people affected by ASDs. Large representative studies are needed to answer questions necessary to determine the potential causes of autism and develop prevention strategies for this disorder.

## Older Fathers More Likely to Have Autistic Children

The risk of developing autism is significantly higher among children born to men who are forty and older than it is among children with fathers under thirty, researchers report.

The reason appears to be genetic, researchers suggest.

Autism is a growing problem, affecting fifty children in every ten thousand, compared with just five in ten thousand only twenty years ago. This increase appears to be partially due to more awareness of the condition and changes in the definition of classic autism to include autism spectrum disorders. However, it could also be that there is an increase in the incidence of autism, experts say.

The condition is marked by social and language problems and repetitive patterns of behavior. Autism spectrum disorder includes pervasive developmental disorder; Rett syndrome, Asperger syndrome, and childhood disintegrative disorder.

The report appears in the September 2006 issue of the *Archives of General Psychiatry*.

There may be several genetic reasons for this finding, said study author Abraham Reichenberg, from Mount Sinai School of Medicine in New York City.

One cause might be mutations in the sperm as men age, Reichenberg said. "Those mutations might be accumulating with age and therefore transmitted from the father to the child," he said. "Another possibility is that mechanisms that the body has to protect itself from mutations are not working that well with age."

It might also be that an improper or defective gene is being activated, Reichenberg noted. These mechanisms operating alone or in concert may be the reason for the association of older parental age and autism, he said.

In their study, Reichenberg's team collected data on the age of the fathers of 318,506 people born during the 1980s in Israel. The age of the mother was known for 132,271 of these people as well. Among these individuals, all the men and three-fourths of the women were assessed by the draft board at age seventeen for any psychiatric disorders.

Among those whose father's age was the only one known, 208 children had a diagnosis of autism spectrum disorder, as did 110 in the group where the age of both parents was known, the researchers found.

When the researchers compared the parents' age when they had their child to the cases of autism among the children, they found thirty-four cases among 60,654 kids born to parents aged fifteen to twenty-nine years old, sixty-two cases among 67,211 kids born to parents aged thirty to thirty-nine years old, thirteen cases among 4,106 kids born to parents aged forty to forty-nine years old, and one case among 190 kids born to parents older than fifty.

Reichenberg's group found the advancing age of fathers was associated with increased risk of autism. In fact, the odds of a child having autism spectrum disorder were nearly six times greater for children of men aged forty and older, compared with men aged twenty-nine years and younger. The older age of mothers was not associated with the risk for autism.

"This phenomenon of older fathers having autistic kids should be explored further, because it might give us a clue about the genetic mechanism that contributes to the development of autism," Reichenberg said.

One expert thinks the finding might be explained by the fathers being mildly autistic, and therefore marrying and having children later.

"The very real possibility that autistic traits in fathers led to older age of marriage and age at childbirth presents a real problem for interpretation of the results," said George M. Anderson, a research scientist at the Child Study Center and Laboratory Medicine at the Yale University School of Medicine. "This critical aspect is downplayed by the authors."

"In the absence of good sociability/integration data in fathers of autistic children, I think one can say little about how much of the reported paternal age effect in autism is due to age-related genetic alterations," Anderson said.

Another expert doesn't think the finding adds much to the understanding of autism.

"Not an especially interesting finding," said Eric Courchesne, director of the Center for Autism Research at the San Diego Children's Hospital.

It is unlikely this finding will have any significant impact on neuroscience research or on early identification or treatment of autism, Courchesne said. "The study says nothing about the brain bases and nothing specific about the genetics or possible environmental factors that may cause the condition," he said.

In fact, Courchesne thinks the finding might be a statistical fluke. "Autism is a heterogeneous disorder, and when you get a huge enough sample, even small and possibly irrelevant statistical associations may be found," he said.

# Part Three

# Conditions That May Accompany Autism Spectrum Disorders

Chapter 12

# Understanding Genetic Disorders That Occur More Frequently in People with Autism

## Chapter Contents

Section 12.1—Tuberous Sclerosis.............................................. 134
Section 12.2—Fragile X Syndrome............................................ 146
Section 12.3—Angelman Syndrome ........................................... 153
Section 12.4—Landau-Kleffner Syndrome .............................. 155
Section 12.5—Prader-Willi Syndrome ..................................... 157
Section 12.6—Williams Syndrome ............................................ 160
Section 12.7—Tourette Syndrome............................................. 163

Section 12.1

# Tuberous Sclerosis

This section begins with text reprinted from "Tuberous Sclerosis Fact Sheet," National Institute of Neurological Disorders and Stroke, National Institutes of Health, NIH Publication No. 07-1846, March 23, 2007. It also includes text reprinted from "Tuberous Sclerosis Complex and Autism Spectrum Disorders," © 2006 Tuberous Sclerosis Alliance. Reprinted with permission.

## Facts about Tuberous Sclerosis

### What is tuberous sclerosis?

Tuberous sclerosis—also called tuberous sclerosis complex (TSC)[1]—is a rare, multisystem genetic disease that causes benign tumors to grow in the brain and on other vital organs such as the kidneys, heart, eyes, lungs, and skin. It commonly affects the central nervous system and results in a combination of symptoms including seizures, developmental delay, behavioral problems, skin abnormalities, and kidney disease.

The disorder affects as many as 25,000 to 40,000 individuals in the United States and about 1 to 2 million individuals worldwide, with an estimated prevalence of one in 6,000 newborns. TSC occurs in all races and ethnic groups, and in both genders.

The name tuberous sclerosis comes from the characteristic tuber or potato-like nodules in the brain, which calcify with age and become hard or sclerotic. The disorder—once known as epiloia or Bourneville disease—was first identified by a French physician more than one hundred years ago.

Many TSC patients show evidence of the disorder in the first year of life. However, clinical features can be subtle initially, and many signs and symptoms take years to develop. As a result, TSC can be unrecognized or misdiagnosed for years.

### What causes tuberous sclerosis?

TSC is caused by defects, or mutations, on two genes—TSC1 and TSC2. Only one of the genes needs to be affected for TSC to be present.

The TSC1 gene, discovered in 1997, is on chromosome 9 and produces a protein called hamartin. The TSC2 gene, discovered in 1993, is on chromosome 16 and produces the protein tuberin. Scientists believe these proteins act in a complex as growth suppressors by inhibiting the activation of a master, evolutionarily conserved kinase called mTOR. Loss of regulation of mTOR occurs in cells lacking either hamartin or tuberin, and this leads to abnormal differentiation and development, and to the generation of enlarged cells, as are seen in TSC brain lesions.

## Is TSC inherited?

Although some individuals inherit the disorder from a parent with TSC, most cases occur as sporadic cases due to new, spontaneous mutations in TSC1 or TSC2. In this situation, neither parent has the disorder or the faulty gene(s). Instead, a faulty gene first occurs in the affected individual.

In familial cases, TSC is an autosomal dominant disorder, which means that the disorder can be transmitted directly from parent to child. In those cases, only one parent needs to have the faulty gene in order to pass it on to a child. If a parent has TSC, each offspring has a 50 percent chance of developing the disorder. Children who inherit TSC may not have the same symptoms as their parent and they may have either a milder or a more severe form of the disorder.

Rarely, individuals acquire TSC through a process called gonadal mosaicism. These patients have parents with no apparent defects in the two genes that cause the disorder. Yet these parents can have a child with TSC because a portion of one of the parent's reproductive cells (sperm or eggs) can contain the genetic mutation without the other cells of the body being involved. In cases of gonadal mosaicism, genetic testing of a blood sample might not reveal the potential for passing the disease to offspring.

## What are the signs and symptoms of TSC?

TSC can affect many different systems of the body, causing a variety of signs and symptoms. Signs of the disorder vary depending on which system and which organs are involved. The natural course of TSC varies from individual to individual, with symptoms ranging from very mild to quite severe. In addition to the benign tumors that frequently occur in TSC, other common symptoms include seizures, mental retardation, behavior problems, and skin abnormalities. Tumors can grow in nearly any organ, but they most commonly occur in the brain, kidneys, heart, lungs, and skin. Malignant tumors are rare in TSC. Those that do occur primarily affect the kidneys.

Kidney problems such as cysts and angiomyolipomas occur in an estimated 70 to 80 percent of individuals with TSC, usually occurring between ages fifteen and thirty. Cysts are usually small, appear in limited numbers, and cause no serious problems. Approximately 2 percent of individuals with TSC develop large numbers of cysts in a pattern similar to polycystic kidney disease[2] during childhood. In these cases, kidney function is compromised and kidney failure occurs. In rare instances, the cysts may bleed, leading to blood loss and anemia.

Angiomyolipomas—benign growths consisting of fatty tissue and muscle cells—are the most common kidney lesions in TSC. These growths are seen in the majority of TSC patients, but are also found in about one of every three hundred people without TSC. Angiomyolipomas caused by TSC are usually found in both kidneys and in most cases they produce no symptoms. However, they can sometimes grow so large that they cause pain or kidney failure. Bleeding from angiomyolipomas may also occur, causing both pain and weakness. If severe bleeding does not stop naturally, there may be severe blood loss, resulting in profound anemia and a life-threatening drop in blood pressure, warranting urgent medical attention.

Other rare kidney problems include renal cell carcinoma, developing from an angiomyolipoma, and oncocytomas, benign tumors unique to individuals with TSC.

Three types of brain tumors are associated with TSC: cortical tubers, for which the disease is named, generally form on the surface of the brain, but may also appear in the deep areas of the brain; subependymal nodules, which form in the walls of the ventricles (the fluid-filled cavities of the brain); and giant-cell tumors (astrocytomas), a type of tumor that can grow and block the flow of fluids within the brain, causing a buildup of fluid and pressure and leading to headaches and blurred vision.

Tumors called cardiac rhabdomyomas are often found in the hearts of infants and young children with TSC. If the tumors are large or there are multiple tumors, they can block circulation and cause death. However, if they do not cause problems at birth—when in most cases they are at their largest size—they usually become smaller with time and do not affect the individual in later life.

Benign tumors called phakomas are sometimes found in the eyes of individuals with TSC, appearing as white patches on the retina. Generally they do not cause vision loss or other vision problems, but they can be used to help diagnose the disease.

Additional tumors and cysts may be found in other areas of the body, including the liver, lungs, and pancreas. Bone cysts, rectal polyps, gum fibromas, and dental pits may also occur.

A wide variety of skin abnormalities may occur in individuals with TSC. Most cause no problems but are helpful in diagnosis. Some cases may cause disfigurement, necessitating treatment. The most common skin abnormalities include the following:

- Hypomelanic macules ("ash leaf spots"), which are white or lighter patches of skin that may appear anywhere on the body and are caused by a lack of skin pigment or melanin—the substance that gives skin its color.

- Reddish spots or bumps called facial angiofibromas (also called adenoma sebaceum), which appear on the face (sometimes resembling acne) and consist of blood vessels and fibrous tissue.

- Raised, discolored areas on the forehead called forehead plaques, which are common and unique to TSC and may help doctors diagnose the disorder.

- Areas of thick, leathery, pebbly skin called shagreen patches, usually found on the lower back or nape of the neck.

- Small fleshy tumors called ungual or subungual fibromas that grow around and under the toenails or fingernails and may need to be surgically removed if they enlarge or cause bleeding. These usually appear later in life, ages twenty to fifty.

- Other skin features that are not unique to individuals with TSC, including molluscum fibrosum or skin tags, which typically occur across the back of the neck and shoulders, café au lait spots or flat brown marks, and poliosis, a tuft or patch of white hair that may appear on the scalp or eyelids.

TSC can cause seizures and varying degrees of mental disability. Seizures of all types may occur, including infantile spasms; tonic-clonic seizures (also known as grand mal seizures); or tonic, akinetic, atypical absence, myoclonic, complex partial, or generalized seizures.

Approximately one-half to two-thirds of individuals with TSC have mental disabilities ranging from mild learning disabilities to severe mental retardation. Behavior problems, including aggression, sudden rage, attention deficit hyperactivity disorder, acting out, obsessive-compulsive disorder, and repetitive, destructive, or self-harming behavior, often occur in children with TSC, and can be difficult to manage.

Some individuals with TSC may also have a developmental disorder called autism.

## How is TSC diagnosed?

In most cases the first clue to recognizing TSC is the presence of seizures or delayed development. In other cases, the first sign may be white patches on the skin (hypomelanotic macules).

Diagnosis of the disorder is based on a careful clinical exam in combination with computed tomography (CT) or magnetic resonance imaging (MRI) of the brain, which may show tubers in the brain, and an ultrasound of the heart, liver, and kidneys, which may show tumors in those organs. Doctors should carefully examine the skin for the wide variety of skin features, the fingernails and toenails for ungual fibromas, the teeth and gums for dental pits or gum fibromas, and the eyes for dilated pupils. A Wood's lamp or ultraviolet light may be used to locate the hypomelanotic macules, which are sometimes hard to see on infants and individuals with pale or fair skin. Because of the wide variety of signs of TSC, it is best if a doctor experienced in the diagnosis of TSC evaluates a potential patient.

In infants TSC may be suspected if the child has cardiac rhabdomyomas or seizures (infantile spasms) at birth. With a careful examination of the skin and brain, it may be possible to diagnose TSC in a very young infant. However, many children are not diagnosed until later in life when their seizures begin and other symptoms such as facial angiofibromas appear.

## How is TSC treated?

There is no cure for TSC, although treatment is available for a number of the symptoms. Antiepileptic drugs may be used to control seizures, and medications may be prescribed for behavior problems. Intervention programs including special schooling and occupational therapy may benefit individuals with special needs and developmental issues. Surgery including dermabrasion and laser treatment may be useful for treatment of skin lesions. Because TSC is a lifelong condition, individuals need to be regularly monitored by a doctor to make sure they are receiving the best possible treatments. Due to the many varied symptoms of TSC, care by a clinician experienced with the disorder is recommended.

Recently much enthusiasm has arisen in regard to the use of rapamycin for treatment of TSC. Rapamycin is a drug that specifically blocks the activity of mTOR. In cell culture experiments and animal models of TSC, rapamycin appears to be very effective. Initial clinical experience with rapamycin and related drugs is also positive, but much additional study is required before these drugs become standard therapy.

## What is the prognosis?

The prognosis for individuals with TSC depends on the severity of symptoms, which range from mild skin abnormalities to varying degrees of learning disabilities and epilepsy to severe mental retardation, uncontrollable seizures, and kidney failure. Those individuals with mild symptoms generally do well and live long, productive lives, while individuals with the more severe form may have serious disabilities.

In rare cases, seizures, infections, or tumors in vital organs may cause complications in some organs such as the kidneys and brain that can lead to severe difficulties and even death. However, with appropriate medical care, most individuals with the disorder can look forward to normal life expectancy.

## What research is being done?

Within the federal government, the leading supporter of research on TSC is the National Institute of Neurological Disorders and Stroke (NINDS). The NINDS, part of the National Institutes of Health (NIH), is responsible for supporting and conducting research on the brain and the central nervous system. NINDS conducts research in its laboratories at NIH and also supports studies through grants to major medical institutions across the country. The National Heart, Lung, and Blood Institute and the National Cancer Institute, also components of the NIH, support and conduct research on TSC.

Scientists who study TSC seek to increase our understanding of the disorder by learning more about the TSC1 and TSC2 genes that can cause the disorder and the function of the proteins—tuberin and hamartin—produced by these genes. Scientists hope knowledge gained from their current research will improve the genetic test for TSC and lead to new avenues of treatment, methods of prevention, and, ultimately, a cure for this disorder.

Research studies run the gamut from very basic scientific investigation to clinical translational research. For example, some investigators are trying to identify all the protein components that are in the same "signaling pathway" in which the TSC1 and TSC2 protein products and the mTOR protein are involved. Other studies are focused on understanding in detail how the disease develops, both in animal models and in patients, to better define new ways of controlling or preventing the development of the disease. Finally, clinical trials of rapamycin are underway (with NINDS and NCI support) to rigorously test the potential benefit of this compound for some of the tumors that are problematic in TSC patients.

### Notes

1. Tuberous sclerosis is often referred to as tuberous sclerosis complex (TSC) in medical literature to help distinguish it from Tourette syndrome, an unrelated neurological disorder.

2. Polycystic kidney disease is a genetic disorder characterized by the growth of numerous fluid-filled cysts in the kidneys.

## Tuberous Sclerosis Complex and Autism Spectrum Disorders

First described in 1943 as a syndrome impacting behavior, autism is typically diagnosed within the first three years of a child's life. The three areas that are evaluated to reach a diagnosis of autism are:

1. An impairment in the ability to interact socially with people; often demonstrating a lack of eye contact and disinterest in physical contact such as hugging or hand-holding;

2. An impairment in the ability to communicate using speech or gestures;

3. A tendency to have narrow patterns of interests and activities coupled with repetitive and obsessive behaviors, and a lack of pretend or imaginative play; often children with autism find it necessary to have rigid and structured routines.

There are a wide range of variants and degree of demonstrated behavior such that autism is often defined as "autistic spectrum disorder" or ASD. Some children have clear signs of ASD in two of the main areas required for diagnosis, but have less obvious features in the third. In these instances, individuals are said to have an atypical form of autism. When the intellectual abilities are normal, early language development is not significantly delayed, and speech is well developed,

140

then individuals may meet criteria for another variant called Asperger syndrome. A third variant, termed pervasive developmental disorder (not otherwise specified) or PDD, describes individuals who have difficulties in all three areas but fail to meet full criteria in any of the areas.

## What is the link between autism spectrum disorder and tuberous sclerosis complex?

Over the years, it has become recognized that between one-fourth and one-half of all children with tuberous sclerosis complex (TSC) develop ASD. The rate of ASD in the general population is substantially lower (around 0.5 or 0.6 percent of the total population), so there is clearly a very substantial increase in the rate of ASD in children with TSC. Likewise, the rate of TSC in children diagnosed with ASD is around 1 percent. Although this is a relatively low rate, it is still clearly much higher than the rate of TSC in the general population, which is about one in six thousand individuals. Either way, the overlap between ASD and TSC is clear.

ASD is usually diagnosed in young children between the ages of two and four, but in individuals with TSC, the diagnosis of ASD may go unrecognized or be delayed due to other developmental disabilities. The importance of an accurate diagnosis of ASD for individuals with TSC is so that the individual can receive appropriate educational services and lifelong support, as needed.

## Why do individuals with TSC frequently develop ASD?

Current research does not definitely answer the questions related to the increase of ASD in individuals with TSC. However, some important leads are beginning to form the basis of an explanation for the link. In general, it is believed the abnormalities in brain development that occur in TSC sometimes interfere with the proper development of brain areas that are important for the development of social communication skills (the ability to appropriately interact with other individuals).

Evidence is beginning to emerge that shows that if cortical tubers (which develop in earlier stages of brain development) in individuals with TSC involve the region of the brain called the temporal lobes, then there is an increased likelihood of an ASD developing. The temporal lobes are important for processing auditory information, especially speech sounds as well as information about faces and facial

141

expressions. Interference with the development of these key skills may then lead to the social communication difficulties that characterize ASD.

It seems, however, that the presence of cortical tubers in the temporal lobes is not sufficient on its own to produce ASD. Instead, it appears that when temporal lobe tubers occur in conjunction with the onset of seizures at a young age, often presenting as infantile spasms, then this combination of factors leads to the much higher chance of ASD. Although the link with early onset epilepsy and infantile spasms raises the possibility that the seizures may play a role in interfering with normal development of brain systems important in social communication, it is possible that the link with early seizures instead reflects the presence of cortical tubers and related structural abnormalities in key locations in the brain. These structural abnormalities may give rise to both the seizures as well as ASD. Further research to try to determine which of these two explanations is correct is required, especially as it has such important implications for treatment.

### *Is it important to diagnose ASD in individuals with TSC?*

Some people express the view that it is enough that an individual has TSC, so another diagnosis such as ASD is unnecessary. Although it makes sense to avoid adding diagnoses and labels, the diagnosis of an ASD is important for several reasons. A diagnosis can often help parents make sense of a range of rather unusual behaviors that otherwise seem extremely puzzling. Often, parents feel that somehow they have been doing something wrong in how they are parenting their child, and that the difficulties that the child is having in relating to others, communicating, or playing is somehow the parents' fault. It can be quite helpful for parents to discover that some of the unusual behaviors their child may be demonstrating are part of the developmental delays a child may be experiencing related to the autistic process.

In addition, the diagnosis is important because children with ASD often benefit from early intervention services that support improvement in speech, language, and behaviors. Early intervention services are available for very young children and their families. These services include physical therapy, speech therapy, and occupational therapy. Early intervention services work with not only the child with ASD, but also the parents and siblings. The goal of early services is to foster the development of children with ASD.

### *How is the diagnosis made?*

The diagnosis of an ASD is based on a report of the child's early development, detailing the way in which he or she acquired skills and the areas in which he or she has struggled, coupled with careful observations and assessments. These evaluations need to be performed by individuals who are experienced in evaluating individuals with complex developmental disabilities and ASD. The assessments are lengthy, and it may be necessary for the evaluator to see the child at home or in the playgroup or nursery setting, often referred to as a functional contextual assessment, before the diagnosis can be confirmed. The diagnosis of ASD is made through a team evaluation, including reports from therapists, pediatricians, teachers, parents, and psychologists.

There are several assessments that are used to reach a diagnosis of ASD; the most commonly used is called the Autism Diagnostic Observation Schedule (ADOS). This assessment should be performed by someone familiar with ASD who is trained to utilize the ADOS.

### *When is diagnosis possible?*

To some extent the answer to this depends on the individual's overall level of ability. In individuals who have the most severe cognitive disabilities, it can sometimes be extremely difficult to make a definitive diagnosis. In general it is hard to make a confident diagnosis before the individual's cognitive age level is at least equivalent to that of an eighteen-month- to two-year-old child. In less affected individuals, it might well be possible to make a diagnosis around the age of two, whereas in the individuals with very significant delays in development it may not be possible until they are much older. Research is continuing to identify the early markers of ASD so early treatments can be implemented.

### *What treatment is suggested?*

Treatment options vary based on the individual's age and ability. The focus of the treatment is often targeted at strengthening skills in individual areas of difficulty. Special education provisions and accommodations are incorporated in a child's individual education plan (IEP). This often includes the individual working with a multidisciplinary team of clinical professionals that provide several different services, including speech and language therapists, developmental and child psychologists, and pediatricians.

According to the Autism Society of America, treatment approaches include the following:

- Applied behavioral analysis (ABA) and discrete trial training
- Treatment of autistic and related communication handicapped children (TEACCH)
- Picture exchange communication system (PECS)

**ABA and discrete trial training:** These methods are often used interchangeably. They include intense repetitive, structured tasks in which good behavior is rewarded and undesirable behavior is ignored. It is time-intensive and focuses on changing current behaviors and does not prepare individuals to respond in new situations. Some individuals with TSC who have ASD have significantly benefited from ABA programs.

**TEACCH (treatment and education of autistic and related communication handicapped children):** This method was developed at the University of North Carolina. TEACCH focuses on adapting the environment to the individual with ASD instead of trying to make the individual adapt to the environment. This is achieved through high structure, organizational charts, and schedules. While many favor this approach, some feel that it is too structured and makes the individual too dependent on charts and other organizational tools.

**PECS (picture exchange communication system):** This method is used to encourage communication. By using pictures, an individual can point to or hand an object to someone to demonstrate what he or she wants.

Options vary and the treatment program needs to be tailored to the individual's age and ability. Treatment is targeted at fostering skills in the three main areas of difficulty—social and communication skills and the development of imaginative play. In addition, treatment aims to ensure that the repetitive or obsessive behaviors do not become too marked or prominent, and do not interfere with family life. Lastly, the treatment aims to help parents foster their child's development and support them during the early, often very demanding, years.

There is growing evidence to suggest that early intervention programs may be one of the most effective current forms of treatment in individuals with ASD, but it is not yet known to what extent the

144

intervention programs of this kind are helpful for children with TSC. Research is needed to evaluate effectiveness of these programs for individuals with TSC who have ASD.

## *What will the future hold?*

Detailed knowledge about the way individuals with TSC and ASD develop is currently being gained through studies in the United States and the United Kingdom, so for now we can be guided only by the development of individuals with ASD who do not have TSC. The range of outcomes here is very great. At one extreme, individuals with ASD are prone to self-injury, particularly if they get upset or frustrated when their routines or activities are interrupted, or if they get frustrated over their communication difficulties.

At the other extreme, individuals with Asperger syndrome or high-functioning ASD can largely outgrow their difficulties and lead an independent or semi-independent life in adulthood. The outcome is to some extent related to the severity of the associated cognitive impairments or a demonstrated level of cognitive disabilities. Individuals who have severe or profound forms of cognitive disability are likely to have persisting difficulties. In addition, the amount of useful speech that the individual acquires indicates how he or she will fare in the future. Lastly, the severity of the social and communication difficulties and behavior problems is also helpful in determining what the outcome will be. The more severe the problems, the more persistent they tend to be.

Section 12.2

# Fragile X Syndrome

"Fragile X Syndrome: The Basics" is excerpted from "Fragile X Syndrome" and reprinted with permission from the University of Michigan Health System, www.med.umich.edu. Copyright 2006 Regents of the University of Michigan. "Fragile X and Autism" is reprinted from "How Do the Behaviors Seen in Persons with Fragile X Relate to Those Seen in Autism?" by Randi Hagerman, M.D. © 2002 National Fragile X Foundation (www.fragilex.org). Reprinted with permission.

## Fragile X Syndrome: The Basics

### What is fragile X syndrome?

Fragile X is the most common inherited form of mental retardation. It affects about 1 in 1,200 males of all racial and ethnic groups. It can cause a range of mental impairment, varying from mild to severe, and can also cause many other typical features and symptoms. Here is some basic information about fragile X.

### What causes fragile X syndrome?

- It is inherited.

- It is caused by mutation of a gene (FMR1) on the X chromosome. Genetic testing for fragile X is possible.

- Mothers may be a carrier of the mutation and pass it on to their children.

- Or, a mother may have a pre-mutation that expands to a full mutation when passed on to the next generation.

- Boys are affected more severely than girls, because girls have another X chromosome, which usually does not have the mutation and can partially compensate for the nonfunctioning one. Boys have only one X chromosome (and one Y chromosome).

- The damaged gene can be passed along silently for generations before a child is affected by fragile X syndrome.

## What are the features of fragile X syndrome?

*Physical Characteristics*

- Prominent ears, large head, prominent forehead, flexible finger joints, high palate, flat feet
- During puberty boys usually develop large testicles (macroorchidism) and a long face.

*Behaviors*

- Intellectual disability, from mild learning disabilities to severe mental retardation and autism
- Developmental delays, especially language
- Attention deficit hyperactivity disorder (ADHD)
- Autistic behaviors, such as hand flapping, hand biting, and chewing on clothes
- Very sensitive to stimuli
- Great sense of humor
- Anxiety
- Excellent memory
- Frequent tantrums

## Who should be tested for fragile X syndrome?

Two types of tests are available to diagnose fragile X syndrome and to test for female carriers. The chromosome test is one. The other is DNA testing, which is more accurate and less expensive. Testing is recommended for:

- Any person with developmental delay, autism, or mental retardation who has any of the physical features or behaviors that are typical in fragile X, a family history of Fragile X, or any relatives with undiagnosed mental retardation;
- Women who have a family history of fragile X or of undiagnosed mental retardation and who are seeking reproductive counseling.

Prenatal testing is possible for fetuses (babies). Pregnant mothers who are known carriers should have their fetuses tested.

## What is the treatment for fragile X syndrome?

There is no cure for fragile X syndrome, but there are many treatments to help your child:

- Early intervention in the preschool years can help your child make better progress.

- To reach full potential, a child may need speech and language therapy, occupational therapy, and physical therapy to help with the many physical, behavioral, and cognitive impacts of fragile X.

- Special education programs should fit your child's individual needs to modify classes and assignments. Children should be integrated into regular education whenever possible.

- Having a regular routine, avoiding overstimulation, and using calming techniques can help reduce behavior problems.

- Medications can be used to help treat the aggression, seizures, hyperactivity, and short attention span that often come along with fragile X syndrome.

- Treatment should be tailored to meet each child's specific needs.

## What do I need to know about the health of my child with fragile X?

Usually children with fragile X do not have a lot of medical problems.

Health problems these kids may have include frequent ear infections, seizures, strabismus, and mitral valve prolapse.

## Fragile X and Autism

Many parents are confused about their child's diagnosis. On the one hand, they've been told that their child has autism, "autistic spectrum disorder," or some degree of autistic-like characteristics. In addition, they may have also been told that their child has fragile X syndrome or that he or she is going to be tested for fragile X.

The association between autism and fragile X was first reported by Brown et al. (1982) and was subsequently confirmed by many others, leading to an extensive field of research. In discussing this association it is important to remember that autism is defined behaviorally using the criteria of the *Diagnostic and Statistical Manual of Mental Disorders, Fourth Edition (DSM IV)*, which include lack of social reciprocity or responsiveness, abnormal use of language and communication, and a restricted repertoire of activities and interests. Autism is a heterogeneous disorder which means that there are several known causes of autism including phenylketonuria (PKU), tuberous sclerosis, and 15q duplications. However fragile X is the most common known cause of autism so far identified. Autism is strongly genetic and it is likely that the inheritance of multiple genes predisposing an individual to autism is necessary in many cases for the full behavioral syndrome to be manifested.

The typical features of fragile X syndrome (FXS)—i.e. hand biting, hand flapping, poor eye contact, shyness, and social anxiety—are probably related to the sensory hyperarousal that has been documented by many investigators including Belser and Sudhalter (1995), Miller et al. (1999), and Roberts et al.(2002). These features are often also referred to as autistic-like features because they can be seen in individuals who have autism without fragile X. Most children with fragile X, however, are interested in social interactions and do not meet the diagnostic criteria for autism.

However, a subgroup of children with fragile X do meet diagnostic criteria for autism. Over the last decade many studies have evaluated this issue and the percentage of children with FXS who have autism has varied from 15 to 33 percent, mainly because the diagnostic criteria for autism has varied and the diagnostic tools used have changed.

Recent work by Don Bailey and colleagues has found that in young boys with FXS, 25 percent met the criteria for autism using the Childhood Autism Rating Scale (CARS) and that their profile of behaviors was very similar to that of children with autism and without fragile X. They also found that children with autism and FXS together had a lower IQ than children with either FXS alone or autism alone (Bailey, Hatton et al. 2001). Furthermore, the level of the fragile X protein (FMRP) did not correlate with the presence or absence of autism (Bailey, Hatton et al. 2000). This suggests that autism with fragile X may relate to additional genetic or environmental factors that could be additive to the FMR1 mutation.

Our studies also agree with this hypothesis. We recently reported a comparison study of preschoolers with FXS, and age matched children (controls) with autism but without fragile X and another set of children (controls) who had developmental disabilities but without autism or FXS. (Rogers, Wehner et al. 2001) We evaluated all of these children with what are the agreed gold standard diagnostic tools for autism including the Autism Diagnostic Observation Schedule-Generic (ADOS-G) and the Autism Diagnostic Interview-Revised (ADI-R) and also utilized the *DSM IV* criteria, IQ, and adaptive behavior measures.

We found that 15 to 33 percent of the children with FXS met the full criteria for autism. Their profile of autistic features was indistinguishable from the children with autism without FXS. Children with FXS who were not autistic had a behavioral profile that was similar to the controls with developmental disabilities. In addition, the group with both FXS and autism were the lowest of all the groups on developmental testing, results similar to the studies of Bailey and colleagues.

The reason why some children with FXS have autism too may relate to additional background gene effects (other genes inherited from their mother and father) and further studies are underway. There also are effects of the fragile X protein deficit that predispose children to autism, including the hyperarousal to stimuli and the shyness and social anxiety. When these problems are severe in FXS, then autism is more likely to occur.

A recent report by Roberts et al. 2002 demonstrated more autonomic dysfunction (problems with the sympathetic or parasympathetic nervous system such as increased heart rate when scared or stressed) and hyperarousal in children with both FXS and autism compared to FXS alone. Also of note is a recent neuroimaging study in females, which demonstrated that the size of the posterior cerebellar vermis (an area of the brain involved in motor function, cognition, and sensory perception) on magnetic resonance imaging (MRI) correlated inversely with the number of autistic features. In addition, the number of autistic features also correlated with the severity of anxiety (Mazzocco, Kates et al. 1997).

More research is needed regarding treatment of children with both FXS and autism. Preliminary studies in autism suggest that early treatment with a selective serotonin reuptake inhibitor (medications like Prozac, Paxil, Luvox, and others) is beneficial for both language and socialization skills (DeLong, Teague et al. 1998) and this possibility needs to be studied in children with FXS and autism. Intensive behavioral interventions are helpful in young children with autism and this too needs to be evaluated in young children with FXS and autism together (Scharfenaker, O'Connor et al. 2002).

Finally, it is important to identify the children with FXS among those who have been diagnosed with autism alone to provide genetic counseling and access to treatments and interventions known to be beneficial for individuals with FXS. Previous screening studies have shown that 2.5 to 6 percent of boys with autism have FXS (Brown, Jenkins et al. 1986; Bailey, Phillips et al. 1996; Hagerman 2002). Therefore, all children with autism or mental retardation should have fragile X DNA testing. Such screening may also identify individuals with the fragile X premutation in association with autism and we are currently evaluating the additive effect of the premutation, which can be associated with mild gene dysfunction (Tassone, Hagerman et al. 2000).

In summary, the association of fragile X syndrome and autism is a strong association that requires assessment in each child and will guide future treatment endeavors.

## References

Bailey, A., W. Phillips, et al. (1996). "Autism: towards an integration of clinical, genetic, neuropsychological, and neurobiological perspectives." *J Child Psychol Psychiatry* 37: 89–126.

Bailey, D. B., Jr., D. D. Hatton, et al. (2000). "Early development, temperament and functional impairment in autism and fragile X syndrome." *J of Autism and Dev Disorders* 30(1): 49–59.

Bailey, D. B., Jr., D. D. Hatton, et al. (2001). "Autistic behavior, FMR1 protein, and developmental trajectories in young males with fragile X syndrome." *Journal of Autism and Developmental Disorders* 31(2): 165–74.

Belser, R. C. and V. Sudhalter (1995). "Arousal difficulties in males with Fragile X Syndrome: A preliminary report." *Developmental Brain Dysfunction* 8: 270–79.

Brown, W. T., E. C. Jenkins, et al. (1986). "Fragile X and autism: a multicenter survey." *American Journal of Medical Genetics* 23(1–2): 341–52.

Brown, W. T., E. C. Jenkins, et al. (1982). "Autism is associated with the fragile-X syndrome." *Journal of Autism & Developmental Disorders* 12(3): 303–8.

DeLong, G. R., L. A. Teague, et al. (1998). "Effects of fluoxetine treatment in young children with idiopathic autism [see comments]." *Developmental Medicine & Child Neurology* 40(8): 551–62.

Hagerman, R. J. (2002). Physical and Behavioral Phenotype. Fragile X Syndrome: Diagnosis, Treatment and Research, 3rd edition. R. J.

Hagerman and P. J. Hagerman. Baltimore: The Johns Hopkins University Press.

Mazzocco, M. M., W. R. Kates, et al. (1997). "Autistic behaviors among girls with fragile X syndrome." *Journal of Autism & Developmental Disorders* 27(4): 415–35.

Miller, L. J., D. N. McIntosh, et al. (1999). "Electrodermal Responses to Sensory Stimuli in Individuals with Fragile X Syndrome: A Preliminary Report." *American Journal of Medical Genetics* 83: 268–79.

Roberts, J., M. L. Boccia, et al. (2001). "Cardiovascular Indices of Physiological Arousal in Boys with Fragile X Syndrome." Developmental Psychobiology 39(2): 107–23.

Rogers, S. J., E. A. Wehner, et al. (2001). "The Behavioral Phenotype in Fragile X: Symptoms of Autism in Very Young Children with Fragile X Syndrome, Idiopathic Autism, and other Developmental Disorders." *Journal of Developmental & Behavioral Pediatrics* 22(6): 409–17.

Scharfenaker, S., R. O'Connor, et al. (2002). An integrated approach to intervention. Fragile X Syndrome: Diagnosis, Treatment and Research, 3rd edition. R. J. Hagerman and P. J. Hagerman. Baltimore: The Johns Hopkins University Press.

Tassone, F., R. J. Hagerman, et al. (2000). "Transcription of the FMR1 gene in individuals with fragile X syndrome." *American Journal of Medical Genetics (Semin. Med. Genet.)* 97(3): 195–203.

# Section 12.3

# *Angelman Syndrome*

"Angelman Syndrome: The Basics" is reprinted from "Angelman Syndrome Information Page," National Institute of Neurological Disorders and Stroke, National Institutes of Health, February 8, 2007. "Angelman Syndrome and Autism" is reprinted from "Angelman Syndrome," by Stephen M. Edelson, Ph.D., © 1995 Center for the Study of Autism, Salem, OR. Reprinted with permission. Reviewed by David A. Cooke, M.D., March 2007.

## *Angelman Syndrome: The Basics*

### *What is Angelman syndrome?*

Angelman syndrome is a genetic disorder that causes developmental delay and neurological problems. The physician Harry Angelman first delineated the syndrome in 1965, when he described several children in his practice as having "flat heads, jerky movements, protruding tongues, and bouts of laughter." Infants with Angelman syndrome appear normal at birth, but often have feeding problems in the first months of life and exhibit noticeable developmental delays by six to twelve months. Seizures often begin between two and three years of age. Speech impairment is pronounced, with little to no use of words. Individuals with this syndrome often display hyperactivity, small head size, sleep disorders, and movement and balance disorders that can cause severe functional deficits. Angelman syndrome results from absence of a functional copy of the *UBE3A* gene inherited from the mother.

### *Is there any treatment?*

There is no specific therapy for Angelman syndrome. Medical therapy for seizures is usually necessary. Physical and occupational therapies, communication therapy, and behavioral therapies are important in allowing individuals with Angelman syndrome to reach their maximum developmental potential.

## What is the prognosis?

Most individuals with Angelman syndrome will have severe developmental delays, speech limitations, and motor difficulties. However, individuals with Angelman syndrome can have normal life spans and generally do not show developmental regression as they age. Early diagnosis and tailored interventions and therapies help improve quality of life.

## What research is being done?

The National Institute of Neurological Disorders and Stroke (NINDS) supports and conducts research on neurogenetic disorders such as Angelman syndrome, to develop techniques to diagnose, treat, prevent, and ultimately cure them.

## Angelman Syndrome and Autism

Angelman syndrome is not considered a subtype of autism, but individuals suffering from this disorder exhibit many behaviors characteristic of autism. They are also sometimes given a secondary diagnosis of autism. In 1965, Harry Angelman, M.D., an English physician, was the first to describe a group of individuals with similar behavioral and physical similarities, which was later termed "Angelman syndrome."

For many of these individuals, a small portion of chromosome 15 is missing; and this appears to be from the maternal side. Interestingly, when a small portion of chromosome 15 is missing and is from the paternal side, the child may suffer from Prader-Willi syndrome.

Similar to autism, individuals with Angelman syndrome display the following behaviors: hand-flapping, little or no speech, attention deficits, hyperactivity, feeding and sleeping problems, and delays in motor development. These individuals may also engage in biting and hair pulling.

In contrast to autism, people with Angelman syndrome are often described as very sociable. They are very affectionate and engage in frequent laughing. The majority of these individuals have abnormal electroencephalograms and epilepsy. Many tend to have a stiff-legged gait and jerky body movements. These individuals also have common facial features, such as a wide smiling mouth, a thin upper lip, and deep-set eyes. More than half have low levels of pigmentation in their eyes, hair, and skin.

The prevalence rate of Angelman syndrome is estimated to be one in twenty-five thousand individuals, and the majority of these individuals are described as severely mentally retarded.

Suggested interventions for Angelman syndrome include behavior modification, speech therapy, and occupational therapy.

## Section 12.4

# Landau-Kleffner Syndrome

"Landau-Kleffner Syndrome: The Basics" is reprinted from "Landau-Kleffner Syndrome Information Page," National Institute of Neurological Disorders and Stroke, National Institutes of Health, February 13, 2007. "Landau-Kleffner Syndrome and Autism" is reprinted from "Landau-Kleffner Syndrome," by Stephen M. Edelson, Ph.D., © 1995 Center for the Study of Autism, Salem, OR. Reprinted with permission. Reviewed by David A. Cooke, M.D., March 2007.

## Landau-Kleffner Syndrome: The Basics

### What is Landau-Kleffner syndrome?

Landau-Kleffner syndrome (LKS) is a rare childhood neurological disorder characterized by the sudden or gradual development of aphasia (the inability to understand or express language) and an abnormal electroencephalogram (EEG). LKS affects the parts of the brain that control comprehension and speech. The disorder usually occurs in children between the ages of five and seven years. Typically, children with LKS develop normally but then lose their language skills for no apparent reason. While many of the affected individuals have seizures, some do not. The disorder is difficult to diagnose and may be misdiagnosed as autism, pervasive developmental disorder, hearing impairment, learning disability, auditory/verbal processing disorder, attention deficit disorder, mental retardation, childhood schizophrenia, or emotional/behavioral problems.

### Is there any treatment?

Treatment for LKS usually consists of medications, such as anticonvulsants and corticosteroids, and speech therapy, which should be started early. A controversial treatment option involves a surgical

155

technique called multiple subpial transection in which the pathways of abnormal electrical brain activity are severed

### *What is the prognosis?*

The prognosis for children with LKS varies. Some affected children may have a permanent severe language disorder, while others may regain much of their language abilities (although it may take months or years). In some cases, remission and relapse may occur. Seizures generally disappear by adulthood.

## *Landau-Kleffner Syndrome and Autism*

Landau-Kleffner syndrome is manifested as a form of aphasia, (loss of language), which usually develops between three and seven years of age. It is twice as common in males than females. Initially, these individuals have a healthy, problem-free development with normal speech and vocabulary. These individuals first lose their ability to comprehend (i.e., receptive speech) and then their ability to speak (i.e., expressive speech). These changes can occur gradually or suddenly.

People with Landau-Kleffner syndrome have abnormal EEG patterns (i.e., brain waves) in the temporal lobe (located on the sides of the brain) and in the temporo-parieto-occipital regions during sleep. Diagnosis of this syndrome usually involves examining the person's EEG patterns during sleep. Approximately 70 percent develop epilepsy; and these seizures are typically infrequent and can be either with or without convulsions.

One common characteristic of Landau-Kleffner syndrome, which is often diagnosed in conjunction with autism, is the failure to respond to sounds. Thus, parents may suspect their child of hearing loss. Autistic characteristics seen in Landau-Kleffner syndrome individuals include pain insensitivity, aggression, poor eye contact, insistence on sameness, and sleep problems.

The cause of Landau-Kleffner syndrome is not known. Some suggested causes have been a dysfunctional immune system, exposure to a virus, and brain trauma. The prognosis is better when the onset is after age six and when speech therapy is started early. Several other treatments have also been shown to be beneficial for many of these individuals, such as anticonvulsant mediations and corticosteroids. There is also a surgical technique in which the pathways of abnormal electrical brain activity are severed.

# Section 12.5

# *Prader-Willi Syndrome*

### *What is Prader-Willi syndrome (PWS)?*

PWS is a complex genetic disorder that typically causes low muscle
tone, short stature, incomplete sexual development, cognitive disabilities, problem behaviors, and a chronic feeling of hunger that can lead
to excessive eating and life-threatening obesity.

### *Is PWS inherited?*

Most cases of PWS are attributed to a spontaneous genetic error
that occurs at or near the time of conception for unknown reasons. In
a very small percentage of cases (2 percent or less), a genetic mutation that does not affect the parent is passed on to the child, and in
these families more than one child may be affected. A PWS-like disorder can also be acquired after birth if the hypothalamus portion of
the brain is damaged through injury or surgery.

### *How common is PWS?*

It is estimated that one in twelve thousand to fifteen thousand
people has PWS. Although considered a "rare" disorder, Prader-Willi
syndrome is one of the most common conditions seen in genetics clinics and is the most common genetic cause of obesity that has been
identified. PWS is found in people of both sexes and all races.

### *How is PWS diagnosed?*

Suspicion of the diagnosis is first assessed clinically, then confirmed
by specialized genetic testing on a blood sample. Formal diagnostic

criteria for the clinical recognition of PWS have been published, as have laboratory testing guidelines for PWS.

### What is known about the genetic abnormality?

Basically, the occurrence of PWS is due to lack of several genes on one of an individual's two chromosome 15s—the one normally contributed by the father. In the majority of cases, there is a deletion—the critical genes are somehow lost from the chromosome. In most of the remaining cases, the entire chromosome from the father is missing and there are instead two chromosome 15s from the mother (uniparental disomy). The critical paternal genes lacking in people with PWS have a role in the regulation of appetite. This is an area of active research in a number of laboratories around the world, since understanding this defect may be very helpful not only to those with PWS but to understanding obesity in otherwise normal people.

### What causes the appetite and obesity problems in PWS?

People with PWS have a flaw in the hypothalamus part of their brain, which normally registers feelings of hunger and satiety. While the problem is not yet fully understood, it is apparent that people with this flaw never feel full; they have a continuous urge to eat that they cannot learn to control. To compound this problem, people with PWS need less food than their peers without the syndrome because their bodies have less muscle and tend to burn fewer calories.

### Does the overeating associated with PWS begin at birth?

No. In fact, newborns with PWS often cannot get enough nourishment because low muscle tone impairs their sucking ability. Many require special feeding techniques or tube feeding for several months after birth, until muscle control improves. Sometime in the following years, usually before school age, children with PWS develop an intense interest in food and can quickly gain excess weight if calories are not restricted.

### Do diet medications work for the appetite problem in PWS?

Unfortunately, no appetite suppressant has worked consistently for people with PWS. Most require an extremely low-calorie diet all their lives and must have their environment designed so that they have very limited access to food. For example, many families have to lock the kitchen or the cabinets and refrigerator. As adults, most affected individuals can control their weight best in a group home designed specifically for people with PWS, where food access can be restricted without interfering with the rights of those who don't need such restriction.

### What kinds of behavior problems do people with PWS have?

In addition to their involuntary focus on food, people with PWS tend to have obsessive-compulsive behaviors that are not related to food, such as repetitive thoughts and verbalizations, collecting and hoarding of possessions, picking at skin irritations, and a strong need for routine and predictability. Frustration or changes in plans can easily set off a loss of emotional control in someone with PWS, ranging from tears to temper tantrums to physical aggression. While psychotropic medications can help some individuals, the essential strategies for minimizing difficult behaviors in PWS are careful structuring of the person's environment and consistent use of positive behavior management and supports.

### Does early diagnosis help?

While there is no medical prevention or cure, early diagnosis of Prader-Willi syndrome gives parents time to learn about and prepare for the challenges that lie ahead and to establish family routines that will support their child's diet and behavior needs from the start. Knowing the cause of their child's developmental delays can facilitate a family's access to important early intervention services and may help program staff identify areas of specific need or risk. Additionally, a diagnosis of PWS opens the doors to a network of information and support from professionals and other families who are dealing with the syndrome.

### What does the future hold for people with PWS?

With help, people with PWS can expect to accomplish many of the things their "normal" peers do—complete school, achieve in their outside areas of interest, be successfully employed, even move away from their family home. They do, however, need a significant amount of support from their families and from school, work, and residential service providers to both achieve these goals and avoid obesity and the serious health consequences that accompany it. Even those with IQs in the normal range need lifelong diet supervision and protection from food availability.

Although in the past many people with PWS died in adolescence or young adulthood, prevention of obesity can enable those with the syndrome to live a normal lifespan. New medications, including psychotropic drugs and synthetic growth hormone, are already improving the quality of life for some people with PWS. Ongoing research offers the hope of new discoveries that will enable people affected by this unusual condition to live more independent lives.

# Section 12.6

# *Williams Syndrome*

"What Is Williams Syndrome?" is reprinted from "What Is Williams Syndrome?" © 2002 Williams Syndrome Association. Reprinted with permission. "Williams Syndrome and Autism" is reprinted from "Williams Syndrome," by Stephen M. Edelson, Ph.D., © 1995 Center for the Study of Autism, Salem, OR. Reprinted with permission. Reviewed by David A. Cooke, M.D., March 2007.

## What Is Williams Syndrome?

Williams syndrome is a rare genetic condition (estimated to occur in 1 in 7,500 births) that causes medical and developmental problems.

Williams syndrome was first recognized as a distinct entity in 1961. It is present at birth, and affects males and females equally. It can occur in all ethnic groups and has been identified in countries throughout the world.

### *What are the common features of Williams syndrome?*

**Characteristic facial appearance:** Most young children with Williams syndrome are described as having similar facial features. These features, which tend to be recognized by only a trained geneticist or birth defects specialist, include a small upturned nose, long philtrum (upper lip length), wide mouth, full lips, small chin, and puffiness around the eyes. Blue- and green-eyed children with Williams syndrome can have a prominent "starburst" or white lacy pattern on their iris. Facial features become more apparent with age.

**Heart and blood vessel problems:** The majority of individuals with Williams syndrome have some type of heart or blood vessel problem. Typically, there is narrowing in the aorta (producing supravalvular aortic stenosis [SVAS]), or narrowing in the pulmonary arteries. There is a broad range in the degree of narrowing, ranging from trivial to severe (requiring surgical correction of the defect). Since there is an increased risk for development of blood vessel narrowing or high blood pressure over time, periodic monitoring of cardiac status is necessary.

**Hypercalcemia (elevated blood calcium levels):** Some young children with Williams syndrome have elevations in their blood calcium level. The true frequency and cause of this problem is unknown. When hypercalcemia is present, it can cause extreme irritability or "colic-like" symptoms. Occasionally, dietary or medical treatment is needed. In most cases, the problem resolves on its own during childhood, but lifelong abnormality in calcium or Vitamin D metabolism may exist and should be monitored.

**Low birth weight/low weight gain:** Most children with Williams syndrome have a slightly lower birth weight than their brothers or sisters. Slow weight gain, especially during the first several years of life, is also a common problem and many children are diagnosed with "failure to thrive." Adult stature is slightly smaller than average.

**Feeding problems:** Many infants and young children have feeding problems. These problems have been linked to low muscle tone, severe gag reflex, poor suck/swallow, tactile defensiveness, and the like. Feeding difficulties tend to resolve as the children get older.

**Irritability (colic during infancy):** Many infants with Williams syndrome have an extended period of colic or irritability. This typically lasts from four to ten months of age, then resolves. It is sometimes attributed to hypercalcemia. Abnormal sleep patterns with delayed acquisition of sleeping through the night may be associated with the colic.

**Dental abnormalities:** Slightly small, widely spaced teeth are common in children with Williams syndrome. They also may have a variety of abnormalities of occlusion (bite), tooth shape, or appearance. Most of these dental changes are readily amenable to orthodontic correction.

**Kidney abnormalities:** There is a slightly increased frequency of problems with kidney structure and/or function.

**Hernias:** Inguinal (groin) and umbilical hernias are more common in Williams syndrome than in the general population.

**Hyperacusis (sensitive hearing):** Children with Williams syndrome often have more sensitive hearing than other children; certain frequencies or noise levels can be painful or startling to the individual. This condition often improves with age.

**Musculoskeletal problems:** Young children with Williams syndrome often have low muscle tone and joint laxity. As the children get older, joint stiffness (contractures) may develop. Physical therapy is very helpful in improving muscle tone, strength, and joint range of motion.

**Overly friendly (excessively social) personality:** Individuals with Williams syndrome have a very endearing personality. They have a unique strength in their expressive language skills, and are extremely polite. They are typically unafraid of strangers and show a greater interest in contact with adults than with their peers.

**Developmental delay, learning disabilities, and attention deficit:** Most people with Williams syndrome have some degree of intellectual handicap. Young children with Williams syndrome often experience developmental delays; milestones such as walking, talking, and toilet training are often achieved somewhat later than is considered normal. Distractibility is a common problem in mid-childhood, which appears to get better as the children get older.

Older children and adults with Williams syndrome often demonstrate intellectual "strengths and weaknesses." There are some intellectual areas (such as speech, long-term memory, and social skills) in which performance is quite strong, while other intellectual areas (such as fine motor and spatial relations) are significantly deficient.

## Williams Syndrome and Autism

Williams syndrome is a genetic disorder characterized by mild mental retardation. It is a rare disorder in which a portion of DNA material on chromosome 7 is missing. The prevalence in the population is somewhere between one out of twenty thousand and one out of fifty thousand births.

Many people with Williams syndrome exhibit autistic behaviors. This includes: developmental and language delays, problems in gross motor skills, hypersensitivity to sounds, being picky eaters, and perseverating.

These individuals differ from the typical autistic individual because they also have cardiovascular abnormalities, high blood pressure, and elevated calcium levels, and are very sociable. They also have unique pixie-like facial features—almond-shaped eyes, oval ears, full lips, small chins, narrow faces, and broad mouths.

## Section 12.7

# *Tourette Syndrome*

Reprinted from "Tourette Syndrome Fact Sheet," National Institute of Neurological Disorders and Stroke, National Institutes of Health, NIH Publication No. 05-2163, February 14, 2007.

### What is Tourette syndrome?

Tourette syndrome (TS) is a neurological disorder characterized by repetitive, stereotyped, involuntary movements and vocalizations called tics. The disorder is named for Dr. Georges Gilles de la Tourette, the pioneering French neurologist who in 1885 first described the condition in an eighty-six-year-old French noblewoman.

The early symptoms of TS are almost always noticed first in childhood, with the average onset between the ages of seven and ten years. TS occurs in people from all ethnic groups; males are affected about three to four times more often than females. It is estimated that two hundred thousand Americans have the most severe form of TS, and as many as one in one hundred exhibit milder and less complex symptoms such as chronic motor or vocal tics or transient tics of childhood. Although TS can be a chronic condition with symptoms lasting a lifetime, most people with the condition experience their worst symptoms in their early teens, with improvement occurring in the late teens and continuing into adulthood.

### What are the symptoms?

Tics are classified as either simple or complex. Simple motor tics are sudden, brief, repetitive movements that involve a limited number of muscle groups. Some of the more common simple tics include eye blinking and other vision irregularities, facial grimacing, shoulder shrugging, and head or shoulder jerking. Simple vocalizations might include repetitive throat clearing, sniffing, or grunting sounds. Complex tics are distinct, coordinated patterns of movements involving several muscle groups. Complex motor tics might include facial grimacing combined with a head twist and a shoulder shrug. Other complex motor tics may actually appear purposeful, including sniffing or touching objects, hopping, jumping, bending, or twisting. Simple vocal tics may include throat clearing, sniffing or snorting, grunting, or barking. More complex vocal tics include words or phrases. Perhaps the most dramatic and disabling tics include motor movements that result in self-harm such as punching oneself in the face or vocal tics including coprolalia (uttering swear words) or echolalia (repeating the words or phrases of others). Some tics are preceded by an urge or sensation in the affected muscle group, commonly called a premonitory urge. Some with TS will describe a need to complete a tic in a certain way or a certain number of times in order to relieve the urge or decrease the sensation.

Tics are often worse with excitement or anxiety and better during calm, focused activities. Certain physical experiences can trigger or worsen tics. For example, tight collars may trigger neck tics, or hearing another person sniff or throat-clear may trigger similar sounds. Tics do not go away during sleep but are often significantly diminished.

### What is the course of TS?

Tics come and go over time, varying in type, frequency, location, and severity. The first symptoms usually occur in the head and neck area and may progress to include muscles of the trunk and extremities.

Motor tics generally precede the development of vocal tics and simple tics often precede complex tics. Most patients experience peak tic severity before the mid-teen years with improvement for the majority of patients in the late teen years and early adulthood. Approximately 10 percent of those affected have a progressive or disabling course that lasts into adulthood.

### Can people with TS control their tics?

Although the symptoms of TS are involuntary, some people can sometimes suppress, camouflage, or otherwise manage their tics in an effort to minimize their impact on functioning. However, people with TS often report a substantial buildup in tension when suppressing their tics to the point where they feel that the tic must be expressed. Tics in response to an environmental trigger can appear to be voluntary or purposeful but are not.

### What causes TS?

Although the cause of TS is unknown, current research points to abnormalities in certain brain regions (including the basal ganglia, frontal lobes, and cortex), the circuits that interconnect these regions, and the neurotransmitters (dopamine, serotonin, and norepinephrine) responsible for communication among nerve cells. Given the often-complex presentation of TS, the cause of the disorder is likely to be equally complex.

### What disorders are associated with TS?

Many with TS experience additional neurobehavioral problems including inattention; hyperactivity and impulsivity (attention deficit hyperactivity disorder, or ADHD) and related problems with reading, writing, and arithmetic; and obsessive-compulsive symptoms such as intrusive thoughts and worries and repetitive behaviors. For example, worries about dirt and germs may be associated with repetitive hand washing, and concerns about bad things happening may be associated with ritualistic behaviors such as counting, repeating, or ordering and arranging. People with TS have also reported problems with depression or anxiety disorders, as well as other difficulties with living, that may or may not be directly related to TS. Given the range of potential complications, people with TS are best served by receiving medical care that provides a comprehensive treatment plan.

## How is TS diagnosed?

TS is a diagnosis that doctors make after verifying that the patient has had both motor and vocal tics for at least one year. The existence of other neurological or psychiatric conditions[1] can also help doctors arrive at a diagnosis. Common tics are not often misdiagnosed by knowledgeable clinicians. But atypical symptoms or atypical presentation (for example, onset of symptoms in adulthood) may require specific specialty expertise for diagnosis. There are no blood or laboratory tests needed for diagnosis, but neuroimaging studies, such as magnetic resonance imaging (MRI), computerized tomography (CT), and electroencephalogram (EEG) scans, or certain blood tests may be used to rule out other conditions that might be confused with TS.

It is not uncommon for patients to obtain a formal diagnosis of TS only after symptoms have been present for some time. The reasons for this are many. For families and physicians unfamiliar with TS, mild and even moderate tic symptoms may be considered inconsequential, part of a developmental phase, or the result of another condition. For example, parents may think that eye blinking is related to vision problems or that sniffing is related to seasonal allergies. Many patients are self-diagnosed after they, their parents, other relatives, or friends read or hear about TS from others.

## How is TS treated?

Because tic symptoms do not often cause impairment, the majority of people with TS require no medication for tic suppression. However, effective medications are available for those whose symptoms interfere with functioning. Neuroleptics are the most consistently useful medications for tic suppression; a number are available but some are more effective than others (for example, haloperidol and pimozide). Unfortunately, there is no one medication that is helpful to all people with TS, nor does any medication completely eliminate symptoms. In addition, all medications have side effects. Most neuroleptic side effects can be managed by initiating treatment slowly and reducing the dose when side effects occur. The most common side effects of neuroleptics include sedation, weight gain, and cognitive dulling. Neurological side effects such as tremor, dystonic reactions (twisting movements or postures), parkinsonian-like symptoms, and other dyskinetic (involuntary) movements are less common and are readily managed with dose reduction. Discontinuing neuroleptics after long-term use must be done slowly to avoid rebound increases in tics and withdrawal dyskinesias. One form of withdrawal dyskinesia called tardive dyskinesia is a movement disorder distinct from TS that may result from the chronic use of neuroleptics. The risk of this side effect can be reduced by using lower doses of neuroleptics for shorter periods of time.

Other medications may also be useful for reducing tic severity, but most have not been as extensively studied or shown to be as consistently useful as neuroleptics. Additional medications with demonstrated efficacy include alpha-adrenergic agonists such as clonidine and guanfacine. These medications are used primarily for hypertension but are also used in the treatment of tics. The most common side effect from these medications that precludes their use is sedation.

Effective medications are also available to treat some of the associated neurobehavioral disorders that can occur in patients with TS. Recent research shows that stimulant medications such as methylphenidate and dextroamphetamine can lessen ADHD symptoms in people with TS without causing tics to become more severe. However, the product labeling for stimulants currently contraindicates the use of these drugs in children with tics or TS and those with a family history of tics. Scientists hope that future studies will include a thorough discussion of the risks and benefits of stimulants in those with TS or a family history of TS and will clarify this issue. For obsessive-compulsive symptoms that significantly disrupt daily functioning, the serotonin reuptake inhibitors (clomipramine, fluoxetine, fluvoxamine, paroxetine, and sertraline) have been proven effective in some patients.

Psychotherapy may also be helpful. Although psychological problems do not cause TS, such problems may result from TS. Psychotherapy can help the person with TS better cope with the disorder and deal with the secondary social and emotional problems that sometimes occur. More recently, specific behavioral treatments that include awareness training and competing response training, such as voluntarily moving in response to a premonitory urge, have shown effectiveness in small controlled trials. Larger and more definitive NIH-funded studies are underway.

## Is TS inherited?

Evidence from twin and family studies suggests that TS is an inherited disorder. Although early family studies suggested an autosomal dominant mode of inheritance (an autosomal dominant disorder is one in which only one copy of the defective gene, inherited from one parent, is necessary to produce the disorder), more recent studies suggest that the pattern of inheritance is much more complex. Although there may be a few genes with substantial effects, it is also possible that many genes with smaller effects and environmental factors may play a role in the development of TS. Genetic studies also suggest that some forms of ADHD and OCD are genetically related to TS, but there is less evidence for a genetic relationship between TS and other neurobehavioral problems that commonly co-occur with TS. It is important for families to understand that genetic predisposition may not necessarily result in full-blown TS; instead, it may express itself as a milder tic disorder or as obsessive-compulsive behaviors. It is also possible that the gene-carrying offspring will not develop any TS symptoms.

The sex of the person also plays an important role in TS gene expression. At-risk males are more likely to have tics and at-risk females are more likely to have obsessive-compulsive symptoms.

People with TS may have genetic risks for other neurobehavioral disorders such as depression or substance abuse. Genetic counseling of individuals with TS should include a full review of all potentially hereditary conditions in the family.

### What is the prognosis?

Although there is no cure for TS, the condition in many individuals improves in the late teens and early twenties. As a result, some may actually become symptom-free or no longer need medication for tic suppression. Although the disorder is generally lifelong and chronic, it is not a degenerative condition. Individuals with TS have a normal life expectancy. TS does not impair intelligence. Although tic symptoms tend to decrease with age, it is possible that neurobehavioral disorders such as depression, panic attacks, mood swings, and antisocial behaviors can persist and cause impairment in adult life.

### What is the best educational setting for children with TS?

Although students with TS often function well in the regular classroom, ADHD, learning disabilities, obsessive-compulsive symptoms, and frequent tics can greatly interfere with academic performance or social adjustment. After a comprehensive assessment, students should be placed in an educational setting that meets their individual needs. Students may require tutoring, smaller or special classes, and in some cases special schools.

All students with TS need a tolerant and compassionate setting that both encourages them to work to their full potential and is flexible enough to accommodate their special needs. This setting may include a private study area, exams outside the regular classroom, or even oral exams when the child's symptoms interfere with his or her ability to write. Untimed testing reduces stress for students with TS.

## *What research is being done?*

Within the federal government, the leading supporter of research on TS and other neurological disorders is the National Institute of Neurological Disorders and Stroke (NINDS). The NINDS, a part of the National Institutes of Health (NIH), is responsible for supporting and conducting research on the brain and central nervous system.

NINDS sponsors research on TS both in its laboratories at the NIH and through grants to major medical institutions across the country. The National Institute of Mental Health, the National Center for Research Resources, the National Institute of Child Health and Human Development, the National Institute on Drug Abuse, and the National Institute on Deafness and Other Communication Disorders also support research of relevance to TS. Another component of the Department of Health and Human Services, the Centers for Disease Control and Prevention, funds professional education programs as well as TS research.

Knowledge about TS comes from studies across a number of medical and scientific disciplines, including genetics, neuroimaging, neuropathology, clinical trials (medication and nonmedication), epidemiology, neurophysiology, neuroimmunology, and descriptive/diagnostic clinical science.

**Genetic studies:** Currently, NIH-funded investigators are conducting a variety of large-scale genetic studies. Rapid advances in the technology of gene finding will allow for genome-wide screening approaches in TS, and finding a gene or genes for TS would be a major step toward understanding genetic risk factors. In addition, understanding the genetics of TS genes will strengthen clinical diagnosis, improve genetic counseling, lead to the clarification of pathophysiology, and provide clues for more effective therapies.

**Neuroimaging studies:** Within the past five years, advances in imaging technology and an increase in trained investigators have led to an increasing use of novel and powerful techniques to identify brain regions, circuitry, and neurochemical factors important in TS and related conditions.

**Neuropathology:** Within the past five years, there has been an increase in the number and quality of donated postmortem brains from TS patients available for research purposes. This increase, coupled with advances in neuropathological techniques, has led to initial findings with implications for neuroimaging studies and animal models of TS.

**Clinical trials:** A number of clinical trials in TS have recently been completed or are currently underway. These include studies of stimulant treatment of ADHD in TS and behavioral treatments for reducing tic severity in children and adults. Smaller trials of novel approaches to treatment such as dopamine agonist and GABAergic medications also show promise.

**Epidemiology and clinical science:** Careful epidemiological studies now estimate the prevalence of TS to be substantially higher than previously thought, with a wider range of clinical severity. Furthermore, clinical studies are providing new findings regarding TS and coexisting conditions. These include subtyping studies of TS and obsessive-compulsive disorder (OCD), an examination of the link between ADHD and learning problems in children with TS, a new appreciation of sensory tics, and the role of coexisting disorders in rage attacks. One of the most important and controversial areas of TS science involves the relationship between TS and autoimmune brain injury associated with group A beta-hemolytic streptococcal infections or other infectious processes. There are a number of epidemiological and clinical investigations currently underway in this intriguing area.

## Notes

1.  These include childhood-onset involuntary movement disorders such as dystonia, or psychiatric disorders characterized by repetitive behaviors or movements (for example, stereotypic behaviors in autism and compulsive behaviors in obsessive-compulsive disorder, or OCD).

# Chapter 13

# *Epilepsy Often Accompanies Autism*

Epilepsy is associated with a variety of developmental and metabolic disorders, including cerebral palsy, neurofibromatosis, pyruvate dependency, tuberous sclerosis, Landau-Kleffner syndrome, and autism. Epilepsy is just one of a set of symptoms commonly found in people with these disorders.

## *What is epilepsy?*

Epilepsy is a brain disorder in which clusters of nerve cells, or neurons, in the brain sometimes signal abnormally. Neurons normally generate electrochemical impulses that act on other neurons, glands, and muscles to produce human thoughts, feelings, and actions. In epilepsy, the normal pattern of neuronal activity becomes disturbed, causing strange sensations, emotions, and behavior, or sometimes convulsions, muscle spasms, and loss of consciousness. During a seizure, neurons may fire as many as five hundred times a second, much faster than the normal rate of about eighty times a second. In some people, this happens only occasionally; for others, it may happen up to hundreds of times a day.

More than two million people in the United States—about one in one hundred—have experienced an unprovoked seizure or been diagnosed with epilepsy. For about 80 percent of those diagnosed with

Excerpted from "Seizures and Epilepsy: Hope Through Research," National Institute of Neurological Disorders and Stroke, National Institutes of Health, NIH Publication No. 04-156, October 25, 2006.

171

epilepsy, seizures can be controlled with modern medicines and surgical techniques. However, about 20 percent of people with epilepsy will continue to experience seizures even with the best available treatment. Doctors call this situation intractable epilepsy. Having a seizure does not necessarily mean that a person has epilepsy. Only when a person has had two or more seizures is he or she considered to have epilepsy.

Epilepsy is not contagious and is not caused by mental illness or mental retardation. Some people with mental retardation may experience seizures, but seizures do not necessarily mean the person has or will develop mental impairment. Many people with epilepsy have normal or above-average intelligence. Famous people who are known or rumored to have had epilepsy include the Russian writer Dostoyevsky, the philosopher Socrates, the military general Napoleon, and the inventor of dynamite, Alfred Nobel, who established the Nobel Prize. Several Olympic medalists and other athletes also have had epilepsy. Seizures sometimes do cause brain damage, particularly if they are severe. However, most seizures do not seem to have a detrimental effect on the brain. Any changes that do occur are usually subtle, and it is often unclear whether these changes are caused by the seizures themselves or by the underlying problem that caused the seizures.

While epilepsy cannot currently be cured, for some people it does eventually go away. One study found that children with idiopathic epilepsy, or epilepsy with an unknown cause, had a 68 to 92 percent chance of becoming seizure-free by twenty years after their diagnosis. The odds of becoming seizure-free are not as good for adults or for children with severe epilepsy syndromes, but it is nonetheless possible that seizures may decrease or even stop over time. This is more likely if the epilepsy has been well controlled by medication or if the person has had epilepsy surgery.

### What are the different kinds of seizures?

Doctors have described more than thirty different types of seizures. Seizures are divided into two major categories—focal seizures and generalized seizures. However, there are many different types of seizures in each of these categories.

**Focal seizures:** Focal seizures, also called partial seizures, occur in just one part of the brain. About 60 percent of people with epilepsy have focal seizures. These seizures are frequently described by the area of the brain in which they originate. For example, someone might be diagnosed with focal frontal lobe seizures.

In a simple focal seizure, the person will remain conscious but experience unusual feelings or sensations that can take many forms. The person may experience sudden and unexplainable feelings of joy, anger, sadness, or nausea. He or she also may hear, smell, taste, see, or feel things that are not real.

In a complex focal seizure, the person has a change in or loss of consciousness. His or her consciousness may be altered, producing a dreamlike experience. People having a complex focal seizure may display strange, repetitious behaviors such as blinks, twitches, mouth movements, or even walking in a circle. These repetitious movements are called automatisms. More complicated actions, which may seem purposeful, can also occur involuntarily. Patients may also continue activities they started before the seizure began, such as washing dishes in a repetitive, unproductive fashion. These seizures usually last just a few seconds.

Some people with focal seizures, especially complex focal seizures, may experience auras—unusual sensations that warn of an impending seizure. These auras are actually simple focal seizures in which the person maintains consciousness. The symptoms an individual person has, and the progression of those symptoms, tend to be stereotyped, or similar every time.

The symptoms of focal seizures can easily be confused with other disorders. For instance, the dreamlike perceptions associated with a complex focal seizure may be misdiagnosed as migraine headaches, which also may cause a dreamlike state. The strange behavior and sensations caused by focal seizures also can be mistaken for symptoms of narcolepsy, fainting, or even mental illness. It may take many tests and careful monitoring by an experienced physician to tell the difference between epilepsy and other disorders.

**Generalized seizures:** Generalized seizures are a result of abnormal neuronal activity on both sides of the brain. These seizures may cause loss of consciousness, falls, or massive muscle spasms.

There are many kinds of generalized seizures. In absence seizures, the person may appear to be staring into space and/or have jerking or twitching muscles. These seizures are sometimes referred to as petit mal seizures, which is an older term. Tonic seizures cause stiffening of muscles of the body, generally those in the back, legs, and arms. Clonic seizures cause repeated jerking movements of muscles on both sides of the body. Myoclonic seizures cause jerks or twitches of the upper body, arms, or legs. Atonic seizures cause a loss of normal muscle tone. The affected person will fall down or may drop his or her head involuntarily. Tonic-clonic seizures cause a mixture of symptoms, including stiffening of the body and repeated jerks of the arms and/or legs as well as loss of consciousness. Tonic-clonic seizures are sometimes referred to by an older term: grand mal seizures.

Not all seizures can be easily defined as either focal or generalized. Some people have seizures that begin as focal seizures but then spread to the entire brain. Other people may have both types of seizures but with no clear pattern.

Society's lack of understanding about the many different types of seizures is one of the biggest problems for people with epilepsy. People who witness a nonconvulsive seizure often find it difficult to understand that behavior which looks deliberate is not under the person's control. In some cases, this has led to the affected person being arrested or admitted to a psychiatric hospital. To combat these problems, people everywhere need to understand the many different types of seizures and how they may appear.

### What are the different kinds of epilepsy?

Just as there are many different kinds of seizures, there are many different kinds of epilepsy. Doctors have identified hundreds of different epilepsy syndromes—disorders characterized by a specific set of symptoms that include epilepsy. Some of these syndromes appear to be hereditary. For other syndromes, the cause is unknown. Epilepsy syndromes are frequently described by their symptoms or by where in the brain they originate. People should discuss the implications of their type of epilepsy with their doctors to understand the full range of symptoms, the possible treatments, and the prognosis.

People with absence epilepsy have repeated absence seizures that cause momentary lapses of consciousness. These seizures almost always begin in childhood or adolescence, and they tend to run in families, suggesting that they may be at least partially due to a defective gene or genes. Some people with absence seizures have purposeless movements during their seizures, such as a jerking arm or rapidly blinking eyes. Others have no noticeable symptoms except for brief times when they are "out of it." Immediately after a seizure, the person can resume whatever he or she was doing. However, these seizures may occur so frequently that the person cannot concentrate in school or other situations. Childhood absence epilepsy usually stops when the child reaches puberty. Absence seizures usually have no lasting effect on intelligence or other brain functions.

Temporal lobe epilepsy, or TLE, is the most common epilepsy syndrome with focal seizures. These seizures are often associated with auras. TLE often begins in childhood. Research has shown that repeated temporal lobe seizures can cause a brain structure called the hippocampus to shrink over time. The hippocampus is important for memory and learning. While it may take years of temporal lobe seizures for measurable hippocampal damage to occur, this finding underlines the need to treat TLE early and as effectively as possible.

Neocortical epilepsy is characterized by seizures that originate from the brain's cortex, or outer layer. The seizures can be either focal or generalized. They may include strange sensations, visual hallucinations, emotional changes, muscle spasms, convulsions, and a variety of other symptoms, depending on where in the brain the seizures originate.

There are many other types of epilepsy, each with its own characteristic set of symptoms. Many of these, including Lennox-Gastaut syndrome and rasmussen encephalitis, begin in childhood. Children with Lennox-Gastaut syndrome have severe epilepsy with several different types of seizures, including atonic seizures, which cause sudden falls and are also called drop attacks. This severe form of epilepsy can be very difficult to treat effectively. Rasmussen encephalitis is a progressive type of epilepsy in which half of the brain shows continual inflammation. It sometimes is treated with a radical surgical procedure called hemispherectomy. Some childhood epilepsy syndromes, such as childhood absence epilepsy, tend to go into remission or stop entirely during adolescence, whereas other syndromes, such as juvenile myoclonic epilepsy and Lennox-Gastaut syndrome, are usually present for life once they develop. Seizure syndromes do not always appear in childhood, however.

Epilepsy syndromes that are easily treated, do not seem to impair cognitive functions or development, and usually stop spontaneously are often described as benign. Benign epilepsy syndromes include benign infantile encephalopathy and benign neonatal convulsions. Other syndromes, such as early myoclonic encephalopathy, include neurological and developmental problems. However, these problems may be caused by underlying neurodegenerative processes rather than by the seizures. Epilepsy syndromes in which the seizures and/or the person's cognitive abilities get worse over time are called progressive epilepsy.

Several types of epilepsy begin in infancy. The most common type of infantile epilepsy is infantile spasms, clusters of seizures that usually begin before the age of six months. During these seizures the infant may bend and cry out. Anticonvulsant drugs often do not work for infantile spasms, but the seizures can be treated with adreno-corticotropic hormone (ACTH) or prednisone.

### How is epilepsy diagnosed?

Doctors have developed a number of different tests to determine whether a person has epilepsy and, if so, what kind of seizures the person has. In some cases, people may have symptoms that look very much like a seizure but in fact are nonepileptic events caused by other disorders. Even doctors may not be able to tell the difference between these disorders and epilepsy without close observation and intensive testing.

**EEG monitoring:** An electroencephalogram (EEG) records brain waves detected by electrodes placed on the scalp. This is the most common diagnostic test for epilepsy and can detect abnormalities in the brain's electrical activity. People with epilepsy frequently have changes in their normal pattern of brain waves, even when they are not experiencing a seizure. While this type of test can be very useful in diagnosing epilepsy, it is not foolproof. Some people continue to show normal brain wave patterns even after they have experienced a seizure. In other cases, the unusual brain waves are generated deep in the brain where the EEG is unable to detect them. Many people who do not have epilepsy also show some unusual brain activity on an EEG. Whenever possible, an EEG should be performed within twenty-four hours of a patient's first seizure. Ideally, EEGs should be performed while the patient is sleeping as well as when he or she is awake, because brain activity during sleep is often quite different than at other times.

Video monitoring is often used in conjunction with EEG to determine the nature of a person's seizures. It also can be used in some cases to rule out other disorders such as cardiac arrhythmia or narcolepsy that may look like epilepsy.

**Brain scans:** One of the most important ways of diagnosing epilepsy is through the use of brain scans. The most commonly used brain scans include CT (computed tomography), PET (positron emission tomography), and MRI (magnetic resonance imaging). CT and MRI scans reveal the structure of the brain, which can be useful for identifying brain tumors, cysts, and other structural abnormalities. PET and an adapted kind of MRI called functional MRI (fMRI) can be used to monitor the brain's activity and detect abnormalities in how it works. SPECT (single photon emission computed tomography) is a relatively new kind of brain scan that is sometimes used to locate seizure foci in the brain.

In some cases, doctors may use an experimental type of brain scan called a magnetoencephalogram, or MEG. MEG detects the magnetic signals generated by neurons to allow doctors to monitor brain activity at different points in the brain over time, revealing different brain functions. While MEG is similar in concept to EEG, it does not require electrodes and it can detect signals from deeper in the brain than an EEG. Doctors also are experimenting with brain scans called magnetic resonance spectroscopy (MRS) that can detect abnormalities in the brain's biochemical processes, and with near-infrared spectroscopy, a technique that can detect oxygen levels in brain tissue.

**Medical history:** Taking a detailed medical history, including symptoms and duration of the seizures, is still one of the best methods available to determine if a person has epilepsy and what kind of seizures he or she has. The doctor will ask questions about the seizures and any past illnesses or other symptoms a person may have had. Since people who have suffered a seizure often do not remember what happened, caregivers' accounts of the seizure are vital to this evaluation.

**Blood tests:** Doctors often take blood samples for testing, particularly when they are examining a child. These blood samples are often screened for metabolic or genetic disorders that may be associated with the seizures. They also may be used to check for underlying problems such as infections, lead poisoning, anemia, and diabetes that may be causing or triggering the seizures.

**Developmental, neurological, and behavioral tests:** Doctors often use tests devised to measure motor abilities, behavior, and intellectual capacity as a way to determine how the epilepsy is affecting that person. These tests also can provide clues about what kind of epilepsy the person has.

### How can epilepsy be treated?

Accurate diagnosis of the type of epilepsy a person has is crucial for finding an effective treatment. There are many different ways to treat epilepsy. Currently available treatments can control seizures at least some of the time in about 80 percent of people with epilepsy. However, another 20 percent—about six hundred thousand people with epilepsy in the United States—have intractable seizures, and another four hundred thousand feel they get inadequate relief from available treatments. These statistics make it clear that improved treatments are desperately needed.

Doctors who treat epilepsy come from many different fields of medicine. They include neurologists, pediatricians, pediatric neurologists, internists, and family physicians, as well as neurosurgeons and doctors called epileptologists who specialize in treating epilepsy. People who need specialized or intensive care for epilepsy may be treated at large medical centers and neurology clinics at hospitals or by neurologists in private practice. Many epilepsy treatment centers are associated with university hospitals that perform research in addition to providing medical care.

Once epilepsy is diagnosed, it is important to begin treatment as soon as possible. Research suggests that medication and other treatments may be less successful in treating epilepsy once seizures and their consequences become established.

**Medications:** When a person starts a new epilepsy drug, it is important to tailor the dosage to achieve the best results. People's bodies react to medications in very different and sometimes unpredictable ways, so it may take some time to find the right drug at the right dose to provide optimal control of seizures while minimizing side effects. A drug that has no effect or very bad side effects at one dose may work very well at another dose. Doctors will usually prescribe a low dose of the new drug initially and monitor blood levels of the drug to determine when the best possible dose has been reached.

Generic versions are available for many antiepileptic drugs. The chemicals in generic drugs are exactly the same as in the brand-name drugs, but they may be absorbed or processed differently in the body because of the way they are prepared. Therefore, patients should always check with their doctors before switching to a generic version of their medication.

Some doctors will advise people with epilepsy to discontinue their antiepileptic drugs after two years have passed without a seizure. Others feel it is better to wait for four to five years. Discontinuing medication should always be done with a doctor's advice and supervision. It is very important to continue taking epilepsy medication for as long as the doctor prescribes it. People also should ask the doctor or pharmacist ahead of time what they should do if they miss a dose.

Discontinuing medication without a doctor's advice is one of the major reasons people who have been seizure-free begin having new seizures. Seizures that result from suddenly stopping medication can be very serious and can lead to status epilepticus. Furthermore, there is some evidence that uncontrolled seizures trigger changes in neurons that can make it more difficult to treat the seizures in the future.

The chance that a person will eventually be able to discontinue medication varies depending on the person's age and his or her type of epilepsy. More than half of children who go into remission with medication can eventually stop their medication without having new seizures. One study showed that 68 percent of adults who had been seizure-free for two years before stopping medication were able to do so without having more seizures and 75 percent could successfully discontinue medication if they had been seizure-free for three years. However, the odds of successfully stopping medication are not as good for people with a family history of epilepsy, those who need multiple medications, those with focal seizures, and those who continue to have abnormal EEG results while on medication.

**Surgery:** When seizures cannot be adequately controlled by medications, doctors may recommend that the person be evaluated for surgery. Surgery for epilepsy is performed by teams of doctors at medical centers. To decide if a person may benefit from surgery, doctors consider the type or types of seizures he or she has. They also take into account the brain region involved and how important that region is for everyday behavior. Surgeons usually avoid operating in areas of the brain that are necessary for speech, language, hearing, or other important abilities. Doctors may perform tests such as a Wada test (administration of the drug amobarbital into the carotid artery) to find areas of the brain that control speech and memory. They often monitor the patient intensively prior to surgery in order to pinpoint the exact location in the brain where seizures begin. They also may use implanted electrodes to record brain activity from the surface of the brain. This yields better information than an external EEG.

A 1990 National Institutes of Health consensus conference on surgery for epilepsy concluded that there are three broad categories of epilepsy that can be treated successfully with surgery. These include focal seizures, seizures that begin as focal seizures before spreading to the rest of the brain, and unilateral multifocal epilepsy with infantile hemiplegia (such as rasmussen encephalitis). Doctors generally recommend surgery only after patients have tried two or three different medications without success, or if there is an identifiable brain lesion—a damaged or dysfunctional area—believed to cause the seizures.

A study published in 2000 compared surgery to an additional year of treatment with antiepileptic drugs in people with longstanding temporal lobe epilepsy. The results showed that 64 percent of patients receiving surgery became seizure-free, compared to 8 percent of those who continued with medication only. Because of this study and other evidence, the American Academy of Neurology (AAN) now recommends surgery for TLE when antiepileptic drugs are not effective. However, the study and the AAN guidelines do not provide guidance on how long seizures should occur, how severe they should be, or how many drugs should be tried before surgery is considered. A nationwide study is now underway to determine how soon surgery for TLE should be performed.

If a person is considered a good candidate for surgery and has seizures that cannot be controlled with available medication, experts generally agree that surgery should be performed as early as possible. It can be difficult for a person who has had years of seizures to fully re-adapt to a seizure-free life if the surgery is successful. The person may never have had an opportunity to develop independence, and he or she may have had difficulties with school and work that could have been avoided with earlier treatment. Surgery should always be performed with support from rehabilitation specialists and counselors who can help the person deal with the many psychological, social, and employment issues he or she may face.

While surgery can significantly reduce or even halt seizures for some people, it is important to remember that any kind of surgery carries some amount of risk (usually small). Surgery for epilepsy does not always successfully reduce seizures and it can result in cognitive or personality changes, even in people who are excellent candidates for surgery. Patients should ask their surgeon about his or her experience, success rates, and complication rates with the procedure they are considering.

Even when surgery completely ends a person's seizures, it is important to continue taking seizure medication for some time to give the brain time to re-adapt. Doctors generally recommend medication for two years after a successful operation to avoid new seizures.

**Devices:** The vagus nerve stimulator was approved by the U.S. Food and Drug Administration (FDA) in 1997 for use in people with seizures that are not well controlled by medication. The vagus nerve stimulator is a battery-powered device that is surgically implanted under the skin of the chest, much like a pacemaker, and is attached to the vagus nerve in the lower neck. This device delivers short bursts of electrical energy to the brain via the vagus nerve. On average, this stimulation reduces seizures by about 20 to 40 percent. Patients usually cannot stop taking epilepsy medication because of the stimulator, but they often experience fewer seizures and they may be able to reduce the dose of their medication. Side effects of the vagus nerve stimulator are generally mild but may include hoarseness, ear pain, a sore throat, or nausea. Adjusting the amount of stimulation can usually eliminate most side effects, although the hoarseness typically persists. The batteries in the vagus nerve stimulator need to be replaced about once every five years; this requires a minor operation that can usually be performed as an outpatient procedure.

Several new devices may become available for epilepsy in the future. Researchers are studying whether transcranial magnetic stimulation (TMS), a procedure which uses a strong magnet held outside the head to influence brain activity, may reduce seizures. They also hope to develop implantable devices that can deliver drugs to specific parts of the brain.

**Diet:** Studies have shown that, in some cases, children may experience fewer seizures if they maintain a strict diet rich in fats and low in carbohydrates. This unusual diet, called the ketogenic diet, causes the body to break down fats instead of carbohydrates to survive. This condition is called ketosis. One study of 150 children whose seizures were poorly controlled by medication found that about one-fourth of the children had a 90 percent or better decrease in seizures with the ketogenic diet, and another half of the group had a 50 percent or better decrease in their seizures. Moreover, some children can discontinue the ketogenic diet after several years and remain seizure-free. The ketogenic diet is not easy to maintain, as it requires strict adherence to an unusual and limited range of foods. Possible side effects include retarded growth due to nutritional deficiency and a buildup of uric acid in the blood, which can lead to kidney stones. People who try the ketogenic diet should seek the guidance of a dietitian to ensure that it does not lead to serious nutritional deficiency.

Researchers are not sure how ketosis inhibits seizures. One study showed that a byproduct of ketosis called beta-hydroxybutyrate (BHB) inhibits seizures in animals. If BHB also works in humans, researchers may eventually be able to develop drugs that mimic the seizure-inhibiting effects of the ketogenic diet.

181

**Other treatment strategies.** Researchers are studying whether biofeedback—a strategy in which individuals learn to control their own brain waves—may be useful in controlling seizures. However, this type of therapy is controversial and most studies have shown discouraging results. Taking large doses of vitamins generally does not help a person's seizures and may even be harmful in some cases. But a good diet and some vitamin supplements, particularly folic acid, may help reduce some birth defects and medication-related nutritional deficiencies. Use of nonvitamin supplements such as melatonin is controversial and can be risky. One study showed that melatonin may reduce seizures in some children, while another found that the risk of seizures increased measurably with melatonin. Most nonvitamin supplements such as those found in health food stores are not regulated by the FDA, so their true effects and their interactions with other drugs are largely unknown.

## Are there special risks associated with epilepsy?

Although most people with epilepsy lead full, active lives, they are at special risk for two life-threatening conditions: status epilepticus and sudden unexplained death.

**Status epilepticus:** Status epilepticus is a potentially life-threatening condition in which a person either has an abnormally prolonged seizure or does not fully regain consciousness between seizures. Although there is no strict definition for the time at which a seizure turns into status epilepticus, most people agree that any seizure lasting longer than five minutes should, for practical purposes, be treated as though it was status epilepticus.

Status epilepticus affects about 195,000 people each year in the United States and results in about 42,000 deaths. While people with epilepsy are at an increased risk for status epilepticus, about 60 percent of people who develop this condition have no previous seizure history. These cases often result from tumors, trauma, or other problems that affect the brain and may themselves be life threatening.

While most seizures do not require emergency medical treatment, someone with a prolonged seizure lasting more than five minutes may be in status epilepticus and should be taken to an emergency room immediately. It is important to treat a person with status epilepticus as soon as possible. One study showed that 80 percent of people in status epilepticus who received medication within thirty minutes of seizure onset eventually stopped having seizures, whereas only 40 percent recovered if two hours had passed before they received medication. Doctors in a hospital setting can treat status epilepticus with several different drugs and can undertake emergency life-saving measures, such as administering oxygen, if necessary.

People in status epilepticus do not always have severe convulsive seizures. Instead, they may have repeated or prolonged nonconvulsive seizures. This type of status epilepticus may appear as a sustained episode of confusion or agitation in someone who does not ordinarily have that kind of mental impairment. While this type of episode may not seem as severe as convulsive status epilepticus, it should still be treated as an emergency.

**Sudden unexplained death:** For reasons that are poorly understood, people with epilepsy have an increased risk of dying suddenly for no discernible reason. This condition, called sudden unexplained death, can occur in people without epilepsy, but epilepsy increases the risk about twofold. Researchers are still unsure why sudden unexplained death occurs. One study suggested that use of more than two anticonvulsant drugs may be a risk factor. However, it is not clear whether the use of multiple drugs causes the sudden death, or whether people who use multiple anticonvulsants have a greater risk of death because they have more severe types of epilepsy.

## What research is being done on epilepsy?

While research has led to many advances in understanding and treating epilepsy, there are many unanswered questions about how and why seizures develop, how they can best be treated or prevented, and how they influence other brain activity and brain development. Researchers, many of whom are supported by the National Institute of Neurological Disorders and Stroke (NINDS), are studying all of these questions. They also are working to identify and test new drugs and other treatments for epilepsy and to learn how those treatments affect brain activity and development.

The NINDS's Anticonvulsant Screening Program (ASP) studies potential new therapies with the goal of enhancing treatment for patients with epilepsy. Since it began in 1975, more than 390 public-private partnerships have been created. These partnerships have resulted in state-of-the-art evaluations of more than twenty-five thousand compounds for their potential as antiepileptic drugs. This government-sponsored effort has contributed to the development of five drugs that are now approved for use in the United States. It has also aided in the discovery and profiling of six new compounds currently in various stages of clinical development. Besides testing for safer, more efficacious therapies, the program is developing and validating new models that may one day find therapies that intervene in the disease process itself as well as models of resistant or refractory epilepsy.

Scientists continue to study how excitatory and inhibitory neurotransmitters interact with brain cells to control nerve firing. They can apply different chemicals to cultures of neurons in laboratory dishes to study how those chemicals influence neuronal activity. They also are studying how glia and other non-neuronal cells in the brain contribute to seizures. This research may lead to new drugs and other new ways of treating seizures.

Researchers also are working to identify genes that may influence epilepsy in some way. Identifying these genes can reveal the underlying chemical processes that influence epilepsy and point to new ways of preventing or treating this disorder. Researchers also can study rats and mice that have missing or abnormal copies of certain genes to determine how these genes affect normal brain development and resistance to damage from disease and other environmental factors. In the future, researchers may be able to use panels of gene fragments, called "gene chips," to determine each person's genetic makeup. This information may allow doctors to prevent epilepsy or to predict which treatments will be most beneficial.

Doctors are now experimenting with several new types of therapies for epilepsy. In one preliminary clinical trial, doctors have begun transplanting fetal pig neurons that produce gamma-aminobutyric acid (GABA) into the brains of patients to learn whether the cell transplants can help control seizures. Preliminary research suggests that stem cell transplants also may prove beneficial for treating epilepsy. Research showing that the brain undergoes subtle changes prior to a seizure has led to a prototype device that may be able to predict seizures up to three minutes before they begin. If this device works, it could greatly reduce the risk of injury from seizures by allowing people to move to a safe area before their seizures start. This type of device also may be hooked up to a treatment pump or other device that will automatically deliver an antiepileptic drug or an electric impulse to forestall the seizures.

Researchers are continually improving MRI and other brain scans. Pre-surgical brain imaging can guide doctors to abnormal brain tissue and away from essential parts of the brain. Researchers also are using brain scans such as magnetoencephalograms (MEG) and magnetic resonance spectroscopy (MRS) to identify and study subtle problems in the brain that cannot otherwise be detected. Their findings may lead to a better understanding of epilepsy and how it can be treated.

### What should you do if you see someone having a seizure?

If you see someone having a seizure with convulsions and/or loss of consciousness, here's how you can help:

- Roll the person on his or her side to prevent choking on any fluids or vomit.

- Cushion the person's head.

- Loosen any tight clothing around the neck.

- Keep the person's airway open. If necessary, grip the person's jaw gently and tilt his or her head back.

- Do **not** restrict the person from moving unless he or she is in danger.

- Do **not** put anything into the person's mouth, not even medicine or liquid. These can cause choking or damage to the person's jaw, tongue, or teeth. Contrary to widespread belief, people cannot swallow their tongues during a seizure or any other time.

- Remove any sharp or solid objects that the person might hit during the seizure.

- Note how long the seizure lasts and what symptoms occurred so you can tell a doctor or emergency personnel if necessary.

- Stay with the person until the seizure ends.

Call 911 if any of the following is true:

- The person is pregnant or has diabetes.

- The seizure happened in water.

- The seizure lasts longer than five minutes.

- The person does not begin breathing again or does not return to consciousness after the seizure stops.

- Another seizure starts before the person regains consciousness.

- The person injures him- or herself during the seizure.

- This is a first seizure or you think it might be. If in doubt, check to see if the person has a medical identification card or jewelry stating that they have epilepsy or a seizure disorder.

After the seizure ends, the person will probably be groggy and tired. He or she also may have a headache and be confused or embarrassed. Be patient with the person and try to help him or her find a place to rest if he or she is tired or doesn't feel well. If necessary, offer to call a taxi, a friend, or a relative to help the person get home safely.

If you see someone having a nonconvulsive seizure, remember that the person's behavior is not intentional. The person may wander aimlessly or make alarming or unusual gestures. You can help by following these guidelines:

- Remove any dangerous objects from the area around the person or in his or her path.

- Don't try to stop the person from wandering unless he or she is in danger.

- Don't shake the person or shout.

- Stay with the person until he or she is completely alert.

## Conclusion

Many people with epilepsy lead productive and outwardly normal lives. Medical and research advances in the past two decades have led to a better understanding of epilepsy and seizures than ever before. Advanced brain scans and other techniques allow greater accuracy in diagnosing epilepsy and determining when a patient may be helped by surgery. More than twenty different medications and a variety of surgical techniques are now available and provide good control of seizures for most people with epilepsy. Other treatment options include the ketogenic diet and the first implantable device, the vagus nerve stimulator. Research on the underlying causes of epilepsy, including identification of genes for some forms of epilepsy and febrile seizures, has led to a greatly improved understanding of epilepsy that may lead to more effective treatments or even new ways of preventing epilepsy in the future.

Chapter 14

# Auditory Processing Disorder in People with Autism

## What is auditory processing?

Auditory processing is a term used to describe what happens when your brain recognizes and interprets the sounds around you. Humans hear when energy that we recognize as sound travels through the ear and is changed into electrical information that can be interpreted by the brain. The "disorder" part of auditory processing disorder (APD) means that something is adversely affecting the processing or interpretation of the information.

Children with APD often do not recognize subtle differences between sounds in words, even though the sounds themselves are loud and clear. For example, the request "Tell me how a chair and a couch are alike" may sound to a child with APD like "Tell me how a couch and a chair are alike." It can even be understood by the child as "Tell me how a cow and a hair are alike." These kinds of problems are more likely to occur when a person with APD is in a noisy environment or when he or she is listening to complex information.

APD goes by many other names. Sometimes it is referred to as central auditory processing disorder (CAPD). Other common names are auditory perception problem, auditory comprehension deficit, central auditory dysfunction, central deafness, and so-called word deafness.

Reprinted from "Auditory Processing Disorder in Children," National Institute on Deafness and Other Communication Disorders, National Institutes of Health, NIH Publication No. 01-4949, February 2004.

187

## What causes auditory processing difficulty?

We are not sure. Human communication relies on taking in complicated perceptual information from the outside world through the senses, such as hearing, and interpreting that information in a meaningful way. Human communication also requires certain mental abilities, such as attention and memory. Scientists still do not understand exactly how all of these processes work and interact or how they malfunction in cases of communication disorders. Even though your child seems to "hear normally," he or she may have difficulty using those sounds for speech and language.

The cause of APD is often unknown. In children, auditory processing difficulty may be associated with conditions such as dyslexia, attention deficit disorder, autism, autism spectrum disorder, specific language impairment, pervasive developmental disorder, or developmental delay. Sometimes this term has been misapplied to children who have no hearing or language disorder but have challenges in learning.

## What are the symptoms of possible auditory processing difficulty?

Children with auditory processing difficulty typically have normal hearing and intelligence. However, they have also been observed to:

- Have trouble paying attention to and remembering information presented orally;

- Have problems carrying out multistep directions;

- Have poor listening skills;

- Need more time to process information;

- Have low academic performance;

- Have behavior problems;

- Have language difficulty (e.g., they confuse syllable sequences and have problems developing vocabulary and understanding language);

- Have difficulty with reading, comprehension, spelling, and vocabulary.

188

## How is suspected auditory processing difficulty diagnosed in children?

You, a teacher, or a day care provider may be the first person to notice symptoms of auditory processing difficulty in your child. So talking to your child's teacher about school or preschool performance is a good idea. Many health professionals can also diagnose APD in your child. There may need to be ongoing observation with the professionals involved.

Much of what will be done by these professionals will be to rule out other problems. A pediatrician or a family doctor can help rule out possible diseases that can cause some of these same symptoms. He or she will also measure growth and development. If there is a disease or disorder related to hearing, you may be referred to an otolaryngologist—a physician who specializes in diseases and disorders of the head and neck.

To determine whether your child has a hearing function problem, an audiologic evaluation is necessary. An audiologist will give tests that can determine the softest sounds and words a person can hear and other tests to see how well people can recognize sounds in words and sentences. For example, for one task, the audiologist might have your child listen to different numbers or words in the right and the left ear at the same time. Another common audiologic task involves giving the child two sentences, one louder than the other, at the same time. The audiologist is trying to identify the processing problem.

A speech-language pathologist can find out how well a person understands and uses language. A mental health professional can give you information about cognitive and behavioral challenges that may contribute to problems in some cases, or he or she may have suggestions that will be helpful. Because the audiologist can help with the functional problems of hearing and processing, and the speech-language pathologist is focused on language, they may work as a team with your child. All of these professionals seek to provide the best outcome for each child.

## What current research is being conducted?

In recent years, scientists have developed new ways to study the human brain through imaging. Imaging is a powerful tool that allows the monitoring of brain activity without any surgery. Imaging studies are already giving scientists new insights into auditory processing. Some of these studies are directed at understanding auditory processing disorders. One of the values of imaging is that it provides an objective, measurable view of a process. Many of the symptoms described as related to APD are described differently by different people.

Imaging will help identify the source of these symptoms. Other scientists are studying the central auditory nervous system. Cognitive neuroscientists are helping to describe how the processes that mediate sound recognition and comprehension work in both normal and disordered systems.

Research into the rehabilitation of child language disorders continues. It is important to know that much research is still needed to understand auditory processing problems, related disorders, and the best interventions for each child or adult. All the strategies undertaken will need to be suited to the needs of the individual child, and their effectiveness will need to be continuously evaluated. The standard for determining if a treatment is effective is that a patient can reasonably expect to benefit from it.

### What treatments are available for auditory processing difficulty?

Much research is still needed to understand APD problems, related disorders, and the best intervention for each child or adult. Several strategies are available to help children with auditory processing difficulties. Some of these are commercially available, but have not been fully studied. Any strategy selected should be used under the guidance of a team of professionals, and the effectiveness of the strategy needs to be evaluated. Researchers are currently studying a variety of approaches to treatment. Several strategies you may hear about include the following:

- Auditory trainers are electronic devices that allow a person to focus attention on a speaker and reduce the interference of background noise. They are often used in classrooms, where the teacher wears a microphone to transmit sound and the child wears a headset to receive the sound. Children who wear hearing aids can use them in addition to the auditory trainer.

- Environmental modifications such as classroom acoustics, placement, and seating may help. An audiologist may suggest ways to improve the listening environment, and he or she will be able to monitor any changes in hearing status.

190

- Exercises to improve language-building skills can increase the ability to learn new words and increase a child's language base.

- Auditory memory enhancement, a procedure that reduces detailed information to a more basic representation, may help. Also, informal auditory training techniques can be used by teachers and therapists to address specific difficulties.

- Auditory integration training may be promoted by practitioners as a way to retrain the auditory system and decrease hearing distortion. However, current research has not proven the benefits of this treatment.

Chapter 15

# Attention Deficit Hyperactivity Disorder and Autism

We are aware that an increasing number of children are being diagnosed as having both attention deficit hyperactivity disorder (AD/HD) and autism/Asperger syndrome. Many parents are understandably confused about the links between the two conditions.

## Diagnosis

There are many reasons for the two conditions being confused in young children. Many children with autism display signs of hyperactivity and inattention when they start school. However, experts are very clear that as the child becomes older the apparent similarities between the two conditions will separate out. The child with autism may become more withdrawn, and given the right environment, their hyperactivity should wane and their difficulties with social skills will emerge. Children with AD/HD, on the other hand, are unlikely to become calmer with age unless they receive medication or high-quality therapeutic interventions. They still develop social and communication skills and are unlikely to have the anxiety levels of a child with autism.

The *Diagnostic and Statistical Manual of Mental Disorders, Fourth Edition* (*DSM-IV*) stipulates that a diagnosis of AD/HD can be made only if the child has shown signs of the condition before the age of seven and has been experiencing the following symptoms to an extent which is developmentally deviant and for a period of at least six months:

- Inattention

- Impulsivity

- Hyperactivity

The condition cannot be diagnosed if it occurs solely within the context of a pervasive developmental disorder such as autism. That is not to say that a child cannot have both conditions. For the reasons mentioned above it is possible that the child with autism will display signs of AD/HD but this should not be considered as an additional diagnosis until their needs relating to their autism are addressed first.

The following hints and tips are intended to be of use whether your child has been diagnosed with both AD/HD and autism or just autism. If you are still not sure why your child has received the diagnosis he or she has then you should go back to the specialist who gave you the original diagnosis for further clarification.

## What Causes AD/HD?

The causes of AD/HD appear to be remarkably similar to those alleged to cause autism. This may be largely because we know so little about both of these conditions. The key similarities are that until recently many professionals thought that AD/HD occurred only as a result of poor parenting. The factors thought to cause AD/HD today range from the biological, such as genetics and brain damage during pregnancy, to the environmental, such as sensitivity to certain foods. It is likely that the causes are actually bioenvironmental—that is, the result of an interaction between both biological and environmental causes.

Some people have suggested that AD/HD belongs on the autistic spectrum, as children with the condition have so much in common with those with autism. However, many children with AD/HD have no difficulties with communication and social skills except where these are the result of their limited functioning in other areas. That is, children with AD/HD may appear to have difficulty interacting with other children at school but this has more to do with their low self-esteem and their difficulty settling to playing or working together in a constructive way rather than an inherent problem with relating to others.

Yet, there are still links between autism and AD/HD. It is clear from the genetic histories of some families that some parents are diagnosed with AD/HD only after their children have been diagnosed with autism. The two conditions are often confused at the time of diagnosis as well.

## Coping with a Combination of AD/HD and Autism

The actual diagnosis that your child has received is irrelevant here. Some children with autism will also display hyperactive behaviors and some children with AD/HD will demonstrate autistic traits. As a result they will need behavioral and other interventions that recognize this combination of needs.

First you can examine what might be causing any hyperactive behaviors.

### Diet

Food additives have long been known to overstimulate some children. It is possible that children with autism are even more sensitive to these substances than other children. However it is fairly straightforward to avoid brightly colored sweets and soft drinks, and many products now advertise themselves as having no artificial colorings or flavorings.

Other stimulants that regularly affect children's behavior include sugar and caffeine. Again, removing these completely from the diet can be a pain but you can take some simple measures to reduce your child's intake of stimulants:

- Switch to decaffeinated tea, coffee, and cola.

- Use carob instead of cocoa to make chocolate-flavored foods.

- Allow your child only small quantities of sugar on a regular basis, rather than giving him or her a huge one-time dose; this should help you avoid sugar highs.

If implementing any of these will involve radical changes to your child's diet then do it as slowly as possible. Switching overnight may be counterproductive, as it is possible that your child has a dependency on these foods.

### Environmental Factors

If your child is especially sensitive to sensory stimuli such as lights, sounds, and textures, then environments where many of these factors interact could be extremely distracting and disturbing for him or her.

195

If your child is frequently calm and only occasionally hyperactive or disruptive then it may be worth charting when and where these incidents occur to see if there is any pattern to your child's behavior. Good examples of places that might overstimulate a child include swimming pools, supermarkets, and fast-food restaurants, and trips to places like these may need careful planning as a result.

## Planning Trips with a Child with AD/HD

First it is important to remember that when your child misbehaves in public it is often the result of his or her own stress and not a desire to be naughty. It can be very hard to keep calm and avoid getting angry even if you know your child is in distress. Planning ahead can reduce some of that stress. However, it is important to remember that long trips are always going to be difficult to manage and the chances are that if you find something stressful then your child probably feels the same way. That should not discourage people from going out, and carefully managed short trips may help your child learn the skills to cope with longer trips later on.

For the more able child you can probably work with him or her to plan the trip so that your child is aware of what incentives there are to keep calm and in control at every stage. Try talking through before each trip exactly what you are planning to do and what you expect. This will make the trip much more predictable for your child, which can, in turn, reduce his or her anxiety levels. You can also write down your plans so that your child can keep them to look at and refer back to. If you write down each stage of the trip on a separate card or sheet of paper then they can then be used as visual prompts to remind your child of what is happening.

An example of a series of flash cards for planning a trip to a swimming pool could read as follows:

- We will go to the swimming pool at a time when there won't be lots of other people there.

- In the car on the way there you can relax and we'll play some quiet music.

- When we get there we have to buy tickets to get in. This won't take more than two or three minutes and then we can go through to the changing rooms.

- The changing rooms can be noisy but we will sit down to relax a for a minute before we get changed.

- While I put our clothes and bags in the lockers you can sit down and wait quietly for me. This will take only a minute.

- We will hold hands while we walk out to the pool.

- I will get into the pool first and then I will help you get in.

- If you want to go then just tell me and we will leave.

## Think About the Worst Possible Outcome

This sounds strange but often people get absorbed by thinking about how difficult the whole trip will be without focusing on the specifics of what might go wrong. For example, in the case of going on the bus, don't think: "This will be so difficult. My child might behave appallingly, and it'll be in public. People might start staring or commenting." Instead, look at what the worst thing that could happen might be: "My child could have a tantrum while we are on the bus." Then plan steps to minimize this possibility:

- If you make sure that your child is next to the window and that you sit next to him or her, then your child won't be able to get out and annoy the other passengers.

- If you take your child's favorite toy or treat with you, then this can be used to placate him or her when necessary.

- If your child does make a lot of noise and people do look, then try to have a stock phrase ready with which to reply to any comments. Something like this might work: "Joe has autism/AD/HD. Lots of stimulation makes him feel anxious. Making these noises helps him to feel calmer."

- If two of you go with the child then you can share responsibility for looking after him or her. This, in turn, will make the experience less intense and exhausting and leave you more able to cope with difficult situations, should they arise.

If you can think of coping strategies for the worst thing you can imagine happening then you can probably cope with any other problems that occur.

## Motivating Your Child to Learn Other Ways of Behaving

If you have a child with a very keen interest in one subject, whatever that is, it is worth encouraging the interest. This can be a valuable motivational tool. It can also help your child to learn concentration skills, and once your child has developed the ability to focus on an enjoyable activity, he or she can begin generalizing this ability to other areas.

Encourage your child to discuss his or her needs with you. Your child may lose interest in an activity and begin wandering after twenty minutes because he or she does not know how to explain what has made him or her lose interest. Children with autism may not realize that their teacher or parent doesn't know how bored they are. Let them know that you are happy for them to move on to something else but that they have to tell you why they want to do this. This need to explain could be very frustrating for them and it is important to avoid putting pressure on them to give a detailed and abstract explanation for their behavior. A simple "Don't understand" or "Bored" is still something to work on.

## Coping with Frustration

Hyperkinetic activity may occur when a child with autism is unusually frustrated or wound up about something. Under these circumstances it is probably not desirable to attempt to contain the activity as the child may then choose to let off steam somewhere else and in a destructive or aggressive way. Even children with low levels of functioning can be supported to do exercises, bounce on a trampoline, punch a punching bag, and run around the yard in order to relieve tension. For more able children, encouraging them to go for a jog or a bicycle ride in order to cool off and release some of that surplus energy might be helpful. This could also be tied in with doing a useful activity like picking up some shopping or doing a paper route so that the need to use up this energy is turned into a useful skill and something your child can feel positive about.

Remember that there are lots of positive things about having plenty of energy, provided that it is channeled in the right directions. However, for families it can also have serious disadvantages. Fundamentally a child with hyperactive behaviors will need certain types of behavioral support whether or not the child has autism as well. Families of such children may also need plenty of respite and support and it is important that families have their support needs addressed even if there are question marks hanging over the diagnosis.

## Drug Treatments for Children with AD/HD

The most widely known drug used to treat AD/HD is Ritalin. This is a stimulant drug that acts to reduce electrical activity in the brain,

198

which in turn reduces hyperactivity. It is widely recognized as useful for children with AD/HD and has also been shown to be of some limited benefit for children with autism.

However, there are many people who advocate against the use of Ritalin. They argue that Ritalin is used to prevent families and schools addressing the real issues of providing appropriate support and education. This is a very valid argument, particularly for children who have Asperger syndrome. Many parents have expressed concern that their children have been misdiagnosed with AD/HD when in fact they are showing hyperactive behaviors as a way of coping with their frustration at school, where their needs are not being met.

Some parents opt to use Ritalin as a way of controlling their child's symptoms for a short time while they address some of the behavioral issues affecting their child. This way of using medication can be very effective provided people are clear that this is what they are doing from the outset.

If you are attempting this it is important to bear the following points in mind:

- Start administering the drug at the lowest dose possible and increase it only after you have found it doesn't work at that level. In this way you can establish the optimum dose—that is, the lowest dose with the best results.

- Set target dates for reducing the dose. If your doctor doesn't provide you with a diary or some other form for monitoring improvements then make one yourself. Note down any aberrant or new behaviors on the chart.

- Keep your child involved in administering and monitoring the medication. Allow him or her to see this as a straightforward medical treatment.

Chapter 16

# Exceptional Abilities in People with Autism

## Chapter Contents

Section 16.1—Hyperlexia: Exceptional Reading
          Abilities in Young Children ............................ 202
Section 16.2—Savant Syndrome: An Extraordinary
          Condition ........................................................ 205

Section 16.1

## Hyperlexia: Exceptional Reading Abilities in Young Children

Reprinted from "Studying Hyperlexia May Unlock How Brains Read," by Shankar Vedantam, *Washington Post*, March 1, 2004. © 2004 *The Washington Post*. Reprinted with permission.

By the time he was a year old, Alex Rosen of Bethesda would spend time at birthday parties thumbing through magazines while other children played with toys. By the time he was three, if his mother's finger skipped a line as she was reading a story, he would place her finger on the correct point in the text. By the time he started school, he was reading like a twelve-year-old.

No one taught him to read, but Alex, who is now eleven, learned on his own to organize letters in alphabetical order while he was still a toddler. He has never had to study for a spelling bee.

"When he was two, I could take him to a really nice restaurant and we would bring a stack of books," said his mother, Ilene Freed Rosen. "He would look through them. People would walk up and say, 'How old is he?' I'd say, 'two,' and they would say, 'My god, my kid would have been running around.'"

Alex has hyperlexia, a condition whose features look like the opposite of the reading and learning disorder dyslexia. The condition endowed him with some unusual abilities, but it also exacted a price: He was slow to begin speaking, and he still has some trouble with verbal communication and difficulty grasping the rapidly changing social rules of eleven-year-old children.

Hyperlexia is extremely rare. About two in every ten thousand children with "autism spectrum disorders" have hyperlexia, and researchers believe that studying Alex's development may help explain why some children naturally pick up reading the same way that others pick up spoken speech. The results, they hope, may also improve the understanding of disorders such as dyslexia and autism, and also help other hyperlexic children.

There is controversy about whether hyperlexia is linked to autism or whether it is a distinct disorder. Georgetown University developmental neuroscientist Peter Turkeltaub, who has studied Alex, said he was not even sure whether to call hyperlexia a disorder or simply a phenomenon.

Understanding hyperlexia may also help explain how normal brains accomplish the feat of reading. Unlike seeing and hearing, skills acquired through evolution, reading is usually not acquired naturally. Humans have been reading for only a few thousand years, and the pressure for everyone to become good readers has become intense in only the past couple of centuries.

Reading involves a complex series of brain activities: Visual centers must first perceive variable, tiny features of printed symbols on a page, then those changes must be mentally converted into strings of sound, and finally the patterns of sound must be interpreted by language centers in the brain to register their meaning.

"Hyperlexia is the antithesis of dyslexia," said Guinevere Eden, director of Georgetown University's Center for the Study of Learning, who has studied Alex. "We spend all our time studying individuals who have a hard time learning to read, and here are these children who acquire reading in a spontaneous way. It's as if they know it already."

In a study conducted when Alex was nine years old, researchers compared his brain function while he was reading with that of other children his age and with children who were older but read at the same level. Alex's reading ability was six years ahead of his age.

In a paper published in the journal *Neuron* in January 2004, the researchers reported that the Bethesda youngster had heightened brain activity in two areas, according to lead author Turkeltaub. One area was the left interior frontal gyrus, located behind the middle of the temple, the other was the left superior temporal cortex, over and behind the ear.

"If you're reading a word that you've never seen before, you need to first translate the letters into sounds, and then put those sounds together to make a whole word," Turkeltaub said in an e-mail. "In your brain, the left superior temporal cortex will translate the letters to sounds, and the left inferior frontal gyrus will put those sounds together to create the whole word."

Alex, it seems, had a very advanced ability to identify individual sounds while reading and then to manipulate those sounds in his head. But paradoxically, even as he incessantly read text, including traffic signs and license plate numbers, Alex had trouble understanding the meaning of what he read. With training, his speaking ability has improved and he has become skilled at reading nonfiction. But he still has difficulty with fiction, in which important aspects of a story, such as a character's inner motivations, are not explicitly described.

The lack of insight into how others think affects Alex's life. If two classmates are not talking to one another, for example, Alex has trouble connecting that behavior to a fight the children had the previous day, his mother said.

"The lessons they need to learn are not in books," Rosen said of children with hyperlexia. "Is a joke funny the second time? Not if you tell it to the same person. It's so difficult to teach someone to be a social human being."

Rosen teaches Alex to pay attention to slang, which is an important part of social communication, especially among children. Rather than fight his natural talent at reading, Rosen has used printed text as a means of communicating with her son. Alex still speaks very formally, mimicking the cadences of written speech. He never uses the interjection "like," the way many youngsters do incessantly, and his sentences are always grammatical and complete.

These skills helped him run for student council president—and win. He is a fearless public speaker, and his mother had to tell Alex that other children are typically nervous in front of an audience.

But Rosen worries that Alex's lack of insight into how other people think may leave him too trusting—his personality is as open as the books he loves. Deception is beyond him, which is why Rosen actually celebrates when Alex tries to manipulate her.

"I love it when you lie to me, Al," she told him in the presence of a visitor last week. "Because it tells me you know what I'm thinking."

Someday, Ilene Freed Rosen sighed, her guileless child would make a fabulous husband.

Section 16.2

# Savant Syndrome: An Extraordinary Condition

The Academy Award–winning movie *Rain Man* made "autistic savant" a household word. But savant skills are not limited to autistic persons, nor are all autistic persons savants. Therefore savant syndrome is a more accurate and inclusive term for this remarkable condition, and savant syndrome includes some persons (about 50 percent) who are autistic with superimposed savant abilities, but also includes persons with other developmental disabilities (the other 50 percent) who have savant abilities as well. With that caveat, since autistic savants are a distinct subgroup in savant syndrome, and often of special interest, this section focuses separately on what we do know about the "autistic savant" as one important part of savant syndrome overall.

Raymond Babbitt, as portrayed so accurately and sensitively by Dustin Hoffman in *Rain Man*, certainly is the world's best-known autistic savant. While a composite character, and not based on the story of one individual, Raymond Babbitt is an accurate portrayal of a high-functioning person who is autistic, with superimposed extraordinary special skills coupled with a prodigious memory. That combination of autistic disorder plus extraordinary special abilities plus remarkable memory is the "autistic savant."

However, not all autistic persons are savants. Approximately one in ten (10 percent) do have some special skills over a spectrum ranging from what are called "splinter skills" to "prodigious" savants. The latter have special skills so spectacular that they would be remarkable even if they were present in a non-handicapped person. Savant skills also occur in other forms of developmental disability, such as mental retardation, but with much less frequency, as low as 1:2000 in a residential population. But since mental retardation is much more common than autistic disorder, and since the frequency of savant skills in that group is much lower than in persons with autism, as it turns out, approximately 50 percent of persons with savant syndrome have autistic disorder, and 50 percent have some other form of developmental disability including mental retardation.

Among the 10 percent of autistic persons who are autistic savant, there is a wide spectrum of savant abilities. Most common are what are called "splinter skills" such as obsessive preoccupation with and memorization of sports trivia, license plates, maps, or things as obscure as vacuum cleaner motor sounds, for example. "Talented" savants are those persons whose special skills and abilities are more specialized and highly honed, making those skills obviously conspicuous when viewed over against overall handicap. Finally there is a group of "prodigious" savants whose skills are so spectacular they would be conspicuous even if they were to occur in a non-handicapped person. There are probably fewer than fifty persons living worldwide who would meet the high-threshold definition of prodigious savants, and approximately one-half of that group would be autistic savants.

This startling juxtaposition of superiority and handicap was originally given the unfortunate name "idiot savant" by Dr. J. Langdon Down (better known for having described Down Syndrome) in 1887. In a series of lectures in London that year, Dr. Down described his thirty-year experience as superintendent of Earlswood Asylum, during which time he was fascinated by the extraordinary paradox of superiority and handicap in the same person. He described ten such cases, including one boy who would come away from an opera with perfect recollection of all of the arias; another could multiply many-digit figures in his head as quickly as they could be written down; another lad had memorized and could recite—backward or forward, albeit with little comprehension—*The Rise and Fall of the Roman Empire*, in its entirety. There is no description in these cases that would permit a diagnosis of autistic disorder as opposed to some other form of developmental disability, but surely some were autistic.

Down made a number of observations that are still valid a century later, and are applicable to the autistic savant today. First, the skills are almost always limited to a very narrow range of special abilities: music; art; mathematics, including lightning calculating and calendar calculating; and mechanical or spatial skills. This narrow range of abilities is particularly intriguing when considering the wide range of abilities in the human repertoire. Second, Down noted that these spectacular special abilities are always linked to a phenomenal memory of a unique type—very narrow but exceedingly deep—often with little understanding or comprehension of that which is so massively stored, a characteristic he called "verbal adhesion" and others have called "memory without reckoning." Third, Down noted that his cases were limited entirely to males. While not that stringent, over time the actual male-to-female ratio has turned out to be approximately six males for every one female savant.

The term "idiot savant" has largely been discarded now, appropriately, and has been replaced by savant syndrome. Actually that original term as used by Down was a misnomer, since almost all reported cases occur in persons with intelligence quotient (IQ) of 40 or more. In Down's time the word "idiot" was an accepted scientific classification for mental retardation with IQ below 25 and he combined that term with the word "savant," derived from the French word "*savoir*," which means "to know" or "knowledgeable person."

The condition of early infantile autism, however, was not described as a separate entity until fifty-six years after Down's original description of savant syndrome. In 1943 Dr. Leo Kanner carefully and accurately described and named a condition he called early infantile autism, now generally referred to as autistic disorder, and sometimes just as autism. Autistic disorder is not a single entity and is more appropriately described as a group of disorders, with a variety of etiologies all with the final common path, cluster, and constellation of symptoms we now call autistic disorder, or autism. Among that group of persons with autistic disorder, approximately one in ten have some savant abilities on the spectrum from splinter skills to prodigious savant. These special skills are superimposed, or grafted on to, the autistic disorder, along with phenomenal memory, as described below.

The skills in the autistic savant continue to be seen within a curiously narrow but remarkably constant range of human abilities: music, usually piano and almost always with perfect pitch; art, typically drawing, painting, or sculpting; lightning calculating, calendar calculating, or other facility with numbers such as computing prime numbers; and mechanical abilities or spatial skills. Unusual language talent—polyglot savant—skills have been reported but are very rare. Other less frequently reported special skills include map memorizing, remarkable sense of direction, unusual sensory discrimination such as enhanced sense of smell or touch, and prefect appreciation of passing time without knowledge of a clock face. A conspicuously disproportionate number of musical savants through this past century, and at the present time, are blind and autistic, demonstrating a curiously recurrent triad of blindness, autism, and musical genius.

In most autistic savants a single special skill exists; in others multiple skills occur. The skills tend to be right hemisphere in type—

nonsymbolic, concrete, directly perceived—in contrast to left-hemisphere type that tend to be more sequential, logical, and symbolic, including language specialization. To the extent imaging studies such as computed tomography (CT), magnetic resonance imaging (MRI), or positron emission tomography (PET) have been carried out, savants, and particularly autistic savants, do demonstrate left hemisphere damage with, presumably, right hemisphere compensatory function. This left hemisphere damage can be from a variety of prenatal, perinatal, and postnatal causes. It is postulated that this left hemisphere damage is coupled with corresponding damage to the higher level cognitive (cortico-limbic) memory circuitry with compensatory takeover of lower level (cortico-striatal) so-called habit or procedural memory. This accounts for the linking of predominantly right brain skills with habit memory so characteristic of autistic savants and savant syndrome more generally. In addition to this idiosyncratic brain circuitry, intense concentration, practice, compensatory drives, and reinforcement by family, teachers, and others play a major role in developing and polishing the savant skills and memory linked so characteristically and regularly in the autistic savant.

CT and MRI scans, impressive as they are, document only brain structure. The real future in unlocking the dynamics and circuitry of savants, and indeed autistic disorder itself, will come from PET and single photon emission computed tomography (SPECT) imaging, which map brain function, not just its architecture. Increasingly in autistic disorder, more and more evidence of left hemisphere dysfunction emerges, and in savant syndrome such left hemisphere dysfunction is likewise increasingly evident, and implicated as an important explanation of savant abilities. There has been only one SPECT functional imaging study reported thus far on an autistic savant, in this case an eleven-year-old autistic artist, D.B. That study showed a distinct abnormality in the left anterior temporal area of the brain. What is so striking about that finding is that it mirrors exactly another recent, far-reaching discovery about savant abilities. Dr. Bruce Miller, a San Francisco neurologist, has described twelve cases now of new savant abilities emerging in elderly, previously nondisabled persons as a particular type of dementia (frontotemporal dementia) proceeded. The SPECT abnormality in these patients was identical to that of the childhood autistic savant. This finding of new savant abilities emerging as a dementia proceeds raises profound questions about hidden potential versus a little Raymond Babbitt, perhaps, within us all.

There have been a number of autistic savants who are quite well known. But there is more to autistic savants than the scientific interests of brain circuits, neurons, and hemispheres. Embedded in the lives of these remarkable people as well are the human interest stories about the power of love, belief, and caring in the families, caretakers, therapists, and teachers that surround the savant, in first discovering, then appreciating, then helping to actualize and realize the savant's full potential beyond deficits. Rather than fearing some dreaded tradeoff of these special gifts as the price of training and teaching the savant broader communication, social, and daily living skills, these remarkable abilities can themselves serve as what I call a "conduit toward normalization" without loss of those unique talents. The century-old debate of whether to "train the talent" or "eliminate the defect" can be convincingly answered now. Training the talent can in fact help ameliorate or lessen the defect. There are now compelling and inspiring examples of such useful application of special skills toward normalization in the classroom, in the workplace, and in the home in a number of well-known autistic savants.

Until we can understand and explain the savant, we cannot fully understand and explain ourselves. For no model of brain function, including memory, will be complete until it can fully incorporate and account for this amazing condition and its remarkable manifestations. And no conclusions about human potential can be finalized either until we fully explore the ramifications of what is seen in the savant. Serious study of savant syndrome, including the autistic savant, can propel us along further than we have ever been in understanding, and maximizing, both brain function and human potential.

# Part Four

# Diagnosing and Evaluating Autism Spectrum Disorders

Chapter 17

# Signs of Autism Spectrum Disorders

All children with autism spectrum disorders (ASD) demonstrate deficits in 1) social interaction, 2) verbal and nonverbal communication, and 3) repetitive behaviors or interests. In addition, they will often have unusual responses to sensory experiences, such as certain sounds or the way objects look. Each of these symptoms runs the gamut from mild to severe. They will present in each individual child differently. For instance, a child may have little trouble learning to read but exhibit extremely poor social interaction. Each child will display communication, social, and behavioral patterns that are individual but fit into the overall diagnosis of ASD.

Children with ASD do not follow the typical patterns of child development. In some children, hints of future problems may be apparent from birth. In most cases, the problems in communication and social skills become more noticeable as the child lags further behind other children the same age. Some other children start off well enough. Oftentimes between twelve and thirty-six months old, the differences in the way they react to people and other unusual behaviors become apparent. Some parents report the change as being sudden, and that their children start to reject people, act strangely, and lose language and social skills they had previously acquired. In other cases, there is a plateau, or leveling, of progress so that the difference between

Excerpted from "Autism Spectrum Disorders (Pervasive Developmental Disorders)," National Institute of Mental Health, National Institutes of Health, NIH Publication No. 04-5511, March 14, 2007.

the child with autism and other children the same age becomes more noticeable.

ASD are defined by a certain set of behaviors that can range from the very mild to the severe. The following possible indicators of ASD were identified on the Public Health Training Network Webcast, Autism Among Us.[1]

## Possible Indicators of Autism Spectrum Disorders

Some possible indicators of autism spectrum disorders are as follows:

- Does not babble, point, or make meaningful gestures by one year of age
- Does not speak one word by sixteen months
- Does not combine two words by two years
- Does not respond to name
- Loses language or social skills
- Poor eye contact
- Doesn't seem to know how to play with toys
- Excessively lines up toys or other objects
- Is attached to one particular toy or object
- Doesn't smile
- At times seems to be hearing impaired

### Social Symptoms

From the start, typically developing infants are social beings. Early in life, they gaze at people, turn toward voices, grasp a finger, and even smile.

In contrast, most children with ASD seem to have tremendous difficulty learning to engage in the give-and-take of everyday human interaction. Even in the first few months of life, many do not interact and they avoid eye contact. They seem indifferent to other people, and often seem to prefer being alone. They may resist attention or passively accept hugs and cuddling. Later, they seldom seek comfort or respond to parents' displays of anger or affection in a typical way. Research has suggested that although children with ASD are attached to their parents, their expression of this attachment is unusual and difficult to "read." To parents, it may seem as if their child is not attached at all. Parents who looked forward to the joys of cuddling, teaching, and playing with their child may feel crushed by this lack of the expected and typical attachment behavior.

Children with ASD also are slower in learning to interpret what others are thinking and feeling. Subtle social cues—whether a smile, a wink, or a grimace—may have little meaning. To a child who misses these cues, "Come here" always means the same thing, whether the speaker is smiling and extending her arms for a hug or frowning and planting her fists on her hips. Without the ability to interpret gestures and facial expressions, the social world may seem bewildering. To compound the problem, people with ASD have difficulty seeing things from another person's perspective. Most five-year-olds understand that other people have different information, feelings, and goals than they have. A person with ASD may lack such understanding. This inability leaves them unable to predict or understand other people's actions.

Although not universal, it is common for people with ASD also to have difficulty regulating their emotions. This can take the form of "immature" behavior such as crying in class or verbal outbursts that seem inappropriate to those around them. The individual with ASD might also be disruptive and physically aggressive at times, making social relationships still more difficult. They have a tendency to "lose control," particularly when they're in a strange or overwhelming environment, or when angry and frustrated. They may at times break things, attack others, or hurt themselves. In their frustration, some bang their heads, pull their hair, or bite their arms.

## Communication Difficulties

By age three, most children have passed predictable milestones on the path to learning language; one of the earliest is babbling. By the first birthday, a typical toddler says words, turns when he hears his name, points when he wants a toy, and when offered something distasteful, makes it clear that the answer is "no."

Some children diagnosed with ASD remain mute throughout their lives. Some infants who later show signs of ASD coo and babble during the first few months of life, but they soon stop. Others may be delayed, developing language as late as age five to nine. Some children may learn to use communication systems such as pictures or sign language.

Those who do speak often use language in unusual ways. They seem unable to combine words into meaningful sentences. Some speak only single words, while others repeat the same phrase over and over. Some ASD children parrot what they hear, a condition called echolalia. Although many children with no ASD go through a stage where they repeat what they hear, it normally passes by the time they are three.

Some children only mildly affected may exhibit slight delays in language, or even seem to have precocious language and unusually large vocabularies, but have great difficulty in sustaining a conversation. The "give and take" of normal conversation is hard for them, although they often carry on a monologue on a favorite subject, giving no one else an opportunity to comment. Another difficulty is often the inability to understand body language, tone of voice, or "phrases of speech." They might interpret a sarcastic expression such as "Oh, that's just great" as meaning it really *is* great.

While it can be hard to understand what ASD children are saying, their body language is also difficult to understand. Facial expressions, movements, and gestures rarely match what they are saying. Also, their tone of voice fails to reflect their feelings. A high-pitched, singsong, or flat, robot-like voice is common. Some children with relatively good language skills speak like little adults, failing to pick up on the "kid-speak" that is common in their peers.

Without meaningful gestures or the language to ask for things, people with ASD are at a loss to let others know what they need. As a result, they may simply scream or grab what they want. Until they are taught better ways to express their needs, ASD children do whatever they can to get through to others. As people with ASD grow up, they can become increasingly aware of their difficulties in understanding others and in being understood. As a result they may become anxious or depressed.

## Repetitive Behaviors

Although children with ASD usually appear physically normal and have good muscle control, odd repetitive motions may set them off from other children. These behaviors might be extreme and highly apparent or more subtle. Some children and older individuals spend a lot of time repeatedly flapping their arms or walking on their toes. Some suddenly freeze in position.

As children, they might spend hours lining up their cars and trains in a certain way, rather than using them for pretend play. If someone accidentally moves one of the toys, the child may be tremendously upset. ASD children need, and demand, absolute consistency in their environment. A slight change in any routine—in mealtimes, dressing, taking a bath, going to school at a certain time and by the same route—can be extremely disturbing. Perhaps order and sameness lend some stability in a world of confusion.<bt>Repetitive behavior sometimes takes the form of a persistent, intense preoccupation. For example, the child might be obsessed with learning all about vacuum cleaners, train schedules, or lighthouses. Often there is great interest in numbers, symbols, or science topics.

## Problems That May Accompany ASD

**Sensory problems:** When children's perceptions are accurate, they can learn from what they see, feel, or hear. On the other hand, if sensory information is faulty, the child's experiences of the world can be confusing. Many ASD children are highly attuned or even painfully sensitive to certain sounds, textures, tastes, and smells. Some children find the feel of clothes touching their skin almost unbearable. Some sounds—a vacuum cleaner, a ringing telephone, a sudden storm, even the sound of waves lapping the shoreline—will cause these children to cover their ears and scream.

In ASD, the brain seems unable to balance the senses appropriately. Some ASD children are oblivious to extreme cold or pain. An ASD child may fall and break an arm, yet never cry. Another may bash his head against a wall and not wince, but a light touch may make the child scream with alarm.

**Mental retardation:** Many children with ASD have some degree of mental impairment. When tested, some areas of ability may be normal, while others may be especially weak. For example, a child with ASD may do well on the parts of the test that measure visual skills but earn low scores on the language subtests.

**Seizures:** One in four children with ASD develops seizures, often starting either in early childhood or adolescence.[2] Seizures, caused by abnormal electrical activity in the brain, can produce a temporary loss of consciousness (a "blackout"), a body convulsion, unusual movements, or staring spells. Sometimes a contributing factor is a lack of sleep or a high fever. An EEG (electroencephalogram—recording of the electric currents developed in the brain by means of electrodes applied to the scalp) can help confirm the seizure's presence.

In most cases, seizures can be controlled by a number of medicines called "anticonvulsants." The dosage of the medication is adjusted carefully so that the least possible amount of medication will be used to be effective.

**Fragile X syndrome:** This disorder is the most common inherited form of mental retardation. It was so named because one part of the X chromosome has a defective piece that appears pinched and fragile when under a microscope. Fragile X syndrome affects about 2 to 5 percent of people with ASD. It is important to have a child with ASD checked for Fragile X, especially if the parents are considering having another child. For an unknown reason, if a child with ASD also has Fragile X, there is a one-in-two chance that boys born to the same parents will have the syndrome.[3] Other members of the family who may be contemplating having a child may also wish to be checked for the syndrome.

A distinction can be made between a father's and mother's ability to pass along to a daughter or son the altered gene on the X chromosome that is linked to fragile X syndrome. Because both males (XY) and females (XX) have at least one X chromosome, both can pass on the mutated gene to their children.

A father with the altered gene for Fragile X on his X chromosome will only pass that gene on to his daughters. He passes a Y chromosome on to his sons, which doesn't transmit the condition. Therefore, if the father has the altered gene on his X chromosome, but the mother's X chromosomes are normal, all of the couple's daughters would have the altered gene for Fragile X, while none of their sons would have the mutated gene.

Because mothers pass on only X chromosomes to their children, if the mother has the altered gene for Fragile X, she can pass that gene to either her sons or her daughters. If the mother has the mutated gene on one X chromosome and has one normal X chromosome, and the father has no genetic mutations, all the children have a 50-50 chance of inheriting the mutated gene.

The odds noted here apply to each child the parents have.[4]

In terms of prevalence, the latest statistics are consistent in showing that 5 percent of people with autism are affected by fragile X and 10 to 15 percent of those with fragile X show autistic traits.

**Tuberous sclerosis:** Tuberous sclerosis is a rare genetic disorder that causes benign tumors to grow in the brain as well as in other vital organs. It has a consistently strong association with ASD. One to 4 percent of people with ASD also have tuberous sclerosis.[5]

## *References*

1.  Newschaffer CJ (Johns Hopkins Bloomberg School of Public Health). Autism Among Us: *Rising Concerns and the Public Health Response* [Video on the Internet]. Public Health Training Network, 2003 June 20. Available from: http://www .publichealthgrandrounds.unc.edu/autism/webcast.htm.

2.  Volkmar FR. Medical Problems, Treatments, and Professionals. In: Powers MD, ed. *Children with Autism: A Parent's Guide, Second Edition*. Bethesda, MD: Woodbine House, 2000, 73–74.

3.  Powers MD. What Is Autism? In: Powers MD, ed. *Children with Autism: A Parent's Guide, Second Edition*. Bethesda, MD: Woodbine House, 2000, 28.

4.  *Families and Fragile X Syndrome*, U.S. Department of Health and Human Services, Public Health Service, National Institutes of Health, National Institute of Child Health and Human Development. 2003

5.  Smalley SI, Autism and tuberous sclerosis. *Journal of Autism and Developmental Disorders*, 1998; 28(5): 407–14.

# Chapter 18

# *The Importance of Early Autism Diagnosis*

Communication remains key to humans' social development. A simple sentence, a shared smile, or a subtle facial expression can convey a great deal of information, and the ability to recognize and master such forms of communication begins in childhood.

But what if a child can't communicate in a typical way?

Each April, the medical community shifts its focus to a developmental disorder that inhibits social and communicative development in children. According to Jane Charles, M.D., assistant professor of pediatrics, the effects of autism can have a significant impact long after childhood, which is why diagnosis and intervention at an early age remain so important.

"With some children, we can make a diagnosis in the waiting room— it's that obvious," Charles said. "But quite often, the symptoms are subtler. Many cases of autism are difficult to diagnose immediately."

The absence of a test for autism further hinders the disorder's diagnosis. Autism can't be detected through blood work or magnetic resonance imaging (MRI), and many of the disorder's symptoms overlap with those of other developmental disorders.

Some of the more prominent symptoms of autism concern a child's mastery of language. Often, autistic children develop language more slowly or do not develop language at all. A child with autism also may develop abnormal language.

"Early Autism Diagnosis, Intervention Important," April 23, 2004, by Michael Baker, Medical University of South Carolina Children's Hospital Public Relations. © 2004 Medical University of South Carolina. Reprinted with permission.

"Autistic children often develop echolalia, a condition that causes them to repeat things they've heard," Charles explained.

For example, immediate echolalia causes a child to mimic another person's speech directly after the other person has finished speaking—like a game of copycat. With delayed echolalia, children repeat words and phrases they've heard in recent days or even months ago.

"In today's culture, delayed echolalia stands out a bit," Charles said. "Many children who come for diagnosis constantly repeat lines from Disney movies. We call it video talk."

Although children typically learn to communicate through listening and repeating what they hear, the difference between autistic and non-autistic children lies in their cognitive processes.

Charles explained the difference in terms of expressive language (language people use to express themselves) and receptive language (language people can understand). In non-autistic children, the capacity for receptive language must be greater than the capacity for expressive language.

"Technically, you can never say more than you know," she explained.

Conversely, autistic children possess a greater capacity for expressive language than for receptive language. So while autistic children may repeat what they've heard, they often lack any context for or understanding of what they're saying.

Autism also affects joint attention, a child's ability to make certain cognitive connections.

"If I were to point to an object in this room, most people would instinctively follow the movement of my hand. It's called gaze direction," Charles said. "But many autistic children can't make that connection."

Similarly, many autistic children don't respond to their names. Some children don't even acknowledge when another person enters the room, even if that person begins to speak. For non-autistic people, it's an almost natural reaction to show signs of alertness when another person begins to speak.

More troubling than the effects of autism is the disorder's growing incidence.

"Three or four children out of one thousand in the United States have autism, and the number rises every year," Charles said.

The reason for the rising rate remains unclear. One factor could be that the guidelines for autism have loosened in recent years. As a result, more children meet the disorder's criteria.

"Traditionally autistic children experienced a significant amount of mental retardation," Charles said. "Now, many people with autism exhibit all the disorder's symptoms while maintaining a normal IQ."

The testing methods for autism have also improved. Two especially accurate methods, the autism diagnostic interview and the autism diagnostic observation schedule, are the "gold standard" for autism diagnosis, according to Charles.

But for all of autism's improved diagnosis techniques and increasingly specific definitions, the disorder's cause still eludes researchers.

The working theory remains genetically oriented. Researchers often identify abnormalities in certain chromosomes, and many speculate that autism contains a link with fragile X syndrome, a disorder that affects the X-chromosome and commonly causes mental retardation in boys.

Furthering suspicion of autism's genetic origins is its occurrence among siblings. Parents of autistic children have a 6 percent chance of giving birth to another child with autism. Fraternal twins have a 10 percent chance of sharing autism, and identical twins share a 90 percent chance of autistic concordance.

The federal government recently endorsed a commitment to autism research using a cooperative between the departments of Education and Health and Human Services. Within the cooperative, the Department of Education focuses on educational intervention, determining the best way to teach children with autism. The Department of Health and Human Services oversees grants by the National Institutes of Health (NIH) and the Centers for Disease Control and Prevention (CDC). The former examines the ideology of autism including the genetic and environmental factors in the disorder's development, while the latter organization conducts research to determine the prevalence of autism in South Carolina and seventeen other states.

Despite the genetic theories and national research, Charles admits that concrete evidence of autism's cause remains absent. "Despite all of the factors and statistics, we can only identify the cause of autism in 10 or 20 percent of the people we see. With the other 80 or 90 percent, we have no clue."

The lack of a starting point for autism has led Charles to assert the importance of timely intervention.

"The important thing to get across is for pediatricians to push for early recognition," she said. "Physicians and parents need to understand how to recognize the symptoms as early as possible."

The First Signs program in New Jersey took a major step in educating the population when it sent a video detailing the early signs of autism to every physician and parent in the state.

Once parents become aware of the warning signs, they need to take action if necessary. If your child exhibits symptoms of autism, Charles suggests immediately consulting a pediatrician. "If your pediatrician blows you off, proceed anyway," she said. Concerned parents can call Baby Net, an organization that will conduct an assessment of the child in question, start speech therapies if necessary, and even refer the child to a clinic for an autism evaluation.

Regardless of where parents turn for help, Charles maintains that time is crucial.

"Autism is a developmental disorder, but children will develop communication skills," she said. "But the extent of their development depends on how soon you recognize the problem."

Chapter 19

# Screening and Diagnosing Autism Spectrum Disorders

## Chapter Contents

Section 19.1—Guidelines for the Screening and Diagnosis
of Autism ............................................................. 226

Section 19.2—Common Autism Screening Tools and Tests .... 232

Section 19.3—Other Assessments Used in the Diagnosis
of Autism ............................................................. 236

Section 19.4—Medical Tests Used in Diagnosing and
Evaluating Autism ............................................. 248

Section 19.1

# Guidelines for the Screening and Diagnosis of Autism

Excerpted from National Guideline Clearinghouse (NGC), *Guideline Summary: Practice Parameter - Screening and Diagnosis of Autism.* In National Guideline Clearinghouse (NGC) http://www.guideline.gov. Rockville (MD): cited September 29, 2006.

## Level One: Evidence-Based Recommendations for Routine Developmental Surveillance and Screening Specifically for Autism

### Clinical Practice Recommendations

1. Developmental surveillance should be performed at all well-child visits from infancy through school age, and at any age thereafter if concerns are raised about social acceptance, learning, or behavior **(Guideline)**.

2. Recommended developmental screening tools include the Ages and Stages Questionnaire, the BRIGANCE® Screens, the Child Development Inventories, and the Parents' Evaluations of Developmental Status **(Guideline)**.

3. Because of the lack of sensitivity and specificity, the Denver-II (DDST-II) and the Revised Denver Pre-Screening Developmental Questionnaire (R-DPDQ) are not recommended for appropriate primary-care developmental surveillance **(Guideline)**.

4. Further developmental evaluation is required whenever a child fails to meet any of the following milestones **(Guideline)**: babbling by twelve months; gesturing (e.g., pointing, waving bye-bye) by twelve months; single words by sixteen months; two-word spontaneous (not just echolalic) phrases by twenty-four months; loss of any language or social skills at any age.

5. Siblings of children with autism should be carefully monitored for acquisition of social, communication, and play skills, and the

occurrence of maladaptive behaviors. Screening should be performed not only for autism-related symptoms but also for language delays, learning difficulties, social problems, and anxiety or depressive symptoms **(Guideline)**.

6.  Screening specifically for autism should be performed on all children failing routine developmental surveillance procedures using one of the validated instruments: the Checklist for Autism in Toddlers (CHAT) or the Autism Screening Questionnaire **(Guideline)**.

7.  Laboratory investigations recommended for any child with developmental delay and/or autism include audiologic assessment and lead screening **(Guideline)**. Early referral for a formal audiologic assessment should include behavioral audiometric measures, assessment of middle ear function, and electrophysiologic procedures using experienced pediatric audiologists with current audiologic testing methods and technologies **(Guideline)**. Lead screening should be performed in any child with developmental delay and pica. Additional periodic screening should be considered if the pica persists **(Guideline)**.

## Level Two: Evidence-Based Recommendations for Diagnosis and Evaluation for Autism

### Clinical Practice Recommendations

1.  Genetic testing in children with autism, specifically high-resolution chromosome studies (karyotype) and DNA analysis for fragile X, should be performed in the presence of mental retardation (or if mental retardation cannot be excluded), if there is a family history of fragile X or undiagnosed mental retardation, or if dysmorphic features are present **(Standard)**. However, there is little likelihood of positive karyotype or fragile X testing in the presence of high-functioning autism.

2.  Selective metabolic testing **(Standard)** should be initiated by the presence of suggestive clinical and physical findings such as the following: if lethargy, cyclic vomiting, or early seizures are evident; the presence of dysmorphic or coarse features; evidence of mental retardation or if mental retardation cannot be ruled out; or if occurrence or adequacy of newborn screening for a birth is questionable.

3.  There is inadequate evidence at the present time to recommend an electroencephalogram study in all individuals with autism. Indications for an adequate sleep-deprived electroencephalogram with appropriate sampling of slow wave sleep include **(Guideline)** clinical seizures or suspicion of subclinical seizures, and a history of regression (clinically significant loss of social and communicative function) at any age, but especially in toddlers and preschoolers.

4.  Recording of event-related potentials and magnetoencephalography are research tools at the present time, without evidence of routine clinical utility **(Guideline)**.

5.  There is no clinical evidence to support the role of routine clinical neuroimaging in the diagnostic evaluation of autism, even in the presence of megalencephaly **(Guideline)**.

6.  There is inadequate supporting evidence for hair analysis, celiac antibodies, allergy testing (particularly food allergies for gluten, casein, Candida, and other molds), immunologic or neurochemical abnormalities, micronutrients such as vitamin levels, intestinal permeability studies, stool analysis, urinary peptides, mitochondrial disorders (including lactate and pyruvate), thyroid function tests, or erythrocyte glutathione peroxidase studies **(Guideline)**.

## *Consensus-Based General Principles of Management*

The following recommendations are based on consensus agreement by the participating organizations involved in the development of this parameter.

**Surveillance and screening:** In the United States, states must follow federal Public Law 105-17: the Individuals with Disabilities Education Act Amendments of 1997—IDEA'97, which mandates immediate referral for a free appropriate public education for eligible children with disabilities from the age of thirty-six months, and early intervention services for infants and toddlers with disabilities from birth through thirty-five months of age.

**Diagnosis:** The diagnosis of autism should include the use of a diagnostic instrument with at least moderate sensitivity and good specificity for autism. Sufficient time should be planned for standardized parent interviews regarding current concerns and behavioral history related to autism, and direct, structured observation of social and communicative behavior and play. Recommended instruments include the following:

- Diagnostic parental interviews
  - The Gilliam Autism Rating Scale
  - The Parent Interview for Autism
  - The Pervasive Developmental Disorders Screening Test-Stage 3
  - The Autism Diagnostic Interview-Revised
- Diagnostic observation instruments
  - The Childhood Autism Rating Scale
  - The Screening Tool for Autism in Two-Year-Olds
  - The Autism Diagnostic Observation Schedule-Generic

**Medical and neurologic evaluation:** Perinatal and developmental history should include milestones; regression in early childhood or later in life; encephalopathic events; attentional deficits; seizure disorder (absence or generalized); depression or mania; and behaviors such as irritability, self-injury, sleep and eating disturbances, and pica. The physical and neurologic examination should include: longitudinal measurements of head circumference and examination for unusual features (facial, limb, stature, etc.) suggesting the need for genetic evaluation; neurocutaneous abnormalities (requiring an ultraviolet [Wood's] lamp examination); gait; tone; reflexes; cranial nerves; and determination of mental status, including verbal and nonverbal language and play.

**Evaluation and monitoring of autism:** The immediate and long-term evaluation and monitoring of autistic individuals requires a comprehensive multidisciplinary approach, and can include one or more of the following professionals: psychologists, neurologists, speech-language pathologists and audiologists, pediatricians, child psychiatrists, occupational therapists, and physical therapists, as well as educators and special educators. Individuals with mild autism should also receive adequate assessments and appropriate diagnoses.

Reevaluation within one year of initial diagnosis and continued monitoring is an expected aspect of clinical practice because relatively small changes in the developmental level affect the impact of autism in the preschool years. In general, there is no need to repeat extensive diagnostic testing; however, follow-up visits can be helpful to address behavioral, environmental, and other developmental concerns.

**Speech, language, and communication evaluation:** A comprehensive speech-language-communication evaluation should be performed on all children who fail language developmental screening procedures by a speech-language pathologist with training and expertise in evaluating children with developmental disabilities. Comprehensive assessments of both pre-verbal and verbal individuals should account for age, cognitive level, and socioemotional abilities, and should include assessment of receptive language and communication, expressive language and communication, voice and speech production, and in verbal individuals, a collection and analysis of spontaneous language samples to supplement scores on formal language tests.

**Cognitive and adaptive behavior evaluations:** Cognitive evaluations should be performed in all children with autism by a psychologist or other trained professional. Cognitive instruments should be appropriate for the mental and chronological age, provide a full range (in the lower direction) of standard scores and current norms independent of social ability, include independent measures of verbal and nonverbal abilities, and provide an overall index of ability. A measure of adaptive functioning should be collected for any child evaluated for an associated cognitive handicap. Consensus-based recommendations for using specific instruments include the Vineland Adaptive Behavior Scales and the Scales of Independent Behavior-Revised.

**Sensorimotor and occupational therapy evaluations:** Evaluation of sensorimotor skills by a qualified experienced professional (occupational therapist or physical therapist) should be considered, including assessment of gross and fine motor skills, praxis, sensory processing abilities, unusual or stereotyped mannerisms, and the impact of these components on the autistic person's life. An occupational therapy evaluation is indicated when deficits exist in functional skills or occupational performance in the areas of play or leisure, self-maintenance through activities of daily living, or productive school and work tasks. Although not routinely warranted as part of all evaluations of children with autism, the sensory integration and praxis tests may be used on an individual basis to detect specific patterns of sensory integrative dysfunction.

**Neuropsychological, behavioral, and academic assessment:**
These assessments should be performed as needed, in addition to the cognitive assessment, to include social skills and relationships, educational functioning, problematic behaviors, learning style, motivation and reinforcement, sensory functioning, and self-regulation. Assessment of family resources should be performed by appropriate psychologists or other qualified health care professionals and should include assessment of parents' level of understanding of their child's condition, family (parent and sibling) strengths, talents, stressors and adaptation, resources and supports, as well as offer appropriate counseling and education.

## Definitions

### Strength of the Recommendations

**Standard:** A principle for patient management that reflects a high degree of clinical certainty (usually requires one or more class I studies that directly address the clinical question, or overwhelming class II evidence when circumstances preclude randomized clinical trials).

**Guideline:** A recommendation for patient management that reflects moderate clinical certainty (usually requires one or more class II studies or a strong consensus of class III evidence).

**Practice option:** Strategy for patient management for which clinical utility is uncertain (inconclusive or conflicting evidence or opinion).

### Quality of the Evidence

**Class I:** Must have all of a through d. (a) Prospective study of a well-defined cohort which includes a description of the nature of the population, the inclusion/exclusion criteria, demographic characteristics such as age and sex, and seizure type. (b) The sample size must be adequate with enough statistical power to justify a conclusion or for identification of subgroups for whom testing does or does not yield significant information. (c) The interpretation of evaluations performed must be done blinded to outcome. (d) There must be a satisfactory description of the technology used for evaluations (e.g., electroencephalogram, magnetic resonance imaging).

**Class II:** Must have a or b. (a) Retrospective study of a well-defined cohort which otherwise meets criteria for class 1a, 1b, and 1d. (b) Prospective or retrospective study which lacks any of the following: adequate sample size, adequate methodology, a description of inclusion/exclusion criteria, and information such as age, sex, and characteristics of the seizure.

**Class III:** Must have a or b. (a) A small cohort or case report. (b) Relevant expert opinion, consensus, or survey. A cost-benefit analysis or a meta-analysis may be class I, II, or III, depending on the strength of the data upon which the analysis is based.

## Section 19.2

# Common Autism Screening Tools and Tests

"Table of All Screening Tools and Rating Scales: Pervasive Developmental Disorder and Autism Spectrum." The following table is reprinted with permission from www.schoolpsychiatry.org, a website for parents, educators, and clinicians that address the needs of children and teens who have mental health conditions. © 2006 by the Massachusetts General Hospital Department of Psychiatry.

The scales described below can help identify a variety of symptoms affecting children and adolescents. Do not assume that a particular "score" on any rating scale or screening tool means a child has a particular disorder—these instruments are only one component of an evaluation. Diagnoses should be made only by a trained clinician after a thorough assessment. Symptoms suggestive of suicidal or harmful behaviors warrant immediate attention by a trained clinician.

### Childhood Autism Test (CHAT)

The CHAT is a screening tool developed for pediatricians to use at the eighteen-month checkup for children. Clinicians complete five items based on observation and ask parents to answer yes/no to an additional nine items. Each section takes an average of five minutes to complete. If parents suspect a pervasive developmental disorder, they can print out this scale, complete the parent items, and take it to their primary care provider. A revised CHAT form is now available that may pick up more cases of autism spectrum disorders (ASD). It is available free at www.firstsigns.org/downloads/m-chat.PDF.

## Autism Screening Instrument for Educational Planning (ASIEP-2)

The ASIEP-2 provides data on five unique components of behavior in individuals from eighteen months of age through adulthood. This tool takes 90–120 minutes to administer. The ASIEP-2 examines behavior in five areas: (a) sensory, relating, body concept, language, and social self-help; (b) vocal behavior; (c) interaction; (d) communication; and (e) learning rate. When combined, these subtests provide a profile of abilities in spontaneous verbal behavior, social interaction, education level, and learning characteristics.

## Pervasive Developmental Disorders Screening Test (PDDST)

The PDDST is designed as a screening test for children between the ages of eighteen months and three years, and includes seventy-one items. The test includes three levels, each of which takes about five minutes to complete.

## Autism Diagnostic Interview-Revised (ADI-R)

A structured interview containing four main factors: the child's communication, social interaction, repetitive behaviors, and age-of-onset symptoms. Because of the time needed to administer the ADI-R by clinically trained personnel (1.5–2.5 hours), this test may not be a practical assessment method in many clinical situations. It contains ninety-three items to be asked of the primary caregiver with children older than two years old.

## Autism Diagnostic Observation Schedule (ADOS)

A standardized instrument for diagnosis of autism, primarily in research settings, designed to detect social and communicative behavior associated with autism and related disorders. It is used with children older than age two. General ratings are provided for four areas: reciprocal social interaction, communication/language, stereotyped/restricted behaviors, and mood and nonspecific abnormal behaviors. Each module requires thirty-five to forty minutes to administer. ADOS measures

233

both nonverbal and pre-verbal communication components, and is conducted by intensively trained clinicians based on the subject's use of language. (It is not used with nonverbal adolescents or adults.)

## Childhood Autism Rating Scale (CARS)

This fifteen-item behavior rating scale helps to identify children, older than age two, with autism, and to distinguish them from developmentally handicapped children who do not have autism. Because it gives a symptom severity rating, the CARS may be useful for periodic monitoring and for assessing response to treatments or interventions. The CARS requires specialized clinical training to administer.

## Autism Behavior Checklist (ABC)

The ABC is part of a broader tool, the Autism Screening Instrument for Educational Planning (ASIEP), that profiles abilities in spontaneous verbal behavior, social interaction, education level, and learning characteristics. The ABC is designed to be completed independently by a parent or a teacher familiar with a child older than age three. It measures target behaviors for intervention, and can be repeated to clarify the impact of treatment interventions. The checklist has fifty-seven questions divided into five categories of behavior: (a) sensory, (b) relating, (c) body and object use, (d) language, and (e) social and self-help.

## Gilliam Autism Rating Scale (GARS)

Designed for use by teachers, parents, and clinicians, the GARS helps to identify and diagnose autism in individuals ages three to twenty-two and to estimate the severity of the problem. The fifty-six items are grouped into four subtests that examine stereotyped behaviors, communication, social interaction, and developmental disturbances for parents to contribute data about their child's development during the first three years of life. The entire scale can be completed in approximately five to ten minutes.

## Autism Research Institute's Form E-2 Checklist

This 109-item diagnostic checklist form rates behaviors frequently seen in autism, and also asks parents to rate the results of any treatments they have tried. It is available in several languages and is used with children ages three to five. Parents who send the completed checklist to ARI will receive scaled test results, interpretive information, and information on autistic spectrum disorders (currently at no charge). The checklist takes fifteen to twenty minutes to complete and is available free at: http://www.patientcenters.com/autism/news/diag _tools.html#ARI

## Social Communication Questionnaire (SCQ)

Previously known as the Autism Screening Questionnaire (ASQ), this forty-item yes/no questionnaire helps evaluate communication skills and social functioning in children and adolescents who may have autism or autism spectrum disorders. The questionnaire can be used to evaluate anyone older than age four, as long as mental age exceeds 2.0 years. Completed by a parent/primary caregiver in less than ten minutes, the SCQ determines whether a child or adolescent should be referred for a complete diagnostic evaluation. Forms can be given directly to the parent, who can answer the questions without supervision.

## Autism Treatment Evaluation Checklist (ATEC)

The Autism Research Institute (ARI) has developed this simple internet scoring instrument (containing seventy-seven items) that provides subscale scores and a summary score. Although designed to evaluate the effectiveness of treatments for autism, it may also prove useful for screening and diagnosis in children ages five to twelve. Since the ATEC is a simple one-page form that can be copied freely and scored immediately (currently at no cost) at the following website, it might be very useful as a diagnostic tool The checklist takes ten to fifteen minutes to complete and can be completed online or printed out at: https://www.autismeval.com/ari-atec/atec_form.pdf

## Pervasive Developmental Disorder Assessment Scale (PDDAS)

An experimental forty-four-item screening scale useful for measuring symptoms of social interaction, speech and language, and play in children ages six to twelve. Since the scale employs mild, moderate, severe, none, and resolved categories, it can be repeated to measure the impact of interventions. It takes five to ten minutes to complete and is available free at: http://www.childbrain.com/pddq6.shtml

Section 19.3

# Other Assessments Used in the Diagnosis of Autism

## Diagnostic Evaluations

**Childhood Autism Rating Scale (CARS):** The CARS is a fifteen-item structured interview and observation instrument that is suitable for use with any child over twenty-four months of age. The objective of CARS is to identify children with autism and to distinguish them from developmentally handicapped children who are not autistic. In addition, it distinguishes mild to moderate from severe autism. Each item uses a seven-point rating scale to indicate the degree to which the child's behavior deviates from an age-appropriate norm. Age range: twenty-four months of age and up. Time: thirty to forty-five minutes.

**The Checklist for Autism in Toddlers (CHAT):** The CHAT is designed to detect core autistic features to enable treatment as early as eighteen months. The CHAT offers clinicians a means of diagnosing autism in infancy so that educational programs can be started months or even years before most autistic symptoms become obvious. Age range: eighteen months and up. Time: thirty minutes.

**Gilliam Autism Rating Scale (GARS-II):** Gilliam Autism Rating Scale is a diagnostic tool helpful in estimating the severity of the child's disorder, based on the definitions of autism adopted by the Autism Society of America and the DSM-IV-TR (2000). The GARS consists of forty-two items describing the characteristic behaviors of persons with autism and includes three subscales: stereotyped behaviors, communication, and social interaction. Ages: three through twenty-two. Time: five to ten minutes.

**Gilliam Asperger's Disorder Scale (GADS):** The GADS is a diagnostic tool consisting of several subscales, including: restricted pattern of behavior, cognitive patterns, pragmatic skills, early development, and key question. Age range: three to twenty-two years. Time: forty-five minutes.

**Autism Diagnostic Interview-Revised (ADI-R):** The ADI-R is a standardized clinical review for caregivers of children and adults. The interview contains 111 items and focuses on behaviors in three content areas: quality of social interaction, (e.g., emotional sharing, offering and seeking comfort, social smiling and responding to other children); communication and language (e.g., stereotyped utterances, pronoun reversal, social usage of language); and repetitive, restricted, and stereotyped interests and behavior (e.g., unusual preoccupations, hand and finger mannerisms, unusual sensory interests). The measure also includes other items relevant for treatment planning, such as self-injury and overactivity. Responses are scored by the clinician based on the caregiver's description of the child's behavior. Age range: Toddler (eighteen months) through adult. Time: 1.5 to 2+ hours.

**Autism Diagnostic Observation Schedule (ADOS):** The ADOS is a semi-structured observation assessment used to evaluate children with no speech to adults who are verbally fluent. The ADOS consists of four modules, and each individual is given just one module, depending on his or her expressive language level and chronological age. Age range: Toddler to adult. Time: thirty-five to forty-five minutes.

## Intelligence Assessments

**Wechsler Preschool and Primary Scales of Intelligence - Third Edition (WPPSI-III):** The Wechsler Intelligence Scales for Children is primarily an IQ test used as a tool in school placement, in determining the presence of a learning disability or a developmental delay, in identifying giftedness, and in tracking intellectual development. Age range: 2 years 6 months to 7 years 3 months. Time: two to three hours.

**Wechsler Intelligence Scale for Children IV - Integrated (WISC-IV-Integrated):** The WISC is a clinical instrument designed to assess cognitive ability and problem-solving processes. The test framework of the WISC is organized into four cognitive domains: verbal, perceptual, working memory, and processing speed. As a psychoeducational tool, the WISC is used to obtain a comprehensive assessment of general cognitive functioning. It is also used as an assessment to identify intellectual giftedness, mental retardation, and cognitive strengths and weaknesses in children with a variety of developmental and neurological conditions. Results are often used as a guide for treatment planning and placement decisions in clinical and educational settings and can provide invaluable clinical information for neuropsychological evaluations and research purposes. Age range: 6 years 0 months to 16 years 11 months. Time: two to three hours.

**Stanford-Binet Intelligence Scale, Fourth Edition (SBIS-IV):** The Stanford-Binet is a battery of fifteen subtests assessing cognitive ability. It measures four areas: verbal reasoning; abstract/visual reasoning; quantitative reasoning; and short-term memory. It is used as a tool in school placement, in determining the presence of a learning disability or a developmental delay, and in tracking intellectual development. In addition, it is sometimes included in neuropsychological testing to assess the brain function of individuals with neurological impairments. Age range: two to twenty-three. Time: forty-five to ninety minutes.

**Bayley Scales of Infant Development, Second Edition (BSID-II):** The BSID-II is a standardized assessment of cognitive and motor development. BSID-II provides infants and children with situations and tasks to capture their interest and produce an observable set of behavior responses for the assessment of current developmental functioning. BSID is often used as one of the first assessments to establish the diagnoses of developmental delay and in planning intervention strategies. Ages: one to thirty-six months. Time: forty-five to sixty minutes.

**Leiter International Performance Scale-Revised (LIPS-R):** The LIPS-R is a nonverbal measure of intellectual ability, memory, and attention often used to assess children, adolescents, and young adults who cannot reliably and validly be assessed with traditional intelligence tests. LIPS-R provides activities that foster attention and allows the examiner to observe the child's approach to problem solving, as well as his or her emotional reactions. Because directions are communicated by pantomime, it is widely used with non-English-speaking subjects, illiterate or disadvantaged individuals, and those with speech, hearing, or other medical disabilities. Age range: 2 years to 20 years, 11 months. Time: two hours.

**Merrill Palmer Scale of Mental Tests (MPSMT):** The MPSMT is widely used as a nonverbal test instrument for assessing visual-spatial skills. MPSMT enables a more detailed assessment of visual-perceptual functioning than is provided by the BSID-II or the WPPSI-III. Ages: 1.6 to 6.0 years. Time: one hour.

**Differential Abilities Scale (DAS):** The DAS measures conceptual and reasoning abilities. It includes a preschool level and a school age level. DAS comprises seventeen cognitive and three achievement subtests. It measures general conceptual ability, verbal and nonverbal ability for the preschool subsets, and verbal, nonverbal reasoning, and spatial ability for the school-age subtests. For language-impaired and non-English-speaking children, a special nonverbal score may be obtained. The DAS is also a measure of basic academic skills. Achievement subtests are basic number skills, spelling, and word reading. Age range: thirty months to seventeen years. Time: three hours.

## Developmental Assessments

**The Developmental Profile II:** The Developmental Profile is a comprehensive assessment of motor, language, personal/self-help, social, and intellectual development. The format is a 186-item inventory designed to assess a child's functional, developmental age level. The test may be administered either in interview format to the parent, as a combination of parent interview and direct testing of the child, or as a self-interview completed by a teacher. Ages: birth to seven years for typically developing children and for developmentally delayed children of any age when their skills are not expected to extend beyond the nine-year ceiling. Time: one hour.

**Brigance Early Development Inventory:** The Brigance Inventory is intended for informal assessment of several aspects of child development and is for children functioning at developmental levels from birth to seven years of age. Major areas assessed include general knowledge and comprehension, speech and language, preacademics, self-help, and psychomotor skills. Within these major areas, there are ninety-eight subtests of sequenced developmental skills. Age: birth to seven years. Time: three hours.

## Adaptive

**Vineland Adaptive Behavior Scales:** The Vineland is a structured interview administered to parents assessing the extent to which their child exhibits behaviors that are needed to cope effectively with the everyday environment. Age range: birth to eighteen years. Time: twenty to sixty minutes.

## Visual Motor

**The Beery-Buktenica Developmental Test of Visual-Motor Integration - 4th Edition (VMI-4):** The VMI assesses visual perception and fine motor coordination necessary for near point copying and handwriting. Low scores on this test may suggest further testing needs to be done to determine if the difficulty lies in the visual perception process, or in the motor response, or in both. Age range: three years to adult. Time: twenty to thirty minutes.

## Psycho-Educational

**Psychoeducational Profile - Revised (PEP-R):** The PEP-R assesses skills and behaviors of children with autism and communicative disabilities who function between the ages of six months and seven years. PEP-R administration graphically represents uneven development, emerging skills, and autistic behavioral characteristics. PEP-R evaluates the learning problems of children with autism spectrum disorder and related communication disorders, and it provides data that can be used to plan behavioral interventions and education programs. It also assesses developmental functioning in the areas of imitation, perception, fine motor, gross motor, eye-hand integration, cognitive performance, cognitive verbal, and behavior. Age ranges: six months to seven years. Time: two hours.

## Speech and Language

**Preschool Language Scale Fourth Edition (PLS-4):** The Preschool Language Scale is a standardized test of auditory comprehension and expressive communication for infants and toddlers. The auditory comprehension subscale assesses basic vocabulary, concepts and grammatical markers in preschool and higher-level abilities such as complex sentences, making comparisons, and inferences in older children. The expressive communication subscale asks preschoolers to name objects, use concepts that describe objects, express quantity, use grammatical markers, etc. It also includes word segmentation, completing analogies, and telling a short story in sequence. Ages: 0 to 6 years, 11 months. Time: fifteen to thirty minutes.

**Goldman-Fristoe-Woodcock Test of Auditory Discrimination:** The Goldman-Fristoe-Woodcock is a systematic means of assessing an individual's articulation of the consonant sounds of standard

American English. It provides a wide range of information by sampling both spontaneous and imitative sound production, including single words and conversational speech. Ages: two to twenty-one years. Time: fifteen minutes.

**Test of Language Development Primary and Intermediate - Third Edition (TOLD-3):** The Test of Language Development identifies language disorders by profiling strengths and deficiencies in basic language abilities, including syntax, semantics, and morphology. The primary form contains nine subtests: picture vocabulary, relational vocabulary, oral vocabulary, grammatic understanding, sentence imitation, grammatic completion, word articulation, phonemic analysis, and word discrimination. The intermediate form contains six subtests: general, malapropisms, picture vocabulary, sentence combining, word ordering and grammatic comprehension. Age range: four to eight years (primary); eight to twelve years (intermediate). Time: forty minutes.

**Clinical Evaluation of Language Fundamentals - Third Edition (CELF-3):** The CELF-3 evaluates expressive and receptive language ability. It focuses on word meanings, word and sentence structure, and recall of spoken language. It uses pictures as stimulus for all three areas of language development. The linguistic concepts subtest evaluates the child's knowledge of modifiers and his or her ability to interpret one-level oral directions. The sentence structure subtest evaluates comprehension of early acquired sentence formation rules and the child's ability to comprehend and respond to spoken sentences. The recalling sentences in context subtest evaluates recall and repetition of spoken sentences. Formulating labels assesses the child's ability to name pictures. The word structure subtest assesses the child's knowledge and use of early acquired morphological rules and forms. Age: six to twenty-one years. Time: three hours.

**Clinical Evaluation of Language Fundamentals - Preschool (CELF-P):** The CELF-P assists in identifying children who have deficits in these language skills: word meanings, word structure, sentence structure, and recall and retrieval. Age: three to six years. Time: two hours.

**Peabody Picture Vocabulary Test-Revised (PPVT-III):** The PPVT measures listening comprehension for spoken words in standard English and a screening test of verbal ability. The purpose of PPVT is to obtain a valid, reliable norm-referenced measure of receptive vocabulary. Its uses include testing preschool children in vocabulary acquisition, an important indicator of a child's linguistic and cognitive development, screening both for giftedness and mental retardation, measuring English language proficiency in individuals for whom English is not a primary language, detecting language impairments, testing persons who have moderate visual disabilities, and research studies. Age range: 2 years 6 months to 90 years. Time: fifteen minutes.

## Pragmatic Language

**Language Processing Test - Revised (LPT-R):** The LPT-R assesses the ability to process, organize, and attach meaning to auditory information using the following subtests: labeling, associations, similarities, multiple meanings, stating functions, categorization, differences, and attributes. Age range: five to eleven years. Time: thirty-five minutes.

**Test of Pragmatic Language (TOPL):** The TOPL contains forty-four items to assess children's ability to effectively use pragmatic language. Subtests include physical setting, audience, topic, purpose, visual-gestural cues, and abstraction. The TOPL is also used with adult remedial, English-as-a-second language, and aphasic children. Age range: five to thirteen years. Time: forty-five minutes.

## Social Skills/Play Assessments

**Social Behavior Assessment Inventory (SBAI):** The SBAI is a 136-item curriculum-based teacher rating instrument that measures the performance level of social behaviors of children in a classroom setting. Four areas of social behaviors are assessed: environmental behavior, interpersonal behaviors, self-related behaviors, and task-related behaviors. Age range: Grades kindergarten to nine. Time: thirty to forty-five minutes.

**Social Skills Rating Scale (SSRS):** The Social Skills Rating Scale allows for a comprehensive evaluation of teacher report, parent report, and child of social behaviors. It includes the areas of social skills (cooperation, assertion, responsibility, empathy, self-control), problem behaviors (external, internal, hyperactivity), and academic competence. Age range: three to eighteen years. Time: twenty-five minutes.

**Social Responsiveness Scale (SRS):** Social Responsiveness Scale is a quantitative measure of autistic social impairment in preschoolers, suitable for assessing treatment response. Age range: four to eighteen years. Time: fifteen to twenty minutes.

**Symbolic Play Scale:** The Symbolic Play Scale provides an overview of the development of symbolic play in children. Age: eighteen months to six years. Time: one hour.

## Executive Functioning/Neuropsychological Testing

**Test of Problem Solving, Elementary and Adolescent-Revised (TOPS-R):** The TOPS-R assesses how children use language to think, reason, and solve problems. It uses age-appropriate tasks to determine strengths and weaknesses in a number of areas: clarifying, analyzing, generating solutions, empathizing, affective thinking, using context cues, and vocabulary comprehension. Age range: six to eleven years (elementary), twelve to seventeen years (adolescent). Time: thirty-five to forty minutes.

**Behavioral Rating Inventory of Executive Functioning - Preschool (BRIEF-P):** The BRIEF-P consists of a single rating form used by parents, teachers, and day care providers to rate a child's executive functions within the context of his or her everyday environments (i.e., home and preschool). The BRIEF-P rating form consists of sixty-three items that measure various aspects of executive functioning, including inhibition, shifting, emotional control, working memory, and planning/organizing. The clinical scales form three broad indexes (inhibitory self-control, flexibility, and emergent metacognition) and one global executive score. Age range: 2 years to 5 years, 11 months.

**Behavior Rating Inventory of Executive Functioning (BRIEF):** The BRIEF consists of two rating forms—a parent questionnaire and a teacher questionnaire designed to assess executive functioning in the home and school environments. Each BRIEF questionnaire contains eighty-six items in eight nonoverlapping clinical scales and two validity scales. These scales form two broader indexes: behavioral regulation and metacognition, as well as a global executive score. Age range: five to eighteen years. Time: thirty minutes.

**Children's Color Trails Test (CCTT):** The Children's Color Trails Test assesses sustained attention, sequencing, and other executive functions while reducing reliance on language and diminishing the effects of cultural bias and parental verbal report. The CCTT is appropriate for testing children within cross-cultural contexts and children with special needs. Time: twenty to thirty minutes.

**The Auditory Sequential Memory Test:** The Auditory Sequential Memory Test is designed to assess ability to repeat from immediate memory an increasing series of digits. Time: twenty minutes.

**The Stroop Test:** The Stroop Test targets inhibition, mental vitality, and flexibility by measuring the speed and accuracy of reading single words (blue, green, yellow), recognizing and naming blocks of color (red, yellow, green), and naming the color that a word is written in regardless of the content of the word (e.g., "green" is presented and the answer is "yellow"—the color that the word is written in). Time: twenty to thirty minutes.

**Tower of Hanoi:** The Tower of Hanoi is a computerized task assessing planning ability within executive functioning. The goal of this task is to move all the discs from the left peg to the right one, moving only one disc at a time, using the smallest number of moves possible. Time: thirty minutes.

**Wisconsin Card Sorting Test:** The Wisconsin Card Sorting Test assesses perseveration and abstract thinking. It allows the clinician to assess the following frontal lobe functions: strategic planning, organized searching, utilizing environmental feedback to shift cognitive sets, directing behavior toward achieving a goal, and modulating impulsive responding. Age range: 6.5 to 89.0 years. Time: twenty to thirty minutes.

**Developmental Neuropsychological Assessment (NEPSY):** The NEPSY is a battery of tests designed to identify neuropsychological deficits that interfere with learning. The NEPSY measures five complex cognitive functional domains: attention/executive, language, sensorimotor, visuospatial processing and memory, and learning. Age range: kindergarten to grade 7. Time: two to three hours.

## Others

**Autism Phenotype Events Questionnaire (APEQ):** The APEQ is a 160-item questionnaire designed to obtain information on the characteristics of the child's presentation and potential environmental exposures that may be related to features of autism. Time: three to four hours.

**Autism Treatment Evaluation Checklist (ATEC):** The ATEC is a one-page form consisting of four subtests. ATEC is designed to assist parents, physicians, and researchers to evaluate various treatments for autism. Time: thirty minutes.

## Repeated Measures

### Subjective Questionnaires

**Aberrant Behavior Checklist (ABC):** The Aberrant Behavior Checklist is a fifty-eight-item rating scale developed for persons with developmental disabilities. It is designed to be used with clients living in the community, often used to assess medication effects on persons with developmental disabilities. Age range: five to fifty-one and up. Time: thirty minutes.

**Clinical Global Impression (CGI):** The Clinical Global Impression scale is a three-item scale designed to assess global severity, improvement, and side effects. It is widely used in clinical drug studies. Time: five minutes.

**Achenbach Child Behavior Checklist (CBCL):** The CBCL is a widely used, standardized assessment of a child's competencies and problems in the social, emotional, and behavioral realms as reported by parents, teachers, and the child. Age range: two to eighteen years. Time: thirty minutes.

**Questions about Behavioral Function (QABF):** The QABF is a checklist designed to assess antecedent behavior and a targeted maladaptive behavior of self-injurious behavior, aggression, or stereotypy in persons with mental retardation and developmental disabilities. Time: fifteen minutes.

**The Parent Stress Index (PSI):** The PSI is a thirty-six-item measure of parents' self-reported stress along several dimensions: parental distress, parent-child dysfunctional interaction, and difficult child. The instrument has established reliability and validity across ethnic/cultural groups representative of the U.S. population. Time: thirty minutes.

**Side Effects and Symptom Questionnaire:** The side effects and symptom questionnaire is a twenty-five-item measure of reported changes in the child's behavior. Time: ten minutes.

## Objective Measures

**Skills assessments:** The number of specific skills acquired (i.e., CARD program data) will be collected during the entire investigation. These skills are subdivided into language, adaptive skills, social skills, play skills, social cognitive and metacognitive skills, gross motor and fine motor skills, executive functioning and school skills. A comprehensive skills assessment will be completed prior to and following intervention. The skills assessment consists of a checklist that identifies specific operants mastered by a child within skill areas that are organized according to developmental age levels. Time: Initial administration: eight hours; subsequent administrations: three hours.

**Natural environment direct observations:** Behavioral observations will be conducted two to three times per week, totaling at least one hour (i.e., six ten-minute sessions per week). Some observations may be videotaped to be scored at a later time with prior parental consent. All behavioral observations will be conducted under a stable and constant condition (i.e., free play situation) for all participants. During this condition, the child participant will be given preferred tangible items or provided with engaging activities with periodic attention from his caregivers. The following target behaviors will be measured. Reliability will be taken in at least 25 percent of the observations:

- Frequency of inappropriate behavior
- Duration in-seat
- Duration of stereotypy (three-second delay to count)
- Engagement (physical contact with toy/task materials)
- Frequency or duration of vocalization
- Number of words uttered
- Frequency of social initiation/reciprocation

**Repeated acquisition:** A defining feature of autism is a global delay in one's ability to learn. Repeated acquisition tasks are commonly used in behavioral pharmacology studies to assess the effect

246

of a drug on the ability of an organism to learn, that is, the efficiency with which the organism's behavior is brought under new forms of stimulus control. Repeated acquisition tasks typically involve the participant learning to respond to a new sequence of positions during each session. For example, four quadrants are presented and the participant must select three quadrants in a particular sequence in order to earn reinforcement. However, the correct sequence is different for every session, and typically one session is conducted per day, so the sequence of responding required to earn reinforcement is different each day. The performance of the participant can be analyzed in a number of ways, including the percentage correct for the entire session, the total number of responses, or the number of errors made until correct responding is reached according to a set criterion.

The complexity of the task can be adjusted by varying either or both of two parameters: 1) the number of response positions present (e.g., number of stimuli present), and 2) the number of responses in the sequence required for reinforcement. For example, ten stimuli could be present but the participant only required to press one particular one out of those ten in order to get reinforcement, versus pressing a sequence of ten which involves each stimuli once, versus having only two stimuli present, etc. The standard degree of complexity in behavioral pharmacology research is having three response options present and requiring the participant to respond to all three in a particular order to earn reinforcement.

**Delayed matching to sample (DMTS):** An additional cognitive process that might be of interest is "short-term memory." A common behavioral measure of short-term memory is a delayed matching to sample procedure. In such procedures, a sample stimulus is presented and then removed and a delay occurs between the removal of the sample stimulus and the presentation of two or more comparison stimuli. The participant earns reinforcement for choosing the correct comparison stimulus. The delay between the removal of the sample stimulus and the presentation of the comparison stimuli can vary from simultaneous, zero, four, eight, sixteen, but typically does not exceed thirty seconds.

The relation between the sample stimulus and the correct comparison stimulus can be varied in order to alter the difficulty of the task. For example, the sample stimulus and the correct comparison stimulus may be identical, often referred to as "identity matching." This is probably the easiest form of delayed matching to sample. Alternatively, the sample stimulus may be related to the correct comparison stimulus in a more abstract way. For example, the sample stimulus may be the written word "vehicle" and the correct comparison stimulus might be a bicycle, with a gorilla and a fork as distracters.

Sessions can be conducted with a fixed delay or the delay can be systematically increased during the session in order to identify a "breaking point" at which the participant is no longer able to respond correctly. For example, on the first trial, the delay may be zero and then the delay may be increased by one second on each subsequent trial, contingent on correct responding on the previous trial. Errors can produce a reduction in the delay by one second. The data are then analyzed to determine the longest delay at which the participant was consistently correct, according to some criterion. This "breaking point" can be considered a measure of the participant's "short-term memory" at the time of the session.

## Section 19.4

# *Medical Tests Used in Diagnosing and Evaluating Autism*

"Diagnosing and Evaluating Autism: Part 1," © 2003 Center for Autism and Related Disabilities, University of Florida–Gainesville (www.card.ufl .edu). Reprinted with permission.

Autism and related disabilities, such as PDD-NOS (pervasive developmental disorder—not otherwise specified), Asperger syndrome, and Rett syndrome, are difficult to diagnose, especially in young children where speech and reasoning skills are still developing. A child may be three years old before the full characteristics of these disabilities are apparent. Typically, medical professionals are not trained extensively in diagnosing and evaluating autism and related disabilities. Doctors will usually rule out other possibilities before mentioning autism.

Although autism is considered a neurological disability, no specific medical test or procedure can confirm a diagnosis of autism. To gather more information that will accurately profile an individual's strengths and needs, a variety of tests, assessments, and evaluations should be administered.

This section includes brief descriptions of some medical tests and evaluations that may be ordered for children suspected of having autism or a related disability.

## Medical Tests

Given the variety of theories about the causes of autism and related disabilities, doctors may use various medical tests and procedures to help with diagnosis.

There is not always a clinical need to do medical tests. Your doctor(s) can recommend when, or if, a test should be done.

The following medical tests may help with diagnosis and possibly suggest changes in an intervention or treatment strategy.

**Hearing:** Various tests such as an audiogram, tympanogram, and the brain stem evoked response can indicate whether a person has a hearing impairment. Audiologists or hearing specialists have methods to test the hearing of any individual by measuring responses such as turning their head, blinking, or staring when a sound is presented. If a hearing impairment is detected, treatment could involve minor surgery, use of hearing aids, or antibiotics.

**Electroencephalogram (EEG):** An EEG measures brain waves that can show seizure disorders. In addition, an EEG may indicate tumors or other brain abnormalities. Additional tests will be needed to make an accurate diagnosis of these conditions. During an EEG, sixteen small sensors are placed at various locations on the scalp to record brain waves that a neurologist interprets. An EEG may take one to twenty-four hours, depending on the doctor's goals when ordering the test. If seizure activity is detected, additional testing may be required and various medications could be prescribed.

**Metabolic screening:** Blood and urine lab tests measure how a person metabolizes food and its impact on growth and development. Some autism spectrum disorders can be treated with special diets.

The following medical tests may help locate neurological factors that can affect typical development and could possibly identify or rule out a cause. Results will probably not change intervention or treatment.

**Magnetic resonance imaging (MRI):** An MRI involves using magnetic sensing equipment to create an image of the brain in extremely fine detail. The patient lies on a sliding table inside a cylinder-shaped magnetic machine and must be still during the procedure. Sometimes patients are sedated in order to complete the MRI.

**Computer assisted axial tomography (CAT SCAN):** An x-ray tube rotates around the patient, taking thousands of exposures that are sent to a computer, where the section of the body that is x-rayed is reconstructed in great detail. CAT scans are helpful in diagnosing structural problems with the brain.

**Genetic testing:** Blood tests look for abnormalities in the genes which could cause a developmental disability.

## Therapy Evaluations

Many individuals with autism and related disabilities require some form of special therapy at some point during their lives. Therapeutic evaluations can help determine if therapy is required to help an individual fulfill their potential.

**Speech-language therapy:** People with autism usually have delays in communication. The most obvious is when they are nonverbal. Yet people who are verbal may also have serious difficulties.

Some individuals can repeat words but can't use language in a meaningful way, which is called echolalia. A speech pathologist who specializes in the diagnosis and treatment of language problems and speech disorders can help a person learn how to effectively communicate.

Speech therapists look for a system of communication that will work for an individual with autism and may consider alternatives to the spoken word such as signing, typing, or a picture board with words.

**Occupational therapy:** Commonly focuses on improving fine motor skills, such as brushing teeth, feeding, and writing, or sensory motor skills that include balance (vestibular system), awareness of body position (proprioceptive system), and touch (tactile system).

After the therapist identifies a specific problem, therapy may include sensory integration activities such as massage, firm touch, swinging, and bouncing.

**Physical therapy:** Specializes in developing strength, coordination, and movement. Therapists work on improving gross motor skills, such as running, reaching, and lifting. This therapy is concerned with improving function of the body's larger muscles through physical activities including exercise and massage.

## Interpreting the Results

Medical tests look for a physical cause of a disability. Autism and related disabilities are not commonly caused by a physical problem. It is important to work with medical professionals that look at your whole child, which includes your child's medical condition as well as his or her behavior, communication, and school environment.

# Chapter 20

# *After the Diagnosis: What Comes Next?*

## Chapter Contents

Section 20.1—Ten Things Parents Need to Do after a
Diagnosis of Autism ............................................ 254

Section 20.2—Moving Forward with Confidence after
Your Child Is Diagnosed with an Autistic
Spectrum Disorder ............................................. 257

Section 20.3—Should You Explain the Diagnosis to Your
Child with Autism or Asperger Syndrome? ...... 260

# Section 20.1

# Ten Things Parents Need to Do after a Diagnosis of Autism

"After the Diagnosis: Ten Things Parents Need to Do When Facing Autism Spectrum Disorders" is reprinted with permission from Mitzi Waltz and First Signs, Inc. © 2001 First Signs, Inc. All rights reserved. First Signs (www.firstsigns.org) is dedicated to early identification and intervention for children with developmental delays and disorders. Reviewed by David A. Cooke, M.D., March 2007.

It's over. The seemingly endless process of doctor visits and testing has ended.

If your child has been diagnosed with an autistic spectrum disorder (autism or pervasive developmental disorder), you may feel that your life as you know it is over, too. You're faced with a barrage of terms you've never heard before, professionals who may or may not seem helpful, and friends and family members who insist on handing you magazine articles about the latest "cure," but who don't really seem to understand what you're going through. Most importantly, you're faced with essential decisions to make about your child's health, education, and future.

Every parent who has walked this road before you has experienced this moment of post-diagnosis paralysis. It really is too much for one or two people to handle alone. It shakes your confidence, and challenges your parenting skills and your personal goals in ways you never expected. It can't be sugarcoated or wished away.

Right after the diagnosis, you're torn between a very real grieving process for the "perfect" child every parent hopes for, anger that your child has been affected by this disorder, fear about the future, and a parent's innate determination to make everything better somehow. Grief, anger, and fear are difficult emotions, and it will take time to work through them. Seek professional counseling and extra support if you need it. But hold on to that core of determination for your child. Along with hope (which you should never let go of, no matter what some doctor, teacher, or relative may tell you), it's going to be your greatest strength.

254

So where will that determination take you from here? In the absence of a medically proven, sure-fire treatment for autistic spectrum disorders, there are many things to consider. The following ten steps will start you on the right path.

1.  Take a deep breath and begin to use the professional guidance you have been given. Begin to communicate and connect with your child and participate in your child's therapy. Begin to understand what is most helpful to your child.

2.  Get organized. Create a filing system for your child's medical, early intervention, and school records, articles and pamphlets, and other items you want to close at hand.

3.  Inform yourself. Read books, surf the internet, and have in-depth conversations with any expert parent or professional you can buttonhole. Find out about print and online resources that can keep you abreast of the latest news about treatments.

4.  Based on what you learn, evaluate treatment possibilities, with a focus on your child's unique characteristics and needs.

5.  Assemble your treatment team. This should include a pediatrician who understands developmental issues and who will be your child's primary care provider. Depending on your child's needs, you may also need a neurologist, neuropsychologist, psychiatrist, speech therapist, occupational therapist, home-based intervention therapist, and others. If your child's needs are especially complex (for example, autism plus epilepsy or cerebral palsy), ask your health maintenance organization (HMO) or county developmental delay services about case management help.

6.  Learn your child's rights, and take steps to secure them. Find out about early intervention programs, regional services, county developmental delay or mental health programs, and special education programs. Start the application process for services for which your child is eligible. Learn about the Individuals with Disabilities Education Act (IDEA), the Americans with Disabilities Act (ADA), the Rehabilitation Act, and other laws that can protect and help your child.

7.  Understand your insurance plan. Find out what it does and doesn't cover. Learn how to get better services for your child, including how to appeal decisions with which you don't agree.

If you are uninsured, find out about Medicaid and state-sponsored plans for uninsured children.

8. Network with other parents. Join a local or national group that can keep you informed. Find other families nearby or online who are coping with the same issues.

9. Take steps to nurture your entire family, including your partner and other children. It's easy, and sometimes necessary, for one child's disability to take precedence over everything else. Most parents have to deliberately make time for giving the rest of the family special attention.

10. Nurture yourself. Do what it takes to maintain your health and well-being by eating right, exercising, taking care of any medical needs, and making sure that you have adequate emotional support.

The worst is over, but the hard work has just begun: You must take the lead in advocating for your child.

Section 20.2

# Moving Forward with Confidence after Your Child Is Diagnosed with an Autistic Spectrum Disorder

"After the Diagnosis: Moving Forward with Confidence" is reprinted with permission from Mitzi Waltz and First Signs, Inc. © 2001 First Signs, Inc. All rights reserved. First Signs (www.FirstSigns.org) is dedicated to early identification and intervention for children with developmental delays and disorders. Reviewed by David A. Cooke, M.D., March 2007.

Usually, a medical diagnosis automatically leads to treatment. Unfortunately, that's often not the case for autistic spectrum disorders (ASDs). As of this writing, the U.S. Food and Drug Administration (FDA) has approved no medications to treat ASDs. Your insurance company or health maintenance organization (HMO) will probably tell you no treatments are covered. Books and websites do present options, but how can you make wise decisions when every day counts?

## Start with the Basics

Some doctors still deliver the diagnosis of autism as if it were an incurable cancer. True, we don't have a cure, but we do have therapies that can help most children with ASDs. Like epilepsy, asthma, and other "incurable" medical conditions, ASDs are eminently treatable. Begin with your child's basic physical health. Many children with ASDs have health problems, such as severe diarrhea or constipation, allergies or food intolerances, or immune-system dysfunction. These may be clues about the actual cause of ASDs, but that's a question for the researchers. Right now, your job is to ensure that your child is not suffering from pain, illness, or poor nutrition. A healthy, comfortable child can benefit most from the other kinds of help that are available.

Next, make sure your child gets a complete multidisciplinary evaluation.

Find out about his strengths and weaknesses and how he learns.

## Evaluating Therapies

Autism is a group of symptoms, not a single medical condition. Just as there may be several reasons for these symptoms to occur, there may be several roads to improvement.

When facing treatment decisions:

* Make sure the interventions you choose are as safe as possible;

* Check the credentials of all healthcare providers, and make sure they are knowledgeable about the latest research;

* Tell your child's primary healthcare provider about everything you try;

* Keep good notes.

I strongly believe, based on both evidence from clinical studies and from talking to many experienced parents, that all young children with ASDs can benefit from a program of intensive, daily, structured, one-to-one interaction. The best-known system is applied behavior analysis (ABA), originally developed at UCLA by Dr. Ivar Lovaas. Floor-time play therapy, an approach developed by Dr. Stanley Greenspan, is also effective for many children. These methods can be tailored to meet each child's individual needs.

Speech therapy, occupational therapy for children with fine motor problems, sensory integration for those under- or oversensitive to sensory information, and physical therapy for delayed gross motor development are also well tested.

Medication for specific symptoms, such as obsessive-compulsive behavior, severe anxiety, or self-injurious behavior, may be helpful. At this time, the most important role for medication is reducing symptoms that prevent the use of interventions like ABA, floor-time play therapy, and speech therapy. Some children also need anti-epilepsy medication, as up to one-fourth of children with autism also have a seizure disorder. A few doctors are experimenting with medications that target the immune or gastrointestinal systems. Always start with the lowest dose possible, make any increases gradually, and communicate regularly with your doctor.

## Biological Interventions

Biological interventions seek to address metabolic or immune-system problems. They include special diets, vitamins, and dietary supplements.

Eliminating the proteins gluten and casein may help with digestive and bowel problems, and may also prevent opiate-like peptides from reaching the brain. Many parents have reported positive benefits from putting their autistic-spectrum child on a gluten-free, casein-free diet. If you're interested, work with a licensed dietitian, and join a diet-focused support group in your area or online.

Supplementation with B vitamins and magnesium has been extensively researched. It's not universally effective, but it does seem to help some. If you want to try vitamins, familiarize yourself with their effects and side effects.

Research on essential fatty acids in autism has just begun. They have shown promise in clinical trials targeting other brain disorders. Other supplements may also be valuable.

Check out alternative healthcare practitioners carefully. Sadly, some are untrained or use false credentials, and some make potentially harmful suggestions. Be especially wary of anyone who both recommends and sells supplements.

## Evaluating New Therapies

The history of autism has been marked by a series of failed "breakthroughs," including dangerous drugs like fenfluramine and even LSD (lysergic acid diethylamide). It seems like every year there's something new, and plenty of families desperate enough to pay thousands for it.

Autism is a complex condition, so miracle cures are unlikely. Like diabetes and asthma, it involves both genetics and environment, and affects multiple systems within the body. Treatment plans must address that complexity. Comprehensive treatment should start as early as possible to help each child achieve his or her greatest potential.

So don't wait for a cure. Get going right away with therapies that have scientific backing, and evaluate other options based on your child's individual needs and symptoms. This generation of children will be the first to benefit from time-tested treatments. There may even be some real breakthroughs! With wise choices and hard work, the chance of a good outcome is excellent.

Section 20.3

## Should You Explain the Diagnosis to Your Child with Autism or Asperger Syndrome?

Excerpted from "Should You Explain the Diagnosis to the Child?" by Tony Attwood, Ph.D. © 2006 Tony Attwood. Reprinted with permission. For additional information, visit www.tonyattwood.com.au. The original article has become part of *The Complete Guide to Asperger's Syndrome* (2006) by Tony Attwood, Jessica Kingsley Publishers (www.jkp.com).

### Should you explain the diagnosis to your child?

The immediate answer is yes. Clinical experience indicates that it is extremely important that the diagnosis is explained as soon as possible and preferably before inappropriate compensatory mechanisms are developed. The child is then more likely to achieve self-acceptance, without unfair comparisons with other children, and be less likely to develop signs of an anxiety disorder, depression, or conduct disorder.

### When and how do you explain the diagnosis?

At what age do you explain the diagnosis? Young children may not consider themselves as particularly different than their peers, and may have difficulty understanding the concept of a developmental disorder as complex as autism. The explanation for young children will need to be age appropriate and provide information that is relevant from the child's perspective. The main themes will be the benefits of programs to help the child make friends and enjoy playing with other children, and to help in learning and achieving success with schoolwork. There can be a discussion and activities to explain the concept of individual differences, for example, those children in the class who find it easy to learn to read, and others who find it more difficult. The clinician or parents can then explain that there is another form of reading, namely reading people and social situations, and that we have programs to help children who have this particular reading difficulty.

## Who else needs to know?

After explaining the diagnosis to the child or adult, it is important to discuss who else needs to know. Children may be concerned about how their peers will respond to the news and any potential negative reaction. Adults will want to know if it is wise to tell friends, prospective employers, and colleagues. The clinician will examine and discuss the issues surrounding disclosure for the client, based on his or her circumstances, the advantages and disadvantages of certain people knowing, and how much information to disclose.

The child's opinion is respected regarding the question of whether or not peers should be told. If the child does want the other children to know, there needs to be an agreement as to how widely the information will be disseminated, who will provide the explanation, how, and whether the child with autism should be present.

An adult who has recently been diagnosed will also need to discuss who to tell and how to explain autism to the family, social network, and work associates. Some adults have a more reserved personality and are very cautious regarding disclosure, deciding to limit the news to carefully selected individuals. Other adults are more open in their disclosure.

## What are the advantages and disadvantages of having a diagnosis?

The advantage to the child of having a diagnosis is not only in preventing or reducing the effects of some compensatory or adjustment strategies, but also to remove worries about other diagnoses, such as being insane, and to be recognized as having genuine difficulties coping with experiences that others find easy and enjoyable. Once the diagnosis is confirmed and understood, there can be a significant positive change in other people's expectations, acceptance, and support. There should be compliments rather than criticism with regard to social competence, and acknowledgement of the child's confusion and exhaustion from learning two curricula at school, the academic curriculum and the social curriculum.

The advantage of acknowledging and understanding the diagnosis for parents is that, at last, they have an explanation for their son's or daughter's unusual behaviors and abilities, and knowledge that the condition is not caused by faulty parenting. The family may then have access to knowledge on autism from literature and the internet, resources from government agencies, and support groups, as well as access to programs to improve social inclusion and emotion management that will greatly benefit the whole family. There may also be greater acceptance of the child within the extended family and among family friends. The parents can now provide an acceptable explanation to other people regarding the child's unusual behavior.

Siblings may have known for some time that their brother or sister was unusual and may have been either compassionate, tolerant, and concerned about any difficulties, or embarrassed, intolerant, and antagonistic. Each sibling will make his or her own accommodations toward the sibling with autism. Parents can now explain to their children why their brother or sister is unusual, and how the family has had to, and will need to, adjust and work cooperatively and constructively to implement the remedial strategies. Parents and professionals can provide the siblings with age-appropriate explanations about their brother or sister to give their friends without jeopardizing their own social networks. Siblings will also need to know how to help their brother or sister at home when friends visit, and be made aware of their role and responsibilities at school and in the neighborhood.

The advantages for school services, especially teachers, is that the child's unusual behavior and profile of social, cognitive, linguistic, and motor skills are recognized as a legitimate disorder that should provide access to resources to help the teacher. Confirmation of the diagnosis should also have a positive effect on the attitudes of other children in the classroom and other staff who have contact with the child. The teacher can access information from textbooks and resource programs specifically developed for teachers of children with autism. The teacher can also explain to other children and staff who teach or supervise the child why he or she behaves and thinks in a different way.

The advantages of the diagnosis for the adolescent or adult with autism can be in terms of support while a student at college or in employment. Acknowledgment of the diagnosis can lead to greater self-understanding and better decision-making with regard to careers, friendships, and relationships. The adult may benefit from joining an adult support group that has local meetings, or an internet support group or chat room. This can provide a sense of belonging to a distinct and valued culture and can enable the person to consult members of the culture for advice. We also know that acceptance of the diagnosis can be an important stage in the development of successful adult relationships with a partner, and invaluable when seeking counseling and therapy from relationship counselors.

There could be disadvantages in having a diagnosis in terms of how the person and others perceive the characteristics. If the diagnostic news is broadcast widely, there will inevitably be some children or adults who misuse this disclosure to torment and despise the person with autism. Children can be quite inventive in stigmatizing differences but more compassionate people may be able to repair some of the damage to the self-esteem of someone with autism who has been ridiculed for being different.

### *Should prospective employers be told about the diagnosis?*

One of the concerns of adults with autism is whether they should include reference to the diagnosis on a job application. If there is considerable competition for a particular vacancy, an applicant having a diagnosis that is unknown to the employer might lead to the application being rejected. A potential solution is for the adult to write a brief, perhaps one page, description of autism and the qualities and difficulties that would be relevant to the job. This personalized brochure could also be used to explain autism to colleagues, juniors, and line managers. A shorter version can be reduced to a business card that can be given to anyone who needs to know about the person's diagnosis.

Having a diagnosis of autism could limit the expectations of others, who may assume that the person will never be able to achieve as well as his or her peers with regard to social, academic, and personal success. The diagnosis should facilitate realistic expectations but not dictate the upper limits of ability.

# Part Five

# Treatments, Therapies, and Interventions for Autism Spectrum Disorders

Chapter 21

# Your Child's Autism Treatment Team

Your child's pediatrician will provide most routine and disability-specific healthcare for your child. He or she may also act as the gatekeeper for other services your child needs, such as speech therapy or psychiatric care. If your current pediatrician isn't up to the job, you might consider a developmental pediatrician, who has extra training in this area. The other members of your child's treatment team will depend on what's needed.

Here's a short list of professionals who may be helpful.

**Developmental pediatrician:** Developmental pediatricians are medical doctors (MDs) who specialize in treating the health problems of children with developmental delays or handicaps. Developmental pediatricians are familiar with neurological problems, medications, and current research on disabilities. They work closely with other specialists, including most of those listed below. (For more information, visit http://www.dbpeds.org).

**Neurologist:** Neurologists are MDs with special expertise in brain disorders, such as epilepsy and cerebral palsy. You can check credentials

"Putting Together Your Child's Treatment Team" is reprinted with permission from Mitzi Waltz and First Signs, Inc. © 2001 First Signs, Inc. All rights reserved. First Signs (www.FirstSigns.org) is dedicated to early identification and intervention for children with developmental delays and disorders. The text of this document is available online at http://www.firstsigns.org/articles/waltz _team.htm; accessed October 2, 2006.

with the American Board of Psychiatry and Neurology (847-945-7900, http://www.abpn.com).

**Psychiatrist:** Psychiatrists are MDs with special expertise in brain disorders that change how a person thinks or behaves, such as attention deficit hyperactivity disorder (ADHD) or clinical depression. They are also credentialed by the American Board of Psychiatry and Neurology.

**Psychologist:** Psychologists can diagnose disorders, provide talk-based therapy, and offer advice on coping skills, education strategies, and behavior management. Licensed psychologists have passed a national examination to receive credentials from the states where they work. They can be certified in a specialty by the American Board of Professional Psychology (573-875-1267, http://www.abpp.org). Limited licensed psychologists have a master's degree (MA) in psychology and operate under supervision. Most school psychologists have a master's degree (MA) only.

**Neuropsychologist:** A neuropsychologist is a psychologist who has completed extra training in the behavioral effects of biologically based mental illnesses, such as autism and epilepsy. They can diagnose disorders, provide talk-based therapy, and offer advice on coping skills, education strategies, and behavior management. Neuropsychologists are credentialed by the American Board of Clinical Neuropsychology (734-936-8269, http://www.theabcn.org).

**Social Worker:** Social workers help people access community resources, provide direct therapy services, or act in other roles. They may have a Bachelor of Arts (BA) in social work or a Masters in Social Work (MSW). Licensed clinical social workers (LCSW) have received a license from their state board (see the Association of Social Work Boards, (800) 225-6880, http://www.aswb.org). Certified social workers (CSW or ASCW) have a master's degree, have passed an examination by the National Association of Social Workers (202-408-8600, http://www.socialworkers.org), and have practiced under supervision for two years.

**Therapist/counselor:** In some places, anyone can call themselves a therapist or counselor. Ask the person you're considering about his or her training and experience. Most states offer a Licensed Professional Counselor (LPC) or Certified Professional Counselor (CPC) credential.

Each state's requirements are different, but most include an MA or Master's of Education (MEd) degree with a major in counseling, a period of supervised practice, and passing a state exam (see the American Association of State Counseling Boards, 703-212-2239, http://www.aascb.org). Counselors may become nationally board-certified through the National Board for Certified Counselors (336-547-0607, http://www.nbcc.org).

**Speech therapist:** Speech therapists help people with communication disorders learn to talk or improve their ability to talk. The American Speech-Language-Hearing Association (800-638-8255, http://www.asha.org) credentials speech therapists, language therapists, and audiologists.

**Occupational therapist:** Occupational therapists (OTs) help people improve their fine-motor skills and may teach them how to perform specific tasks (such as holding a pencil for writing). Some are trained to provide sensory integration therapy, a specialty that helps people with over- or undersensitivity to touch, sound, smell, or taste. The National Board for Certification in Occupational Therapy (301-990-7979, http://www.nbcot.org) credentials OTs.

**Physical therapist:** Physical therapists help people develop or improve gross-motor skills, such as walking, running, and climbing. They have a bachelor's (BA) or higher degree in physical therapy and have passed a state licensing exam (see https://www.apta.org for more information).

**Behavior therapist:** Behavior therapists are specialists in behavior modification techniques. They can come from a number of different educational backgrounds. Some design or oversee behavior modification programs to be carried out by others. Others provide direct services to people at home, particularly those who offer applied behavioral analysis (ABA) programs for children with autism. Most behavior therapists have at least a BA in an appropriate specialty. Some states require a special credential for ABA practitioners.

**Assistive technology specialist:** Assistive technology (AT) specialists help find devices and technologies that can extend a person's physical abilities, such as talking computers. They can come from a variety of different educational backgrounds, so ask about training and expertise. Many are also occupational or speech therapists.

Your pediatrician may be able to recommend good people. Other parents can offer ideas. You can also get information through a county health or mental health department, a crisis line, or a local support and advocacy group. Once you have some names to choose from and have checked their credentials, here are some questions you may want to ask:

- Are you accepting new clients?

- Do you charge for an initial consultation?

- What is your approach to working with people who have my child's diagnosis?

- How and when will treatment goals be set?

- How will family members be involved in my child's treatment?

- Do you accept my insurance plan, or charge an affordable rate for out-of-pocket payment?

- Do you have sliding-scale rates?

Once you have found your team members, help them work well together. Make sure everyone who helps your child knows who the other members of the treatment team are, and how to reach them. Ensure that important information, test results, and reports are shared.

Chapter 22

# Evaluating Autism Treatments: Rules of Thumb and Questions to Ask

## Red Flags and Rules of Thumb for Evaluating Treatments

1.  Be suspicious of any treatment which makes grandiose claims, using words like "miraculous," "amazing breakthrough," "recovery," or "cure." Legitimate medical and educational professionals show respect for the uniqueness of each individual with autism and the feelings of that individual's family, and therefore never indulge in overstatements and boasts about what they will be able to accomplish. When they are particularly successful in helping a person, they do not solicit testimonials from the person's family or encourage parents to make grandiose promises and claims to others.

2.  Be suspicious of professionals who publicize and promote their method or program as if it were a packageable commodity. Since autism is not a "thing" a person "has," but an attempt to capture in a single label a wide range of behavioral adaptations to a wide range of sensory and movement regulatory differences, there

The first part of this chapter is reprinted from "Red Flags and Rules of Thumb for Evaluating Treatments," © 2003 Autism National Committee. Reprinted with permission. "Questions to Ask when Considering a Treatment," is excerpted from "Autism Spectrum Disorders (Pervasive Developmental Disorders)," National Institute of Mental Health, National Institutes of Health, NIH Publication No. 04-5511, March 14, 2007.

can be no such thing as a general treatment "for autism." Likewise, beware of parent support groups dedicated to the promotion of a particular "miraculous" method. Enthusiastic testimonials from people who claim they have been helped by a product or treatment are no substitute for the evidence gathered through careful, unbiased investigation, and for considering the unique developmental profile of your individual child. Run for the hills if you are ever made to feel guilty or inadequate for failing to buy into a treatment or for questioning the eager rhetoric surrounding it.

3.  Remember that many treatments are composed of an eclectic mix of active and inactive ingredients. The more clarity we can achieve about what really helps, the less time, energy, and money we will waste on inactive, incidental, and occasionally harmful treatment components. It is helpful to note the common features in many effective interventions, across many different disciplines:

    - Using environmental accommodations which slow down interactions, setting a consistent pattern paced to the person's unique rhythms

    - Eliminating unnecessary stimuli and distractions which may overwhelm and confuse

    - Giving the person, on a daily basis, as much uninterrupted time and attention as possible

    - Following the person's lead by building on his or her own enthusiasms and interests

    - Utilizing typical home and community settings, and the friendship and support of typically developing peers

    - Last but not least, sharing with the person a belief in their competence and delight in their companionship

## Questions to Ask when Considering a Treatment

There is no single best treatment package for all children with autism spectrum disorders (ASDs). One point that most professionals agree on is that early intervention is important; another is that most individuals with ASD respond well to highly structured, specialized programs.

Before you make decisions on your child's treatment, you will want to gather information about the various options available. Learn as much as you can, look at all the options, and make your decision on your child's treatment based on your child's needs. You may want to visit public schools in your area to see the type of program they offer to special needs children.

Guidelines used by the Autism Society of America include the following questions parents can ask about potential treatments:

- Will the treatment result in harm to my child?

- How will failure of the treatment affect my child and family?

- Has the treatment been validated scientifically?

- Are there assessment procedures specified?

- How will the treatment be integrated into my child's current program?

Do not become so infatuated with a given treatment that functional curriculum, vocational life, and social skills are ignored.

The National Institute of Mental Health suggests a list of questions parents can ask when planning for their child:

- How successful has the program been for other children?

- How many children have gone on to placement in a regular school and how have they performed?

- Do staff members have training and experience in working with children and adolescents with autism?

- How are activities planned and organized?

- Are there predictable daily schedules and routines?

- How much individual attention will my child receive?

- How is progress measured? Will my child's behavior be closely observed and recorded?

- Will my child be given tasks and rewards that are personally motivating?

- Is the environment designed to minimize distractions?

- Will the program prepare me to continue the therapy at home?

- What is the cost, time commitment, and location of the program?

# Chapter 23

# *Autism Treatment Options: An Overview*

## *What Are Your Treatment Options?*

Discovering that your child has an autism spectrum disorder (ASD) can be an overwhelming experience. For some, the diagnosis may come as a complete surprise; others may have had suspicions and tried for months or years to get an accurate diagnosis. In either case, a diagnosis brings a multitude of questions about how to proceed. A generation ago, many people with autism were placed in institutions. Professionals were less educated about autism than they are today and specific services and supports were largely nonexistent. Today the picture is much clearer. With appropriate services and supports, training, and information, children on the autism spectrum will grow, learn, and flourish, even if at a different developmental rate than others.

While there is no known cure for autism, there are treatment and education approaches that may reduce some of the challenges associated with the condition. Intervention may help to lessen disruptive behaviors, and education can teach self-help skills that allow for greater independence. But just as there is no one symptom or behavior that identifies individuals with ASD, there is no single treatment that will be effective for all people on the spectrum. Individuals can learn to function within the confines of ASD and use the positive aspects of their condition to their benefit, but treatment must begin as early as possible and be tailored to the child's unique strengths, weaknesses, and needs.

Throughout the history of the Autism Society of America (ASA), parents and professionals have been confounded by conflicting messages regarding what are, versus what are not, appropriate treatment approaches for children and adults on the autism spectrum.

The purpose of this text is to provide a general overview of a variety of available approaches, not specific treatment recommendations. Keep in mind that the word "treatment" is used in a very limited sense. While typically used for children under three, the approaches described herein may be included in an educational program for older children as well.

It is important to match a child's potential and specific needs with treatments or strategies that are likely to be effective in moving him or her closer to established goals and greatest potential. ASA does not want to give the impression that parents or professionals will select one item from a list of available treatments. A search for appropriate treatment must be paired with the knowledge that all treatment approaches are not equal, what works for one will not work for all, and other options do not have to be excluded. The basis for choosing any treatment plan should come from a thorough evaluation of the strengths and weaknesses observed in the child.

### Understanding Your Options

Treatment approaches are constantly evolving as more is learned about the autism spectrum. There are many therapeutic programs, both conventional and complementary, that focus on replacing dysfunctional behaviors and developing specific skills.

As a parent, it's natural to want to do something immediately. The literature states time and time again the importance of early treatment for individuals on the autism spectrum However, it is important not to rush in with changes. It does no good to push ahead with a treatment that is not appropriate for the individual or one that may be harmful. You also must consider the larger implications of beginning a new treatment. A child may have already learned to cope with his or her current environment and sudden changes or unexpected different expectations could be stressful and confusing. Various treatment approaches should be investigated and information gathered concerning various options before proceeding with any child's treatment.

Parents will encounter numerous accounts from other parents about successes and failures with many of the treatment approaches mentioned. Professionals also differ in their theories of what they feel is the most successful treatment for autism. It can be frustrating! Parents do learn to sift through the information, examine options with a critical eye, and make rational, educated decisions on what is appropriate given the individual circumstance. Parents live with the individual on the spectrum every day and best know his or her needs and the unique ways that autism impacts their lives. Parents must be empowered to trust their instincts as various options are explored, considered, and implemented.

The descriptions of treatment approaches provided here are for informational purposes only. They serve as overviews and should always be followed by contact with qualified professionals and should be discussed with parents or individuals on the spectrum who have personal experience. The Autism Society of America does not endorse any specific treatment or therapy.

While doing research, parents and professionals will hear about many different treatment approaches, such as auditory training, discrete trial training, vitamin therapy, anti-yeast therapy, facilitated communication, music therapy, occupational therapy, physical therapy, and sensory integration. These approaches can generally be broken down into three categories:

- Learning approaches

- Biomedical and dietary approaches

- Complementary approaches

Some of these treatment approaches have research studies that support their efficacy; others may not. Some parents will want to try only treatment methods that have undergone research and testing and are generally accepted by the professional community. Keep in mind, however, that scientific studies are often difficult to do since each individual on the autism spectrum is different.

For others, formal testing might not be a prerequisite for them to try a treatment with their child. Even for those with "scientific" proof, the Autism Society of America recommends that all available options are investigated to determine the approach that is most appropriate.

Experts agree, though, that early intervention is important in addressing the symptoms associated with ASD. The earlier treatment is started, the more opportunity for the individual to reach his or her highest potential. Many of the approaches described can be used on children as young as age two or three. They may also continue to be used in conjunction with special education programs or traditional elementary school for children who are mainstreamed.

## Programs for Children under Three

If a child is younger than three years old, he or she is eligible for "early intervention" assistance. This federally funded program is available in every state, but may be provided by different agencies. Contact the local chapter of the Autism Society of America in your area for more specific information, search program listings in Autism Source™, located on the internet at www.autismsource.org, or obtain a state resource sheet from the National Information Center for Children and Youth with Disabilities.

This early education assistance may be available in two forms: home-based or school-based. Home-based programs generally assign members of an early intervention team to come to the home to train parents or caregivers to educate the child on the spectrum. School-based programs may be in a public school or a private organization. Both of these programs should be staffed by teachers and other professionals who have experience working with children with disabilities, and specifically autism. Related services should also be offered, such as speech, physical, or occupational therapy, depending on the needs of each child. The program may be only for children with disabilities or it may also include typically developing peers.

## Programs for School-Aged Children

From the age of three through the age of twenty-one, every child diagnosed on the autism spectrum is guaranteed a free appropriate public education supplied by the local education agency. The Individuals with Disabilities Education Act (IDEA) is a federal mandate that guarantees this education. Whatever the level of impairment, the educational program for an individual on the autism spectrum should be based on the unique needs of the student and thoroughly documented in the IEP (Individualized Education Program). If this is the first attempt by the parents and the school system to develop the appropriate curriculum, conducting a comprehensive needs assessment is a good place to start. Consult with professionals who are well versed in the spectrum of autism and related conditions about the best possible educational methods that will be effective in assisting the student to learn and benefit from his or her school program. Educational programming for students with ASD often addresses a wide range of skill development, including academics, language, social skills, self-help skills, behavioral issues, and leisure skills.

Parents can and should be an active and equal participant in deciding on an appropriate educational plan for their child. Parents know the child best and can provide valuable information to teachers and other professionals who will be providing educational services. Collaboration between parents and professionals is essential; open communication will certainly lead to better evaluation of progress and improved outcomes for the student.

To learn about other services specific to an area, contact resources in the community, such as the local ASA chapter, a local university-affiliated program for developmental disabilities, or the local Easter Seals or parent training and information center. Be persistent, but be patient. It may take days or weeks to find the information you need. If a local resource is not able to provide the information or services sought, ask for a referral to another agency or local resource that may be helpful.

## *Evaluating Approaches*

Because no two children on the autism spectrum have the exact same symptoms and behavioral patterns, a treatment approach that works for one child may not be successful with another. This makes evaluating different approaches difficult and that much more essential. There is little comparative research between treatment approaches. Primarily this is because there are too many variables that have to be controlled. So, it's no wonder that parents might be confused about what to do.

The Autism Society of America has long promoted the empowerment of individual consumers (including people on the spectrum, parents, and professionals) to critically examine a variety of available options and be forearmed with a set of parameters under which they can better determine associated threats and opportunities and, therefore, make informed decisions. Further, better-educated consumers will help control the embracing of unproven notions that may distract from effective courses of treatment for individuals with ASD.

In the article "Behavioral and Educational Treatment for Autistic Spectrum Disorders" (*Autism Advocate*, volume 33, no. 6), Bryna Siegel, Ph.D., suggests thinking about "each symptom as an autism specific learning disability" that tells "something about a barrier to understanding." Using this model, what the student can and cannot do well can be evaluated. "Take stock of which autistic learning disabilities are present," and "then select treatments that address that particular child's unique autism learning disability profile."

Understanding these learning differences is the first step in assessing whether a specific treatment approach may be helpful; understanding a child's strengths is equally important. For example, some children are good visual learners, while other children may need written, rather than oral, cues.

### Finding Treatment Programs in Your Area

Once familiar with the treatments that are available and appropriate for individuals with ASD, parents begin to think about where they can receive these services. Treatments may be obtained through either the medical or educational community, depending on the nature of the treatment. There are also a variety of resources useful in finding qualified professionals or service providers in your area. There are several state agencies established to provide this type of information and support, including protection and advocacy agencies, developmental disabilities councils, vocational rehabilitation centers, parent training centers, and educational resources. Local chapters of the Autism Society of America are run by parents of individuals on the autism spectrum and have been established to provide guidance, advice, and referrals to programs and professionals in a specific geographic region.

## Learning Approaches

The behaviors exhibited by children on the autism spectrum are frequently the most troubling aspect of the condition for parents and caregivers. These behaviors may be socially inappropriate, repetitive, aggressive and/or dangerous, and may include the following:

- Hand flapping
- Finger snapping
- Rocking
- Placing objects in one's mouth
- Head banging

Children with ASD may also engage in self-injurious behavior, such as eye-gouging or biting their arms; they may show little or no sensitivity to burns or bruises and may physically attack someone with no discernible provocation. The reasons for these behaviors are complex, but some professionals think that sensory integration issues contribute to them.

Communication skills, both the spoken and written word, are also an issue for some children on the autism spectrum. An individual might have difficulty understanding how typical communication works and may have difficulty with reciprocal conversation. Many children with ASD also have language difficulties, either being nonverbal or having delayed speech. Some children use language in unusual ways, such as repeating the words or sentences said to them (echolalia) or using only single words to communicate. Language difficulties may contribute to behavioral problems for a child with autism because of an inability to use language to communicate his or her needs.

Many treatment approaches have been developed to address the range of social, language, sensory, and behavioral difficulties that may accompany the condition.

## Applied Behavior Analysis (ABA)

Many of the interventions used to treat children on the autism spectrum are based on the theory of applied behavior analysis (ABA)—that behavior rewarded is more likely to be repeated than behavior ignored. Although ABA is a theory, many people use the term to describe a specific treatment approach with subsets that include discrete trial training or the Lovaas method. While the terms "discrete trial" and "Lovaas" have been used interchangeably, only practitioners who are affiliated with Dr. O. Ivar Lovaas from UCLA can be said to implement the Lovaas approach.

In discrete trial training, every task given to the child consists of a request to perform a specific action, a response from the child, and a reaction from the therapist. It is not just about correcting behaviors but is designed to teach skills from basic, such as sleeping and dressing, to more involved, such as social interaction. Discrete trial training is an intensive approach. Children usually work for thirty to forty hours a week one-on-one with a trained professional. Tasks are broken down into short simple pieces, or trials. When a task has been successfully completed, a reward is offered, reinforcing the behavior or task. This method is not without controversy. Some practitioners feel it is emotionally too difficult for some children with ASD, that the time requirement of thirty to forty hours a week is too intensive and intrusive on family life, and that while it may change a particular behavior, it does not prepare a child to respond to new situations. However, research has shown that ABA techniques show consistent results in teaching new skills and behaviors to children on the autism spectrum.

## Treatment and Education of Autistic and Related Communication Handicapped Children (TEACCH)

The first statewide program for treatment and services for people with autism, TEACCH was developed at the School of Medicine at the University of North Carolina in the 1970s. TEACCH uses a structured teaching approach based on the idea that the environment should be adapted to the child with ASD, not the child to the environment. It uses no one specific technique, but rather a program based around the child's functioning level. The child's learning abilities are assessed through the Psycho Educational Profile (PEP), and teaching strategies are designed to improve communication, social, and coping skills. Rather than teach a specific skill or behavior, the TEACCH approach aims to provide the child with the skills to understand his or her world and other people's behaviors. For example, some children with autism scream when they are in pain. The TEACCH approach would search for the cause of the screaming and then teach the child how to signal pain through communication skills.

There have been criticisms that the TEACCH approach is too structured, that children with ASD, particularly those individuals who are less affected, become too focused on the charts, organizational aids, and schedules, and that it discourages mainstream behavior (meaning that they may respond only to specific stimuli as taught in their curriculum and not everyday situations). Others feel that, in an environment conducive to learning, ultimately the child with ASD understands what is expected and how to respond.

## Picture Exchange Communication Systems (PECS)

One of the main areas affected in individuals on the autism spectrum is the ability to communicate; some will develop verbal language, while others may never talk. An augmented communication program, such as picture exchange communication systems (PECS), is helpful to get language started as well as to provide a way of communicating for those children that do not talk.

PECS was developed at the Delaware Autistic Program to help children and adults with ASD to acquire functional communication skills. It uses ABA-based methods to teach children to exchange a picture for something they want—an item or activity.

The advantage to PECS is that it is clear, intentional, and initiated by the child. The child hands you a picture, and his or her request is immediately understood. It also makes it easy for the child with ASD to communicate with anyone—all they have to do is accept the picture.

## Pivotal Response Treatment (PRT)

Pivotal response treatment is a naturalistic intervention model producing positive changes in critical behaviors, leading to generalized improvement in communication, social, and behavioral areas. Rather than targeting individual behaviors one at a time, PRT targets pivotal areas of a child's development, such as motivation, responsivity to multiple cues, self-management, and social initiations. By targeting these critical areas, PRT results in widespread, collateral improvements in other social, communicative, and behavioral areas.

The underlying motivational strategies of PRT are incorporated throughout intervention as often as possible, and they include child choice, task variation, interspersing maintenance tasks, rewarding attempts, and the use of direct and natural reinforcers. The child plays a crucial role in determining the activities and objects that will be used in the PRT exchange. For example, intentional attempts at functional communication are rewarded with a natural reinforcer (e.g., if a child attempts a request for a stuffed animal, the child receives the animal, not a piece of candy or other unrelated reinforcer). Pivotal response treatment is used to teach language, decrease disruptive/self-stimulatory behaviors, and increase social, communication, and academic skills.

## Floor-Time/DIR Method

An educational model developed by child psychiatrist Stanley Greenspan, the DIR (Developmental, Individual-Difference, Relationship-Based)/floor-time approach provides a comprehensive framework for understanding and treating children challenged by autism spectrum and related disorders. It focuses on helping children master the building blocks of relating, communicating, and thinking, rather than on symptoms alone. Floor-time is much like play therapy, in that it builds an increasingly larger circle of interaction between a child and an adult in a developmentally based sequence. Greenspan has described six stages of emotional development that children meet to develop a foundation for more advanced learning—a developmental ladder that must be climbed one rung at a time. Children with ASD may have trouble with this developmental ladder for a number of reasons, such as over- and under-reacting to senses, difficulty processing information, or difficulty in getting their bodies to do what they want.

Through the use of DIR/floor-time, parents and educators can help the child move up the developmental ladder by following the child's lead and building on what the child does to encourage more interactions. The approach does not treat the child with autism in separate pieces for speech development or motor development, but rather addresses the emotional development, in contrast to other approaches that tend to focus on cognitive development. It is frequently used for a child's daily playtime in conjunction with other methods such as ABA.

### Social Stories

Social stories were developed in 1991 by Carol Gray as a tool for teaching social skills to children with ASD. They address "theory of mind" deficits, that is, the ability to understand or recognize feelings, points of view, or plans of others. Through a story developed about a particular situation or event, the child is provided with as much information as possible to help him or her understand the expected or appropriate response. The stories typically have three sentence types: descriptive sentences addressing the where, who, what, and why of the situation; perspective sentences that provide some understanding of the thoughts and emotions of others; and directive sentences that suggest a response. The stories, which can be written by anyone, are specific to the child's needs, and are written in the first person and present tense. They frequently incorporate the use of pictures, photographs, or music.

Before developing and using social stories, it is important to identify how the child interacts socially and to determine what situations are difficult and under what circumstances. Situations that are frightening, produce tantrums or crying, or make a child withdraw or want to escape, are all appropriate for social stories. However, it is important to address the child's misunderstanding of the situation. A child who cries when his or her teacher leaves the room may be doing so because he or she is frightened or frustrated. A story about crying won't address the reason for the behavior. Rather, a story about what scares the child and how he or she can deal with those feelings will be more effective.

## *Relationship Development Intervention (RDI)*

RDI is a program based upon the model of experience sharing developed by Steven Gutstein, Ph.D. The program educates and coaches parents of children with ASD and others who interact and work with the child. A primary focus for RDI consultants is on helping parents systematically teach their children with ASD the motivation for and skills of experience sharing interaction. The RDI program provides a path for people on the autism spectrum to learn friendship, empathy, and love of sharing their world with others. People with ASD learn to tolerate and accept change and transition. Clinicians are certified by The ConnectionsCenter to serve as consultants to parents and help them customize and implement their RDI programs. Certified consultants use information from the relationship development assessment to develop clear, specific, developmentally appropriate treatment objectives and customized activities.

## *Sensory Integration*

Individuals on the autism spectrum frequently have sensory difficulties. They may be hypo- or hyper-reactive or lack the ability to integrate the senses. Sensory integration therapy, usually done by occupational, physical, or speech therapists, focuses on desensitizing the child and helping him or her to reorganize sensory information. For example, if a child has difficulties with the sense of touch, therapy might include handling a variety of materials with different textures.

Temple Grandin, Ph.D., who herself has autism, developed a "squeeze machine," a device that delivers deep touch pressure to help her learn to tolerate touching and to reduce anxiety and nervousness. The "squeeze machine" applies lateral, inwardly directed pressure to both lateral aspects of a person's entire body, by compressing the user between two foam-padded panels. Clinical observations and several studies suggest that deep touch pressure may be beneficial for individuals with ASD and probably children with ADHD.

Auditory integration therapy is used in individuals who have an oversensitivity to sound. It may involve having the child listen to a variety of different sound frequencies coordinated to the level of impairment.

Before proceeding with any sensory integration therapy, it is important that the therapist observe the child and have a clear understanding of his or her specific sensitivities.

## Facilitated Communication

Facilitated communication (FC) was developed in the 1970s in Australia. It is based on the idea that the person is unable to communicate because of a movement disorder, not because of a lack of communication skills. FC involves a facilitator who, by supporting an individual's hand or arm, helps the person communicate through the use of a computer or typewriter. It has not been scientifically validated; critics claim that the communication may be influenced by the thoughts of the facilitator. FC is very controversial and some have adopted formal positions opposing the acceptance of FC. As with any treatment you consider, do your research and learn the pros and cons, find out how practitioners are trained and considered competent to administer the treatment, weigh the benefits and risks (including time and cost) for the family and the individual on the spectrum, consult with trusted professionals, and talk to others who have used the treatment approach.

## Complementary Approaches

While early educational intervention is key to improving the lives of individuals with ASD, some parents and professionals believe that other treatment approaches may play an important role in improving communication skills and reducing associated behavioral symptoms. These complementary therapies may include music, art, or animal therapy and may be done on an individual basis or integrated into an educational program. All of them can help by increasing communication skills, developing social interaction, and providing a sense of accomplishment. They can provide a nonthreatening way for a child on the autism spectrum to develop a positive relationship with a therapist in a safe environment.

Art and music are particularly useful in sensory integration, providing tactile, visual, and auditory stimulation. Music therapy is good for speech development and language comprehension. Songs can be used to teach language and increase the ability to put words together. Art therapy can provide a nonverbal, symbolic way for the child to express him- or herself.

Animal therapy may include horseback riding or swimming with dolphins. Therapeutic riding programs provide both physical and emotional benefits, improving coordination and motor development, while creating a sense of well-being and increasing self-confidence. Dolphin therapy was first used in the 1970s by psychologist David Nathanson. He believed that interactions with dolphins would increase a child's attention, enhancing cognitive processes. In a number of studies, he found that children with disabilities learned faster and retained information longer when they were with dolphins, compared to children who learned in a classroom setting.

Again, as with all other therapy or treatment approaches, it is important to gather information and make an informed decision. Keep in mind, however, that with most complementary approaches there will be little scientific research that has been conducted to support the particular therapy.

## Biomedical and Dietary Approaches

Autism is a spectrum disorder with a variety of options for treatment for individuals across the lifespan. Professionals and families have found that a combination of approaches may be effective in treating symptoms and behaviors that make it hard for individuals with autism to function. These treatment options may include psychosocial and pharmacological interventions.

While there are no drugs, vitamins, or special diets that can correct underlying neurological problems associated with autism, parents and professionals have found that some drugs used for other disorders are sometimes effective in treating some aspects of behaviors associated with autism.

Changes to diet and the addition of certain vitamins or minerals may also help with behavioral issues. For more then a decade, there have been claims by parents and some professionals that adding essential vitamins such as $B_6$ and $B_{12}$ and removing gluten and casein from a child's diet may improve digestion, allergies, and sociability. Not all researchers and experts agree about whether these therapies are effective or scientifically valid.

### Medications

There are a number of medications, developed for other conditions, that have been found effective in treating some of the symptoms and behaviors frequently found in individuals with autism spectrum disorders (ASD). Some of these behaviors include: hyperactivity, impulsivity, attention difficulties, and anxiety. The goal of medications is to reduce these behaviors to allow the individual with ASD to take advantage of educational and behavioral treatments.

When medication is being discussed or prescribed, it's important to ask about the safety of its use in children on the autism spectrum. The following questions might be helpful:

• What is the appropriate dosage?

• How is it administered (pills, liquid)?

• What are the long-term consequences?

• Are there possible side effects?

• How will monitoring occur and by whom?

• What laboratory tests are required before starting the drug and during treatment?

• Are there possible interactions with other drugs, vitamins, or foods?

Given the complexity of medications, drug interactions, and the unpredictability of how each patient may react to a particular drug, parents should seek out and work with a medical doctor with an expertise in the area of medication management and experience with individuals with ASD.

### What Medications Are Available?

The Autism Society of America (ASA) does not endorse any specific medication or type of treatment approach. ASA recommends that all options available are investigated to determine the approach that is most appropriate. People on the spectrum, parents, and professionals must be empowered to critically examine the wide variety of options available to determine associated threats and opportunities and, therefore, make informed decisions. The information provided here is meant as an overview of the types of medications sometimes prescribed. Be sure to consult a medical professional for more information.

There are a number of medications that are frequently used for individuals with autism to address certain behaviors or symptoms. Some have studies to support their use, while others do not.

Serotonin re-uptake inhibitors have been effective in treating depression, obsessive-compulsive behaviors, and anxiety that present in some individuals with ASD. Researchers who have consistently found elevated levels of serotonin in the bloodstream of one-third of individuals with autism feel that these drugs could potentially reverse some of the symptoms of serotonin dysregulation in autism. Three drugs that have been studied are clomipramine (Anafranil), fluvoxamine (Luvox), and fluoxetine (Prozac). Studies have shown that they may reduce the frequency and intensity of repetitive behaviors, and may decrease irritability, tantrums, and aggressive behavior. Some children have also shown improvements in eye contact and responsiveness.

Other drugs, such as Elavil, Wellbutrin, Valium, Ativan, and Xanax, have not been studied as much but may have a role in treating the behavioral symptoms. However, all these drugs have potential side effects, which should be discussed with qualified professionals before treatment is started.

Anti-psychotic medications have been the most widely studied of the psychopharmacologic agents in autism over the past thirty-five years. Originally developed for treating schizophrenia, these drugs have been found to decrease hyperactivity, stereotypical behaviors, withdrawal, and aggression in individuals with autism. Four that have been approved by the Food and Drug Administration (FDA) are clozapine (Clozaril), risperidone (Risperdal), olanzapine (Zyprexa), and quetiapine (Seroquel). Only risperidone has been investigated in a controlled study of adults with autism and was approved in 2006 by the FDA for the treatment of autism. Like the antidepressants, these drugs all have potential side effects, including sedation, which need to be carefully monitored by a qualified professional with experience in autism.

Stimulants, such as Ritalin, Adderall, and Dexedrine, used to treat hyperactivity in children with attention deficit hyperactivity disorder (ADHD), have also been prescribed for children with ASD. Although few studies have been done, anecdotal evidence shows these medications may increase focus and decrease impulsivity and hyperactivity in autism, particularly in children who are not as severely affected as others. However, dosages need to be carefully monitored, because behavioral side effects are often dose-related.

Increased use of medications to treat autism spectrum disorders has highlighted the need for more studies of these drugs in children. The National Institute of Mental Health has established a network of Research Units on Pediatric Psychopharmacology (RUPPs) that combine expertise in psychopharmacology and psychiatry.

If you are considering the use of medications, contact a medical professional experienced in treating individuals on the autism spectrum to learn of possible side effects and discuss potential benefit. People with ASD may have very sensitive nervous systems and normally recommended dosage may need to be adjusted. Even the use of large doses of vitamins should be done under the supervision of a medical doctor.

## Vitamins and Minerals

Over more then a decade, claims have been made that vitamin and mineral supplements may improve the symptoms of autism in a natural way. While not all researchers agree about whether these therapies are scientifically proven, many parents, and an increasing number of physicians, report improvement in people with ASD when using individual or combined nutritional supplements.

Malabsorption problems and nutritional deficiencies have been addressed in several as-of-yet unreplicated studies. A few studies suggest that intestinal disorders and chronic gastrointestinal inflammation may reduce the absorption of essential nutrients and cause disruptions in immune and general metabolic functions that are dependent upon these essential vitamins. Other studies have shown that some children on the autism spectrum may have low levels of vitamins A, $B_1$, $B_3$, $B_5$, as well as biotin, selenium, zinc, and magnesium, while others may have an elevated serum copper to plasma zinc ratio, suggesting that people on the autism spectrum may benefit by avoiding copper and taking extra zinc to boost their immune system. Other studies have indicated a need for more calcium. There are several laboratories that test for nutritional deficiencies but many insurance companies will not pay for these tests.

Perhaps the most common vitamin supplement used for individuals with ASD is vitamin B, which plays an important role in creating enzymes needed by the brain. In eighteen studies or more on the use of vitamin B and magnesium (which is needed to make vitamin B effective), almost half of the individuals with autism showed improvement. The benefits include decreased behavioral problems, improved eye contact, better attention, and improvements in learning. Other research studies have shown that other supplements may help symptoms as well. Cod liver oil supplements (rich in vitamins A and D) have resulted in improved eye contact and behavior of children with autism. Vitamin C helps in brain function and deficiency symptoms like depression and confusion. Increasing vitamin C has been shown in a clinical trial to improve symptom severity in children with ASD.

## Using Vitamins and Minerals

If you are considering the addition of vitamins or minerals to your child's diet, a laboratory and clinical assessment of nutritional status is highly recommended. The most accurate method for measuring vitamin and mineral levels is through a blood test. It is also important to work with someone knowledgeable in nutritional therapy. While large doses of some vitamins and minerals may not be harmful, others can be toxic. Once supplements are chosen, they should be phased in slowly (over several weeks) and then the effects should be observed for one to two months.

## Dietary Interventions

Individuals with ASD may exhibit low tolerance or allergies to certain foods or chemicals. While not a specific cause of autism, these food intolerances or allergies may contribute to behavioral issues. Many parents and professionals have reported significant changes when specific substances are eliminated from the child's diet.

Individuals on the autism spectrum may have trouble digesting proteins such as gluten. Research in the United States and England has found elevated levels of certain peptides in the urine of children with ASD, suggesting the incomplete breakdown of peptides from foods that contain gluten and casein. Gluten is found in wheat, oats, and rye, and casein in dairy products. The incomplete breakdown and the excessive absorption of peptides may cause disruption in biochemical and neuroregulatory processes in the brain, affecting brain functions. Until there is more information as to why these proteins are not broken down, the removal of the proteins from the diet is the only way to prevent further neurological and gastrointestinal damage.

It is important not to withdraw gluten/casein food products at once from a child's diet, as there can be withdrawal symptoms. Parents wishing to pursue a gluten/casein free diet should consult a gastroenterologist or nutritionist, who can help ensure proper nutrition. For information about implementing a gluten/casein free diet, go to www .gfcfdiet.com. Additional information about gluten-free foods can be found at www.celiacsociety.org. The Autism Society of America's magazine, *Autism Advocate*, also has a regular feature of recipes for those with special dietary needs.

Some hypothesize that children with ASD have what is referred to as a "leaky gut"—tiny holes in their intestinal tract that may be caused by an overgrowth of yeast. Some believe that this overgrowth may contribute to behavioral and medical problems in individuals on the spectrum, such as confusion, hyperactivity, stomach problems, and fatigue. The use of nutritional supplements, anti-fungal drugs and/ or a yeast-free diet may reduce the behavioral problems. However, caution should be paid to the fact that just as antibiotics can lead to bacterial resistance, anti-fungals can lead to fungal resistance.

Chapter 24

# Behavioral Interventions

## Chapter Contents

Section 24.1—Improving Behavior in Children with
      Autism Spectrum Disorders ............................ 294
Section 24.2—Applied Behavioral Analysis (ABA)................... 297
Section 24.3—Social Stories: Helping People with Autism
      Interpret Social Situations ............................ 300

Section 24.1

# *Improving Behavior in Children with Autism Spectrum Disorders*

Reprinted from "A Guide to Improving Behaviors in Children with Autism Spectrum Disorders." This article was written by Laurie Stephens, Ph.D., the Director of Autism Spectrum Disorders Programs, The Help Group, www.thehelpgroup.org. Reprinted with permission from The Help Group, *HelpLetter*, Spring 2006.

Children with autism spectrum disorders (ASD) experience the world in a very different way than other children. For these children, behaviors considered to be inappropriate, such as outbursts, tantrums, or "meltdowns," may be their only way to communicate their needs, wants, and frustrations. Sadly, these actions may result in children with ASD doing poorly in school and community events and experiencing difficulty maintaining friendships, and can cause family problems at home. These difficulties often lead to a child being referred for treatment. This section helps parents, family members, educators, and health care professionals understand potential causes of behavioral difficulties for children with ASD and provides guidelines to improve behaviors.

## *Potential Causes for Inappropriate Behaviors*

**Communication delays:** Children with ASD may not always understand what is being said to them or asked of them, due to their communication delays. They may lack the language to adequately express their wants and needs. Acting out, or throwing a tantrum, is a good way to get attention and often is the only way the children can express themselves.

**Sensory dysfunctions:** Sensory dysfunctions can also be a primary cause of behaviors. A common feature of ASD is oversensitivity to sounds, texture, smell, and lights. For the child, it can be as bad as experiencing his or her environment as a jarring alarm going off constantly, a strobe light flashing, a putrid smell everywhere, a feeling of clothing being overly tight and itchy, and being asked questions in a foreign language and getting in trouble when the answer is wrong. Very few people would be able to keep their behavior in check under such circumstances, but this is often an everyday reality for children with ASD.

**Need for routine:** A core feature of ASD is the need for sameness or routine. When children impose a high level of rigidity and structure on their environment, they are setting up unrealistic expectations. When these expectations are not met, it leads to an increase in anxiety and frustration, which, in turn, leads to an increase in behaviors.

## Tips to Avoid Behavioral Difficulties in Children with ASD

**Focus on the positive:** The best way to eliminate negative behaviors is to reinforce the positive behaviors children engage in throughout the day. This will increase the likelihood they will repeat those behaviors. For example, praising children for homework they've already completed is more effective than yelling at them to finish it. Use motivating statements like, "Wow, I see you've been working hard on your homework. I'll bet you'll be finished in no time at all." When children finish a task, it is important to give some kind of reinforcement, such as a treat, a token, or praise.

**Tell the child what to do instead of what not to do:** It is more effective to give children direct commands. This is particularly true for children with ASD, as they often take language literally. When we tell kids what not to do, we assume they know what the appropriate alternative behavior is. For instance, if you tell a child with ASD not to jump in a puddle, he or she may not understand that means to go around the puddle; he or she may think it is fine to splash in the puddle, walk through the puddle, and so on. Saying, "walk around the puddle" makes expectations clear and reduces behavioral outbursts.

**Avoid too much language:** Children with ASD often have communication deficits. When frustrated or anxious, they may be even less able to understand spoken language than usual. Rather than trying to reason with a child in the middle of a tantrum, try to use few words and concrete language. Statements such as, "It is time to get in the car" are more easily understood and followed than if you explain why the child needs to get in the car, how you are going to be late, and what will happen if he or she doesn't get in the car.

**Warn of upcoming changes or transitions:** While it may not always be possible, it is best to tell children with ASD about any change that may be occurring and give them plenty of time to adjust. If you are buying new furniture, share pictures or bring your child to the showroom to see and touch it. Ask for help to decide where to place the furniture. This prepares the child for change and reduces anxiety.

**Use visual schedules or reminders:** Structure and consistency are two keys to improving behaviors. A fun way to do this is to develop simple visual reminders or schedules. This can be as simple as putting a picture of your child's teacher on the calendar for every day that he or she needs to go to school, or as complex as having a full schedule written out for every step for getting ready to go to school, along with the expected times of completion.

**Teach calming techniques:** Often, we tell children to "calm down" when they are feeling anxious or upset. The problem is that we only use the word "calm" when a child is upset! It is important to identify for children what it means to be relaxed or "calm" so that they know the feeling we want them to experience. Try different relaxation techniques, such as counting to ten, taking deep breaths, yoga, and music, to see which ones works best for the child. What calms any child will be highly individualized.

**Beware of sensory overload:** It is always important to look at the environment that the child is in and determine if it is overstimulating. A child may throw a tantrum in the grocery store because it is too bright or the "beep-beep" of the price scanners is bothersome. The tantrum may be the only way the child knows to quickly get parents out of the store. If you think your child has sensory issues, devise coping strategies, such as letting him or her wear sunglasses in the shop or listen to music to drown out upsetting sounds.

**Use "time-outs" effectively:** The use of techniques, such as "time-outs," needs to be used with careful consideration in a child with ASD. This common punishment removes a child from an enjoyable activity. This may not be effective in children with ASD because what other children consider an enjoyable activity may not be fun for them. For example, a child may be held back from recess because she hasn't finished her work. However, if the child finds recess too loud, too unstructured, and too crowded, he or she will actually prefer staying in over going to recess, and may even stop doing school work in an effort to avoid recess. The teacher in this case has mistakenly reinforced the negative behavior by assuming that the child wanted to go to recess.

These strategies can be used in any environment by parents, family members, health care professionals, and educators. Consistent and regular use to of these tips can prevent or reduce inappropriate behaviors. It's important to always keep in mind that children with ASD are not necessarily being manipulative or stubborn when they are having behavioral difficulties. They may not have any other way to express what they are experiencing. If we learn to listen to behaviors, we'll be able help them handle them in a more effective and productive manner.

## Section 24.2

## *Applied Behavioral Analysis (ABA)*

Applied behavioral analysis is a discipline devoted to the understanding and improvement of human behavior. But there are other disciplines with similar intent. What sets applied behavioral analysis apart? The answer lies in its focus, goals, and methodology. Applied behavioral analysis focuses on objectively defined, observable behaviors of social significance; it seeks to improve the behavior under study while demonstrating a reliable relationship between the procedures employed and the behavioral improvement; and it uses the methods of science—description, quantification, and analysis.

Autism spectrum disorder exists on a continuum (i.e., some children with autism are more impacted than others). Autistic spectrum disorders are characterized by deficits in language and social interaction, and by restricted, repetitive, and stereotypical patterns of behavior, interests, and activities. There are no treatments which are accepted by everyone as "the" approach to use, but the applied behavioral analysis (ABA) approach to teaching language and social skills, which is based on B. F. Skinner's research into the principles of learning and which is useful in any condition for which remedial education is required, seems to be meeting with considerable success.

## Discrete Trial Teaching

Discrete trial teaching (DTT; often referred to as applied behavioral analysis, or ABA) is an intensive behavioral therapy, used to help children with autism learn. It is based on Skinner's (1938) *Analysis of Nonverbal Behavior*. The basic premise is that a command is given, a response is evoked, and a consequence reinforces the response. This cycle consists of a trial. How many times that trial needs to be done (in most cases a good starting point is ten) is determined by the consultant (often referred to as rate of learning, or ROL). If the child complies, he or she is positively reinforced; if the child does not comply, he or she is physically prompted through the trial, and then positively reinforced. The program relies solely on positive reinforcement. Every set of trials (determined by the ROL) is considered to be a drill. A child's individual program could have fifteen to twenty-five drills per session, depending on ROL and age. A session usually lasts two to three hours. Our program utilizes a work-break-play model. Depending on ROL and age, a child works for five minutes, then has a one-minute break to do whatever he or she wants, then two minutes of structured play (to begin to generalize the skill learned in work). The model keeps repeating itself. Lastly and most importantly, parents need to be involved to help generalize the skills the children are doing in their sessions.

## Fluency Teaching

Fluency is a relatively new technique that is based on the premise that if known skills are practiced repeatedly, they become more fluent. If known skills become more fluent, it will be easier for children to generalize those skills and learn new skills.

As the child masters skills he or she is put into "fluency drills" to help the child become more "fluent" in retrieving information. Consider the following example: In third grade we have to memorize times tables. We are tested and drilled to know these facts "fluently." The reason for this is because in fourth grade we are introduced to division. While performing the operation of division, we need to use other operations that have been previously mastered. If these mastered skills are not "fluent," the new operation (division) we are trying to learn is much more difficult. The reason it is more difficult is because we are essentially performing two operations.

When a skill is "fluent" it is not thought about, it is just performed. The founders of this new method of teaching children with autism believe that if we can help children become more "fluent" with actions and labels, they will be more likely to learn higher-level skills with ease. They are also more likely to interact with their environments if they are more "fluent" with their language.

## Verbal Behavior

Verbal behavior (often referred to as applied verbal behavior, or AVB) is an extension of the intensive behavioral therapy (DTT) used to help children with autism learn. It is based on B. F. Skinner's (1957) *Analysis of Verbal Behavior*. This extension has resulted in a classification system that allows for the identification of functionally different types of language. Based on this system, Skinner (1957) identified and named verbal relations. Verbal behavior programs rely heavily on communication (manding), teaching in the natural environment, pairing therapists with reinforcement, and teaching with a procedure referred to as "errorless teaching."

Section 24.3

# Social Stories: Helping People with Autism Interpret Social Situations

"Social Stories," © The Illinois Autism/PDD Training and Technical Assistance Project. Reprinted with permission. The text of this document is available online, at http://www.illinoisautismproject.org/fact_sheets/Social%20Story%20Fact%20Sheet%20_2_.pdf; accessed April 26, 2007.

## What Are Social Stories?

Individuals with autism spectrum disorder (ASD) have trouble interpreting social situations. Social stories are developmentally appropriate short stories, typically written for a specific individual with ASD, that provide the individual with the means to understand and respond to various social situations. Because individuals with ASD are primarily visual learners, social stories allow them to learn social behaviors that they would otherwise struggle to understand.

## Why Use Social Stories?

There are a number of reasons to use social stories:

- To teach basic social skills (sharing, asking a friend to play, etc.)
- To teach understanding, interpretation, and appropriate response in social situations (predicting outcomes, preparing for change, coping, problem solving, etc.)

## How to Create a Social Story

1. Have the individual with autism be the main character.

2. Personalize the story so that the individual with autism feels at home.

3. Be specific about the setting(s) in the story.

4. Be specific in describing other characters in the story.

5. Write actual, realistic dialog appropriate to the ability of the individual with autism.

6. Repeat the important points in the story.

7. Involve the individual with autism when you write the story.

8. Have the individual with autism illustrate the story with drawings or use photographs or icons.

9. When using social stories for learning, expose the individual with autism to the story frequently.

## Use the Four Sentence Types

Carole Gray recommends two to five descriptive or control sentences for every directive sentence in the story.

The four different types of sentences you should use are as follows:

- **Descriptive:** Provides information about the child or adolescent, the environment, and what will take place in the social situation.

- **Directive:** Describes how the child or adolescent should respond in the social situation.

- **Perspective:** Identifies the feelings or reactions of others in the social situation.

- **Control:** Provides analogies of similar situations using nonhuman references.

Here is an example of a social story:

When school is over, the bell rings. This always makes me smile.
I like to put my paper and pencils in my bag, and say goodbye to my teacher.
When I walk down the hall, I like to stop and talk to the people I see. I do not have a lot of time so I will try to just wave.
When I leave the building, I will get on the bus and sit in my assigned seat. Now I am on my way home!!

## Additional Resources

### Articles

Crozier, S. & Sileo, N. (2005). Encouraging Positive Behavior With

Social Stories: An Intervention For Children With Autism Spectrum Disorder. *Teaching Exceptional Children* 37(6): 26–31.

Swaggart, B. L., Gagnon, E., Bock, S. J., Earles, T. L., Quinn, C., Myles, B. S., and Simpson, R. L. (1995). Using social stories to teach social and behavioral skills to children with autism. *Focus on Autistic Behavior* 10(1): 1–15.

### Books

Gray, C. (2000). *The New Social Story Book*. Arlington, TX: Future Horizons.

Baker, J. (2001). *The Social Skills Picture Book*. Arlington, TX: Future Horizons.

Chapter 25

# Communication Therapies

## Chapter Contents

Section 25.1—Communication and Interaction in
　　　　　Children with Autism Spectrum Disorders ...... 304
Section 25.2—Picture Exchange Communication System ....... 314
Section 25.3—Facilitated Communication: A Largely
　　　　　Discredited Therapy ........................................... 317

## Section 25.1

## Communication and Interaction in Children with Autism Spectrum Disorders

Communication happens when one person sends a message to another person either verbally or nonverbally. Interaction happens when two people, for example, an adult and a child, respond to one another—a two-way communication.

Most children with an autistic spectrum disorder (ASD) will have difficulty interacting with others. This is because in order to be successful at interaction the child needs to respond to others when he or she is approached by them or be able to initiate interactions. Although many children with an ASD are able to do this when they want something, they tend not to use interaction to show people things or to be sociable.

It is important to remember that communication and interaction do not have to involve the use of language and speech. Many children with an ASD are delayed in their use of language and shy away from using speech. Therefore, other methods of communication need to be established before speech and language will follow.

### Understanding the Communication of a Child with an ASD

Often parents and caregivers of children with an ASD feel that they are unable to communicate and interact with their child and are unsure of how to do so. The child may appear not to hear what is said to him or her, fail to respond to their his or her name, or be indifferent to any attempts of communication that are made. The use of everyday opportunities and play can encourage communication and interaction in a child with ASD.

The way in which the child communicates needs to be observed in order to develop his or her communicative strengths and needs. For example, if the child is not using any sound or speech, rather then communicating with him or her through words, try using gestures. The child with an ASD may use some of the following to communicate with others: crying, taking the adult's hand to the desired object, looking at the desired object, reaching, using pictures, and echolalia.

Echolalia is the repetition of other people's words and is a common feature of the child with an ASD. Initially when the child uses echolalia it is likely that he or she is repeating words that he or she does not understand and is doing so with no communicative intent. However, echolalia is a good sign, as it shows that the child's communication is developing—in time, the child will begin to use the repeated words and phrases to communicate something significant. For example, children may memorize the words that were said to them when they were asked if they would like a drink, and use them later, in a different situation, to ask a question of their own.

Being successful in communication with the child with an ASD involves an understanding not only of how he or she communicates but also of why he or she communicates. In understanding the purpose of the child's communication you can help the child find more ways and more reasons to communicate.

There are two main different types of communication:

- **Pre-intentional communication:** This is when the child says or does things without intending them to affect those around him or her. This type of communication can be used by the child to calm him- or herself, focus him- or herself, or as a reaction to an upsetting or fun experience.

- **Intentional communication:** This is when the child says or does things with the purpose of sending a message to another person. This type of communication can be used to protest about what the child is being asked to do and to make requests.

Intentional communication is easier for children once they have learned that their actions have an effect on other people—the move from pre-intentional communication to intentional communication is a big step for children with an ASD.

Sussman (1999) believes that it is helpful to view children with an ASD as being on a continuum in terms of their intentional communication, at one end of the continuum are children who communicate mainly to get the things they want; "at the other end are children who communicate for many reasons, such as to ask questions, comment on something, or be sociable."

## The Four Different Stages of Communication (as Defined by the Hanen Program)

The stage of communication that the child has reached depends on three things:

- The child's ability to interact with another person

- How and why the child communicates

- The child's understanding

**Stage one—The own agenda stage:** A child at this stage of communication will appear uninterested in the people around him or her and will tend to play alone. His or her communication will be mainly pre-intentional. The majority of children first diagnosed with an ASD are at this stage.

**Stage two—The requester stage:** At this stage the child has begun to realize that his or her actions have an affect on other people. The child is likely to communicate to the adult his or her wants and what he or she enjoys by pulling the adult toward objects, areas, or games.

**Stage three—The early communicator stage:** At this stage the child's interactions will begin to increase in length and become more intentional. The child may also begin to echo some of the things that he or she hears to communicate needs. Gradually the child will begin to point to things that he or she wants to show the adult and begin to shift his or her gaze. This is a sign that child is beginning to engage in a two-way interaction.

**Stage four—The partner stage:** When the child reaches this stage he or she has become a more effective communicator. The child will be using speech to talk and will be able to carry out a simple conversation. While the child may appear confident and capable when using communication in familiar environments (e.g., at home), the child may struggle when he or she enters unfamiliar territory (e.g., at a new nursery or school). In this situation the child may use memorized phrases and can often appear to be ignoring his or her communication partners by speaking over them and ignoring the rules of turn taking.

## Ways That Adults Can Affect the Communication of the Child with ASD

**Take on the role of a helper and teacher:** When the child is unable to communicate his or her needs it is tempting to help the child by constantly doing things for him or her. For example, fetching shoes and tying shoelaces. However, in doing this the opportunities for children to show that they can do such things for themselves are reduced. When the child is at the own agenda stage it is particularly difficult to decipher how much to do for the child. In this instance it is appropriate to ask the child if he or she needs help, wait, and then ask a second time before adding the help.

**Instead of letting the child do his or her own thing, encourage the child to do things with others:** It is tempting to believe that the child is merely showing independence when he or she shows no interest in interacting with the adult. However, it is important that the child does learn to interact and is not just left to his or her own devices. In this instance the key is to persevere with joining in with whatever activity the child is engaged in, whether this is playing with a piece of string or taking toys in and out of the toy box. If the child shows anger and aggression when this is tried, still persevere. Anger is a type of interaction and is better than no interaction at all. As this interaction is continued with the child, he or she may begin to realize in time that interaction with another person can be fun.

**Slow down the pace and give the child a chance to communicate:** Caring for a child with an ASD can be hard work and time consuming. There is often the temptation to rush the child when he or she is performing daily tasks such as eating breakfast and getting dressed. A child with ASD will benefit from a few minutes extra time when engaged in these tasks, to help the child understand what is happening around him or her and to think about what he or she can say during these activities.

**When playing with the child take on the role of a partner rather than a leader:** As the child becomes more capable at communicating, he or she needs less direction—if the child is given too many questions and suggestions it can become difficult for him or her to initiate his or her own conversations. It is important to follow the child's lead and respond to what he or she does.

**Present the child with feedback:** It is important to reward the child when he or she attempts to understand and communicate. By doing this you can increase the likelihood that the child will try and do it again. By using simple descriptive praise that comments on what the child has achieved, you can help the child to make a connection between his or her own actions and your specific words.

## Giving the Child with ASD a Reason to Communicate

If the child with ASD has no difficulty getting what he or she wants, that child will have no reason to communicate and interact. Therefore, on many occasions the adult will need to engineer a situation in order to create a communicative opportunity for the child and encourage interaction.

**Encourage requests:** This can be achieved by placing the child's favorite toy, food, or video in a place where the child can see it but is unable to reach it, for example, a high shelf. Alternatively, place the child's favorite object in a container that the child will find difficult to open, such as an old ice-cream tub or an old jam jar. This will encourage the child to ask for help and result in an interaction between adult and child.

**Give the child a toy that is difficult to operate:** Wind-up toys and games that need to be squeezed to make them work will be difficult for the child to operate alone but will also interest the child. Once the child has been given the toy or game, allow him or her some time to establish how to use it. When the child becomes frustrated at his or her inability to work the toy or game, the adult can step in and help. Examples of this type of toy include Jack-in-the-boxes, spinning tops, and music boxes.

**Give the child a toy that is "high interest":** Balloons and bubbles are high-interest toys and can be easily adapted to involve two people. Simple games such as blowing up a balloon and then letting it go so that it flies up in the air may appeal to the child. Blowing up the balloon part way and waiting for a response from the child before blowing it up to its full capacity is also a clever way to enhance interaction between adult and child. A similar thing can be achieved with bubbles: blow a few bubbles toward the child, and once his or her attention has been captured, close the container and wait for a response from him or her before you blow any more.

**Give things to the child gradually:** If the child is given everything that he or she wants, the child will have no reason to ask the adult for anything else. By staggering how much food or how many toys are given to the child, he or she is provided with opportunities to interact by expressing wants and needs. For example, if the child wants a cookie, break it into small pieces, initially giving the child one piece and then gradually giving him or her more once he or she has communicated a request for it.

**Let the child decide when to end an activity:** Once the child is engaged in an activity with the adult, carry on with that activity until the child indicates that he or she has had enough. Look out for facial grimaces or the child pushing away the activity. This way, the child is forced to communicate that he or she is ready to finish the activity. If the child does not use language to indicate he or she has finished, accompany the child's form of communication with words such as "had enough" and "stop" to encourage language development.

## Increasing Interaction by Following the Child's Lead

Following the child's lead rather than directing him or her will enable the child to learn to communicate while he or she does things with another person, hence increasing interaction. The child that leads is more likely to pay attention to the activity, is more likely to focus on the same thing as the adult, and will learn how to make choices for him- or herself.

When following the child's lead it is beneficial to be in a position where the adult is face-to-face with the child; this way the adult can easily observe what it is that the child is interested in. It will also help the child to make eye contact—something that can often be difficult for the child with an ASD. Being level with the child will also ensure that he or she is in a position to see the variety of facial expressions that are used in communication. A child with an ASD will often fail to pick up on these nonverbal communicative behaviors during conversation; therefore, it is important to draw attention to them where possible. It is hoped that the child will eventually become used to the adult playing with him or her at the child's level and begin to anticipate the adult's presence, fetching the adult if he or she is not there.

Imitating the child's actions and words will help the child become involved in two-way interactions. If the child bangs the spoon on the table, and the adult does the same, it is likely that the child will pay attention to the adult. This idea can also be used with sounds that the child makes or with the child's sensory behaviors, for example, hand flapping and spinning. Once the child has established that the adult is imitating his or her actions, the child may begin to imitate back. This creates the opportunity for the adult to add something new to the exchange for the child to duplicate.

When the child with an ASD is disinterested in playing with any of the toys presented, or prefers to line toys up rather then play with them, there are still communication and interaction opportunities available. For example, if the child is lining up the cars in a row, the adult can join in the activity by handing the child the cars one by one. This way, the adult plays a part in the game and the child has to include the adult in what he or she is doing. If the child is interested only in throwing the toys on the floor, the adult could use a basket to collect them before giving them back to the child, thus establishing a pattern of interaction and communication with the child.

## Ways That Adults Can Help the Child With an ASD Understand What Is Said

A child with an ASD will find processing information a difficult thing to do. This is because the child may find it difficult to understand the world around him or her. Even when the child with an ASD does understand a situation, he or she may not understand the words that go with that situation. Sometimes it is easy to assume that the child understands what is being said to him or her because the child appears to follow instructions. However, the likelihood is that the child will know what to do when instructions are given in certain contexts because he or she has been in those situations numerous times previously.

There are several ways in which to enhance a child's comprehension of what people are saying to him or her.

**Say less and say it slowly:** The adult can limit the amount of words he or she uses to communicate with the child but still communicate the relevant information. Use key words that are specific to the context of the situation, repeat and stress them, and use gesture, such as pointing, to accompany them. Sussman (1999) uses the following rhyme as a reminder of how an adult can make it easier for a child with an ASD to understand: "Say less and stress, go slow and show!"

If the child has only recently begun to use speech as a means of communication, the adult should use single words to communicate with him or her. For example, label favorite toys and food. When using this method of communication it is important to label things immediately after they are given to the child. If the child's attention has shifted onto something else, the word will lose its meaning.

Pausing in between spoken words and phrases can also help the child with an ASD to understand what is being said to him or her. The adult should use pauses to give the child time to process what has been said and to give the child an opportunity to think of a response.

Using gestures to accompany language can also encourage the child to understand what is being said. For example, when offering the child a drink the adult should imitate the action of drinking by pretending to hold a glass in one hand and bringing it to his or her mouth as if taking a sip. A similar gesture can be used for eating. Over-exaggerated facial expressions can also be used along with shaking the head for "yes" and "no" and waving the hand for "hello" and "goodbye." When talking to the child about people (for example, "grandma is staying"), it helps to present the child with a photo of the person who is being spoken about.

Other visual methods that can be used to increase understanding include picture timetables, line drawings, cue cards, and object/picture schedules.

## Using Augmentative and Alternative Communication (AAC) Supports

AAC describes any form of language other than speech that assists a child in social-communicative interactions. There is a large range of AAC devices available for children who have no speech, and these children themselves are very diverse. Therefore, it is essential that a team of appropriate individuals evaluate different AAC options with the parents of a child with ASD before a decision about their use is made. Criteria that need to be discussed before an AAC device is implemented include cognitive and motor abilities, learning style, communication needs, and literacy ability.

The use of AAC devices for children with ASD can be particularly helpful. Those children with ASD who have no spoken language often resort to challenging behaviors to meet their needs and express their feelings. The use of an AAC device can give them a primary means of social communicative interactions with others. If it is decided that an

AAC device is appropriate for the child, it is the responsibility of those around the child to model the system.

Different types of AAC devices that are suitable for the child with ASD include the following:

- Picture exchange communication system (PECS, Frost and Bondy, 1994)
- Sign language
- Interactive communication boards
- Communication cue cards
- Conversation books
- Voice output communication aids

**Sign language:** There are several difference sign language systems. When using sign language with a child with an ASD, it can be beneficial to use a total communication approach. Total communication is the use of combined speech and sign so that the same language structure is modeled for the child in two modalities. The use of total communication helps to highlight key word meanings and assists in language comprehension.

**Interactive communication boards:** Interactive communication boards contain visual symbols organized by topic. They can be created in different sizes and formats depending on the activity and environment for which they are needed. They can be both portable and stationary—one board is designed to stay in one location. The selection and organization of the symbols that are used need to be motivating and chosen to enhance functional communication for the child.

**Cue cards:** Cue cards are primarily used with verbal children. They are used to remind the child what to say and to provide the child with an alternative means of communication. They can contain one or more messages in pictorial or written form and can replace verbal prompts. They are, therefore, particularly useful for children who are reliant on verbal prompts. Cue cards can work well in situations where the child with an ASD needs to express a message in a stressful situation.

**Conversation books:** A conversation book can be pictorial or consist of a written summary of conversation topics used for increasing conversational abilities. The conversational topics are organized in a small book, wallet, or something similar and are used as a focus of conversation with an adult. It is important that the book is age-appropriate and that the topics chosen are meaningful to the child. This can often be best achieved by using photographs—especially for the younger child. Conversation books organize the conversation for the child. They provide a concrete, visual means to share and maintain topics.

**Voice output communication aids:** Speech output devices give nonverbal children a "voice." A team of relevant professionals should determine the most appropriate technology option. Once this has been established, the team then needs to decide on an appropriate vocabulary selection, the layout of the device, the size of the symbols, and the principal situations in which to encourage the child to use the device. There are a wide range of devices available, including simpler ones for people who do not understand visual symbols. In order to use these devices, the child will need an understanding of cause and effect.

The combined use of AAC, social supports, organizational supports, and visually cued instruction can enhance the social communicative interactions in children with autism.

## References

Gray, C. (2002) *My Social Stories Book*. London: Jessica Kingsley Publishers.

Leicestershire County Council and Fosse Health Trust (1998) *Autism: How to Help Your Young Child*. London: National Autistic Society.

Moor, J. (2002) *Playing, Laughing and Learning with Children on the Autistic Spectrum: A Practical Resource of Play Ideas for Parents and Carers*. London: Jessica Kingsley Publishers.

Potter, P. and Wittaker, C. (2001) *Enabling Communication in Children with Autism*. London: Jessica Kingsley Publishers.

Sussman, F. (1999) *More than Words*. Canada: The Hanen Programme

## Section 25.2

# *Picture Exchange Communication System*

"Picture Exchange Communication System," © The Illinois Autism/PDD Training and Technical Assistance Project. Reprinted with permission. The text of this document is available online at http://www.illinoisautismproject .org/fact_sheets/PECS%20Fact%20Sheet.pdf; accessed March 22, 2007. Original images from Mayer Johnson, redrawn with permission by Alison DeKleine for Omnigraphics, Inc.

## *What Is the Picture Exchange Communication System?*

The Picture Exchange Communication System (PECS) is a type of augmentative alternative communication (AAC) originally developed for children with autism. The primary purpose of PECS is to teach individuals with autism to initiate communication. Individuals are taught to initiate by handing a picture to a communication partner in exchange for a desired item.

## *Why Use PECS?*

PECS allows individuals with autism to communicate by using pictures instead of, or in conjunction with, speech. PECS provides a functional outlet of expression for individuals who otherwise have difficulty communicating with others. It can be used, beginning as early as age two, to initiate conversation and to communicate wants or needs to another person and has also successfully been taught to adults with similar communication needs. Lastly, oftentimes as individuals with autism increase their ability to communicate, their behavior tends to lessen.

## *How Does PECS Work?*

After being taught the phase six system, an individual using PECS chooses a picture from a variety of pictures available, then gives the picture to a communication partner. Knowing the individual's request, the partner can then provide the desired item or fulfill a desired need.

## The Six Phases of PECS

**Phase I. Purpose—To initiate communication:** The individual with autism sees a desired item. He is physically guided by a prompter to pick up a picture of that item from the table and place it into the communication partner's hand in exchange for the desired item. Physical guidance by the prompter is faded as soon as possible.

cookies

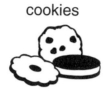

**Phase II. Purpose—To teach distance and persistence:** A communication book is provided with one picture on the front of the book at a time. The individual with autism is taught to locate his or her communication book and travel to the communication partner to exchange a picture for the desired object.

**Phase III. Purpose—To discriminate between pictures or symbols:** The individual with autism is presented with a picture of a highly preferred item and a picture of a nonpreferred item on his or her communication book. The individual exchanges a picture and receives the corresponding item. If the individual selects the preferred item then he or she is given the item with animated social reinforcement. If he or she exchanges the undesirable item then an error correction sequence is introduced. Once the individual begins to discriminate between the items, correspondence checks are completed to ensure that the individual's actions correspond to his or her requests. Discrimination training continues by adding multiple desired items and increasing the number of pictures on the front of the book.

cookies          paper towel

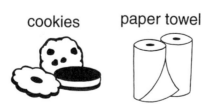

**Phase IV. Purpose—To begin using sentence structure:** The individual is introduced to a new icon "I want" to begin teaching the individual to use a sentence starter. A sentence strip is added to the front of the communication book and the individual learns to build and exchange the phrase by attaching the "I want" picture to the strip, attaching the picture of the desired item to the strip, removing the strip, and exchanging the strip. The communication partner then turns the strip toward the individual with autism and reads the phrase and provides the individual with the desired item.

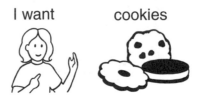

**Phase V. Purpose—To answer a direct question:** The individual is taught to answer the question "What do you want?"

**Phase VI. Purpose—To begin to develop commenting:** The individual learns to communicate more than just his or her wants and needs. He or she learns to comment about the environment. Icons such as "I see" and "I hear" are introduced one at a time on the communication board in a systematic fashion.

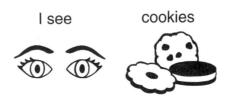

## Resources

Frost, L., and Bondy, A. (2002). *The Picture Exchange Communication System Training Manual.* Newark, DE: Pyramid Educational Products, Inc.

# Section 25.3

# *Facilitated Communication: A Largely Discredited Therapy*

## What Is Facilitated Communication?

Facilitated communication (FC) began in Australia in the 1970s. Rosemary Crossley, an aide at an institution for people with severe multiple disabilities, encouraged a young woman who had cerebral palsy to communicate by acting as her facilitator (Crossley and MacDonald 1980).

The facilitator normally supports a client's hand, wrist, or arm while that person uses a communicator to spell out words, phrases, or sentences.

Crossley went on to establish the DEAL Communication Centre in Melbourne in 1986, which aimed to "assist people with no speech or with dysfunctional speech to find alternative means of communication." Use of FC with people with autism is centered on the notion that many of the difficulties faced are due to a movement disorder rather than social or communication deficits. Much of the philosophy of the DEAL Centre was based upon the premise that the language skills (as opposed to speech skills) of people with autism and other communication disorders were generally less impaired than previous research had indicated. The assumption is that the problem of communication for people with autism is essentially a difficulty with expression. Interest in FC quickly spread to other countries—in particular the United States, Canada, and Denmark, and recently it has been used within the United Kingdom with some people with autism.

There have been highly publicized claims for its effectiveness. Many are now communicating . . . and producing language of such complexity

317

as to challenge commonly held beliefs about the language of people diagnosed as autistic or significantly intellectually impaired (Crossley and Remington-Gurley 1992).

## Research into FC

Alongside the enthusiasm there has been significant criticism of the approach. There has been some reluctance by advocates of FC to put it forward for independent evaluation on the basis that such evaluation would be artificial and interfere with the relationship of trust between facilitator and client.

Nevertheless, experimenters have over recent years built up a useful body of research. Howlin (1997) in her review of forty-five controlled trials of FC involving over 350 subjects found confirmation of independent communication in only 6 percent of subjects. In more than 90 percent of cases the responses were found to be influenced unwittingly by the facilitators rather than the clients.

Bebko, Perry, and Bryson (1996) found some evidence of independent communication in nine (of twenty) subjects. However, among students who were capable of responding independently, their responses were worse under facilitated conditions than they were unsupported.

Meanwhile in the United States, in an unprecedented move, five major national professional bodies have now adopted a formal position of opposing the acceptance of FC as a valid mode of enhancing expression for people with disabilities. These bodies include the American Association on Mental Retardation, the American Academy of Child and Adolescent Psychiatry, and the American Speech-Language-Hearing Association.

The research review on educational interventions commissioned by the Department for Education and Employment (Jordan, Jones, and Murray 1998) concluded that it would be hard to justify further research on FC. There have already been a large number of anecdotal and ethnographic case study reports detailing the technique's supposed benefits, followed by an even greater number of controlled scientific studies, all showing that the phenomenon fails to materialize once facilitator effects have been controlled.

Mostert (2001), in his review of studies into FC since 1995, confirms that their conclusions support those of earlier studies that claims are largely unsubstantiated and that its use as an intervention for people with communication impairments should not be recommended.

## Alleged Abuse

A further concern about facilitated communication has been around accusations of abuse. There has been some use of this unproven technique in court cases in the United States. It is suggested that this has been possible only by courts evading their state's test of scientific admissibility (Gorman 1999).

## References

American Academy of Child and Adolescent Psychiatry. *Policy statement on facilitated communication*, approved by Council 20 October 1993.

Attwood, T. Movement disorders and autism: a rationale for the use of facilitated communication. *Communication*, 1992, 26(3): 27–29.

Bebko, J. M., Perry, A., and Bryson, S. Multiple method validation study of facilitated communication: II Individual differences and subgroup results. *Journal of Autism and Developmental Disorders*, 1996, 26: 19–42.

Bettison, S. Informal evaluation of Crossley's facilitated communication. *Journal of Autism and Developmental Disorders*, 1991, 21(4): 561–63.

Biklen, D. Communication unbound: autism and praxis. *Harvard Educational Review*, 1990, 60: 291–315.

Biklen, D. *Communication unbound: how facilitated communication is challenging traditional views of autism and ability/disability*. New York: Teachers College Press, 1993.

Biklen, D. and Schubert, A. New words: the communication of students with autism. *Remedial and Special Education*, 1991, 12(6): 46–57.

Crossley, R. and McDonald, A. *Annie's coming out*. New York: Penguin Books, 1980.

Crossley, R. and Remington-Gurley, J. Getting the words out: facilitated communication training. *Topics in Language Disorders*, 1992, 12: 29–45.

Edelson, S. M. et al. Evaluation of a mechanical hand-support for facilitated communication. *Journal of Autism and Developmental Disorders*, 1998, 28(2): 153–57.

319

Emerson, A. Facilitated communication. *Communication Matters*, April 1994, 20–23.

Emerson, A. Facilitated communication: a practitioner's personal account. *Communication*, Spring 1996, 16–19.

Facilitated communication reports generate heated controversy. *Autism Research Review International*, 1991, 5(1): 1–2.

Gorman, B. J. Facilitated communication in America: eight years and counting. *Skeptic*, 1998, 6(3): 64–77.

Gorman, B. J. Facilitated communication: rejected in science, accepted in court a case study and analysis of the use of FC evidence under Frye and Daubert. *Behavioral Sciences and the Law*, 1999, 17(4): 517–41.

Gould, J. Facilitated communication: an overview. *Communication*, 1993, 27(2): 9–15.

Grayson, A. Can the physical support given in facilitated communication interactions help to overcome problems associated with executive function? In: *Living and Learning with Autism*. Sunderland, Autism Research Unit, 1997, 231–42.

Green, G. and Shane, H. C. Science, reason and facilitated communication. *Journal of the Association for Persons with Severe Handicaps*, 1994, 19(3): 151–72.

Happé, F. The autobiographical writings of three Asperger syndrome adults: problems of interpretation and implications for theory In: U. Frith, ed., *Autism and Asperger Syndrome*, Cambridge: Cambridge University Press, 1991, 207–47.

Howlin, P. Autism: preparing for adulthood. London: Routledge, 1997, 5–6.

Howlin, P. Facilitated communication and autism: are the claims for success justified? *Communication*, 1994, 28(2): 10–12.

Howlin, P. and Jones, D. P. H. An assessment approach to abuse allegations made through facilitated communication. *Child Abuse and Neglect*, 1996, 20(2): 103–10.

Jones, D. P. H. Autism, facilitated communication and allegations of child abuse and neglect. *Child Abuse and Neglect*, 1994, 18(6): 461–93.

Jordan, R., Jones, G., and Murray, D. *Educational interventions for children with autism: a literature review of recent and current research*. London: Department for Education and Employment, 1998.

Kerrin, R. G. et al. Who's doing the pointing? Investigating facilitated communication in a classroom setting with students with autism. *Focus on Autism and other Developmental Disabilities*, 1998, 13(2): 73–79.

Kezuka, E. The role of touch in facilitated communication. *Journal of Autism and Developmental Disorders*, 1997, 27(5): 571–93.

Konstantareas, M. M. Allegations of sexual abuse by nonverbal autistic people via facilitated communication: testing of validity. *Child Abuse and Neglect*, 1998, 22(10): 1027–41.

Konstantareas, M. M. and Gravelle, G. Facilitated communication: the contribution of physical, emotional and mental support. *Autism*, 1998, 2(4): 389–414.

Mostert M. P. Facilitated communication since 1995: a review of published studies. *Journal of Autism and Developmental Disorders*, 2001, 31(3): 287–313.

Myles, B. et al. Collateral behavioral and social effects of using facilitated communication with individuals with autism. *Focus on Autism and Other Developmental Disabilities, 1996*, 11(3): 163–69.

Perry, A. et al. Brief report: degree of facilitator influence in facilitated communication as a function of facilitator characteristics, attitudes and beliefs. *Journal of Autism and Developmental Disorders*, 1998, 28(1): 87–90.

Prior, M. and Cummins, R. Questions about facilitated communication and autism. *Journal of Autism and Developmental Disorders*, 1992, 22(3): 331–36.

Richer, J. Facilitated communication: a response by child protection. *Child Abuse and Neglect*, 1994, 18(6): 531–37.

Rimland, B. Facilitated communication: problems, puzzles and paradoxes: six challenges for researchers. *Autism Research Review International*, 1991, 5(4): 3.

Rimland, B. Facilitated communication: a light at the end of the tunnel? *Autism Research Review International*, 1993, 7(3): 3.

Routh, D. K. Facilitated communication as unwitting ventriloquism. *Journal of Pediatric Psychology*, 1994, 19(6): 673–75.

Rumbelow, H. Autistic son's language aid led to abuse charge. *The Times*, 13 July 2000, 9.

Siegel, B. Brief report: assessing allegations of sexual molestation made through facilitated communication. *Journal of Autism and Developmental Disorders*, 1995, 25(3): 319–26.

Twachtman-Cullen, D. *A passion to believe: autism and the facilitated communication phenomenon*. Oxford: Westview Press, 1997.

Williams, D. Invited commentary: in the real world. *Journal of the Association for Persons with Severe Handicaps*, 1994, 19(3): 196–99.

Chapter 26

# Sensory Interventions

## Chapter Contents

Section 26.1—Sensory Integration and Motor Therapies ........ 324
Section 26.2—Auditory Integration Training .......................... 326

Section 26.1

# *Sensory Integration and Motor Therapies*

Many people with autism have sensory problems, such as hypersensitivity or hyposensitivity to stimulation. They may also have difficulty being able to integrate senses. These problems can be mild or severe.

Sensory integration focuses on the vestibular sense (i.e., motion, balance), on the tactile sense (i.e., touch), and on proprioception (e.g., joints, ligaments). Techniques usually focus on stimulating these senses in order to make them less or more sensitive and to help a child to recognize sensory information.

Sensory integration therapy is usually given by specially trained occupational, physical, or speech therapists who observe the child carefully to gain a clear understanding of his or her particular sensitivities. Experts and researchers disagree about whether these kinds of therapies really work or if they are scientifically valid. Some people have found that when the sensory needs of autism are met, learning is more focused, progress is better, and people are better able to cope with day-to-day situations. Addressing sensory issues may be a very long process.

In addition, physical therapy and exercise can be helpful for people with autism who have limited gross and fine motor skills.

Following are some examples of sensory integration and motor therapies.

**Berard Auditory Integration Training (called Berard AIT or AIT):** This involves listening to processed music for a total of ten hours (two half-hour sessions per day, over a period of ten to twelve days). AIT is believed to improve auditory processing, decrease or eliminate sound sensitivity, and reduce behavioral problems in some autistic children.

**Computer-based auditory interventions:** These include Earobics and Fast ForWord. These programs may be helpful for children who have delays in language and have difficulty discriminating speech sounds.

**Irlen lenses:** This involves wearing ambient (prism) lenses. People who benefit from these lenses are often hypersensitive to certain types of lighting, such as fluorescent lights and bright sunlight; hypersensitive to certain colors or color contrasts; and/or have difficulty reading printed text. Irlen lenses may reduce sensitivity to these lighting and color problems as well as improve reading skills and increase attention span.

**Oculomotor exercises:** This involves performing eye movement exercises to reorganize and normalize the visual system.

**Swinging:** Swinging a child on a swing can help normalize the vestibular sense.

**Deep pressure:** Dr. Temple Grandin developed a hug machine, which provides deep pressure to help in learning to tolerate touch and which appears to have a calming effect.

**The Wilbarger Protocol:** Some children have a tendency to respond to certain harmless sensations as if they were dangerous or painful. This is called sensory defensiveness (SD). The child with SD may misperceive the world as dangerous, alarming, or at the very least irritating. When left untreated, SD can have a negative influence on every aspect of life. The protocol uses frequent application of firm/deep pressure touch input to various parts of the body. This is followed by gentle joint compression.

**Weighted vest:** The concept of the weighted vest is based on the technique of deep pressure. Deep pressure is used to assist the child to self-calm and relax so that sensory stimuli can be processed. The use of a weighted vest is thought to provide the child with unconscious information from the muscles and joints. Children who are easily distracted, hyperactive, and lacking in concentration are said to respond positively to the additional weight a vest provides.

Section 26.2

# *Auditory Integration Training*

## *What Is Auditory Integration Training (AIT)?*

Dr. Guy Bérard (now retired) was an ear, nose, and throat specialist in Annecy, France, who invented and developed a special auditory training device that has proved to be useful in the treatment of hyperacusis (or excessive auditory sensitivity). Dr. Bérard began developing this in the early 1980s, when he learned that he himself was becoming deaf. He conceived of the idea of developing an electronic machine that would exercise the entire hearing apparatus—the eardrum, the small bones in the ear, the cochlear membrane, and so on as a form of physical therapy, in a manner somewhat similar to that in which deteriorating joints and muscles can be rejuvenated by proper physical therapy and exercise.

This technique was used with many of Dr. Bérard's patients, some of whom had autism, and many others with a variety of auditory difficulties. In relation to autism, Bérard thought that sound sensitivity and consequent behavioral disturbance could result from distortions in hearing. Dr. Bérard states that "Auditory Integration Training cannot be called a cure for autism, but many (people) benefit greatly from the treatment" (Bérard 1997).

The device consists of a machine containing a number of electronic elements, including a variety of auditory filters, which makes the sound emanating from the machine modifiable to be appropriate for the individual person, in accordance with their auditory sensitivities and deficiencies as determined by audiometric testing. In use, the child or adult sits before the machine, wearing earphones, while specially selected music is played into the machine. The machine filters and amplifies the music as necessary and feeds the resulting modified music to each ear independently. The volume is set as loud as is possible without discomfort.

Dr. Bernard Rimland (from the Autism Research Institute) has been in touch with a number of parents of children with autism who have taken their children to be treated by Dr. Bérard. The mother of one of these children has written a book about the experience (Stehli 1992).

## Research into AIT

So far there is not a great deal of data on which to evaluate AIT, but two studies have been carried out in the United States and Australia. An initial pilot project conducted by Drs. Rimland and Edelson at Portland State University in 1990 offered some interesting results and so a second study was undertaken that examined several specific issues of the AIT procedure.

Another research project carried out at the Autism Research Institute in Sydney (Bettison 1996) indicated that although Auditory Training (AT) did lead to a significant improvement in sound sensitivity in general, a structured listening (SL) program led to about the same amount of improvement. (The structured listening program was a simplified version of the AT procedure, and omitted the input of the special equipment used in AT.) Bettison stresses, however, that her results do not prove that AT and SL were the actual cause of the children's improvements, nor, if the interventions were beneficial, which aspects were having the beneficial effect. She concludes that both SL and AT appear to help in reducing sound sensitivity in many, but not all, children with autism who are sound sensitive.

## References and Further Reading

Bérard, G. *Hearing equals behavior*. New Canaan, CT: Keats Publishing Inc., 1993.

Bérard, G. Auditory Integration Training (Bérard's Method). In: *Approaches to autism*. 3rd ed. London: The National Autistic Society, 1997, 11.

Bettison, S. The long-term effects of auditory training on children with autism. *Journal of Autism and Developmental Disorders*, 1996, 26(3): 361–74.

Bettison, S. Auditory integration training some observations of the effects on individuals. *Autism News*, 1999, December, 4–5.

Brown, M. M. Auditory integration training and autism: two case studies. *British Journal of Occupational Therapy*, 1999, January, 62(1): 13–18.

Collins, M. *Auditory integration therapy (AIT): research summaries.* Listen to Learn Centre, 2000.

Edelson, S. M. et al. Auditory integration training: a double-blind study of behavioral and electrophysiological effects in people with autism. *Focus on Autism and other Developmental Disabilities*, 1999, 14(2): 73–81.

Gillberg, C. et al. Auditory integration training in children with autism: a brief report of an open pilot study. *Autism*, 1997, 1(1): 97–100.

Gillberg, C. et al. Auditory integration training in children with autism: Reply to Rimland and Edelson. *Autism*, 1998, 2(1): 93–94. Rimland and Edelson had disagreed with the interpretation of the results of a pilot study of auditory integration training that Gillberg et al had conducted. Gillberg et al now respond stating they still conclude that their overall findings from an open pilot study of nine children being given AIT do not provide clear support for the positive effect on core autistic features, but that a moderate reduction in sensory problems may have occurred.

Howlin, P. *A visit to the Light and Sound Therapy Centre.* London: The National Autistic Society, 1996.

Kirby, W. J. Abstract: The effects of auditory integration training on children diagnosed with attention deficit/hyperactivity disorder: a pilot study. *Sound Connection*, 2000, 7(3): 4–5.

Link, H. M. Auditory integration training (AIT): sound therapy? Case studies of three boys with autism who received AIT. *British Journal of Learning Disabilities*, 1997, 25: 106–10. The progress of three boys with autism receiving AIT was closely monitored. Few if any beneficial effects on behavior were observed. Sound hypersensitivity remained unchanged. The paper also questions the validity of the AIT techniques used, and highlights the need for an AIT watchdog.

Mudford, O. Auditory integration training: recent UK research. *Autism*, 2000, 4(3): 337–38.

Mudford, O. Auditory integration training for children with autism: no behavioral benefits detected. *American Journal on Mental Retardation*, 2000, 105(2): 118–29.

Randall, T. Harvey's auditory integration training: a parent's view. *The Autism File*, 1999, 1: 7–9.

Rimland, B. and Edelson, S. M. *Auditory integration training in autism: a pilot study.* San Diego, CA: Autism Research Institute, 1992. (ARI Publication No. 112)

Rimland, B. and Edelson, S. M. The effects of auditory integration training on autism. *American Journal of Speech-Language Pathology*, 1994, 3(2): 16–24.

Rimland, B. and Edelson, S. M. Brief report: a pilot study of auditory integration training in autism. *Journal of Autism and Developmental Disorders*, 1995, 25(1): 61–70.

Rimland, B. and Edelson, S. M. Letter about auditory integration training. *Autism*, 1998, 2(1): 91–92. Letter disagreeing with the conclusion of Gillberg et al. in *Autism*, 1997, 1(1), that the results of a pilot study of auditory integration training referred to do not provide any support for a positive effect on autistic symptoms. According to Rimland and Edelson, both statistical analysis and visual inspection clearly show positive effects.

Rimland, B. and Edelson, S. M. Response to Howlin on the value of auditory integration training. *Journal of Autism and Developmental Disorders*, 1998, 28(2): 169–70. Rimland and Edelson state that Howlin's negative evaluation of auditory integration training is in large part a consequence of her "obvious unfamiliarity with the various outcome scales used in the two studies she cites." They point out, among other things, that the maximum possible score range on the ABC is not 0–58, as Howlin assumes, but 0–3, making the difference of 0.38 reported a meaningful proportion of the range and of both clinical and statistical significance. Howlin is also criticized for basing her comments on Rimland and Edelson's pilot study (n = 19) rather than the much larger (n = 445) controlled study. Having regard to the nine studies that have been conducted, Rimland and Edelson consider that "research data collected to date favor the use of AIT."

Stehli, A. *The sound of a miracle: a child's triumph over autism.* Doubleday, 1991.

Chapter 27

# Dietary Interventions

## Chapter Contents

Section 27.1—Diet and Vitamins in the Treatment of
Autism ................................................................. 332
Section 27.2—Secretin for Autism: Hope and
Disappointment ................................................. 345
Section 27.3—Is Eliminating Casein and Gluten from a
Child's Diet a Viable Treatment for Autism? ... 348

# Section 27.1

# *Diet and Vitamins in the Treatment of Autism*

## *Introduction*

Since the 1960s, when interest in the effects of diet and vitamins on the treatment of autism began, there has been much research carried out in this area, although not necessarily into all diets and vitamins that could be of use. As with all approaches to treating autism, it is important to remember that some will work with varying degrees of success in one person, while not having any effect at all for another. It is also important to stress that while experimenting with vitamins and supplements is unlikely to result in any serious side effects, consultation with a doctor or professionally qualified dietitian on any change of diet is strongly recommended. Please note that some vitamins and supplements can be toxic in high doses. There are several organizations that can help with a decision to use vitamins or diets in treating autism and Asperger syndrome and it would be useful to consult these.

## *Vitamin $B_6$/Magnesium*

### *Who could benefit?*

Since the 1960s when Rimland initiated research into the use of a high dose of vitamin $B_6$ alongside a normal dose of magnesium, a high proportion of people on the autistic spectrum have benefited from taking more vitamin $B_6$. It is important however, to recognize that only those on the autistic spectrum with a need for vitamin $B_6$ in particular will benefit from this treatment.

## How successful has this diet proved? Have any studies been carried out?

There have been around twenty published studies since 1965 and vitamin $B_6$ has proved beneficial to around 50 percent of those involved. It is not fully understood why vitamin $B_6$ is useful in this way. If the treatment is going to be useful then it should have an effect within a few days, but if there is no change in three to four weeks it should be stopped.

### Is this treatment safe?

Thousands of children with autism have been administered vitamin $B_6$ since the 1960s without any signs of significant side effects. However, in 1983, Schaumburg reported a small number of patients as suffering from numbness and tingling in the hands and feet due to peripheral neuropathy. It should be noted that these children were not taking magnesium, which should always be used when taking such high doses of vitamin $B_6$ so as to prevent side effects due to vitaminotherapy such as irritability, sound sensitivity, and enuresis. Also, once the vitamin treatment was discontinued or markedly reduced, all adverse symptoms disappeared completely. However, it should be noted that the British National Formulary (British Medical Association and the Royal Pharmaceutical Society of Great Britain 2005) states that concerns regarding possible toxicity resulting from prolonged use of pyridoxine (vitamin $B_6$) at high dosage have not yet been resolved.

### Where can I get them?

Health food shops and pharmacies supply vitamin $B_6$ and magnesium supplements.

## Vitamin C

### Who could benefit?

Vitamin C helps us all by enabling our brains to function properly, although how it does this is still unknown. The symptoms of vitamin C deficiency include depression and confusion, both of which are symptoms common in people with autism. Therefore, the idea is that people with autism would in some cases benefit from vitamin C supplements.

### How successful has this diet proved? Have any studies been carried out?

Most people know that vitamin C is capable of fighting viruses and bacteria, but these are not the only benefits. Two studies into the effects of vitamin C supplements in children with autism are of particular interest. The first ever test was carried out in 1967 by Rimland, where $B_3$, $B_5$, $B_6$, and C were administered. In this test, the benefits of using vitamin C in autism were overshadowed by the apparent effectiveness of vitamin $B_6$. However, the dosage for vitamin C was very low (1 to 3 grams per day) and therefore it would be wrong to draw conclusions from this test.

A second study of vitamin C in autism was initiated by Dolske et al. in 1993. The study involved a thirty-week double-blind placebo-controlled trial of 52 mg/lb per day in eighteen children with autism. The much higher dosage produced more favorable results.

More recently, Adams and Holloway (2004) conducted a randomized, double-blind, placebo-controlled three-month study of moderate dose multivitamin/mineral supplement for twenty children with autistic spectrum disorder. A Global Impressions parental questionnaire found that the supplement group reported statistically significant improvements in sleep and gastrointestinal problems compared to the placebo group. Vitamin C levels were measured at the end of the study, and the authors report that the placebo group had levels that were significantly below average for typical children, whereas the supplement group had near-average levels.

### Is this treatment safe?

Vitamin C has been taken in quite high doses without any major side effects. However, it can have a laxative effect and if this should happen then it should stop being administered. As with all these treatments it is essential that a medical professional is consulted.

### Where can I get them?

Pleasant-tasting vitamin C can be bought in most pharmacies.

## Dimethylglycine (DMG)

### Who could benefit?

DMG is a food supplement and therefore a prescription is not required.

It is naturally found in some foods such as rice and liver, although only in small amounts. It has appeared to be helpful to children with communication problems, particularly those with minimal speech development.

### *How successful has this diet proved? Have any studies been carried out?*

No official studies or trials have been carried out on DMG in autism or any other disorder. However, Rimland has noted the results of various people who have used the supplement. The first time DMG was discovered to have a positive effect was in 1965, when two Russians, M. G. Blumena and T. L. Belyakova (Rimland 1990, 3), wrote about improvements in the speech of twelve out of fifteen children with learning disabilities following use of calcium pangamate (also known as pangamic acid, and whose essential factor is DMG). As well as improved vocabulary and the use of simple sentences, there was a marked improvement in their general mental state. Following this, the psychiatrist Allan Cott tried pangamic acid on a number of his patients, some of whom had autism and many of which responded to the treatment in the same way as those in Russia.

DMG has also been known to improve the behavior of some children and adults. Rimland has written of a father who gave his son one DMG tablet per day, which led to a much-improved behavior report from the child's school.

If DMG is used, then the effects should be apparent within a week, although it should be tried for up to a month to make sure your child doesn't respond in a different way.

### *Is it safe?*

Rimland (1997) reports that a small proportion of children who have received DMG have become hyperactive and states that this is because they are lacking folic acid, a possible adjunct to DMG. Administering this could help to stop hyperactivity.

## *Gluten- and Casein-Free Diet*

### *Who could benefit?*

Further research is needed in order to establish which individuals with autism are likely to benefit. To date benefits have been reported for individuals with urinary peptide abnormalities.

## How successful has this diet proved? Have any studies been carried out?

Knivsberg et al. (2003) provide a report of findings to date, stating that dietary interventions yielding positive results have been reported in surveys, case studies, and studies of groups of children with autism. Researchers have also noted positive feedback from parents who have tried the gluten- and casein-free diet on their children.

Knivsberg et al (2003) carried out (to their knowledge) the first controlled, randomized study with an intervention period of one year to evaluate the effect of the gluten- and casein-free diet on children with autism. They report that urinary peptide abnormalities, partly attributable to gluten (present in grains and cereals) and casein (present in milk and milk products) have been detected in some individuals with autism. Knivsberg et al (2003) propose that these abnormalities reflecting opioid effect processes may explain behaviors displayed by people with autism. The research, comprising two sets of observations and tests carried out on a diet group and a control group at a one-year interval, reported a significant reduction of autistic behaviors for participants in the diet group.

Further research is required to ascertain whether dietary intervention is more beneficial to some children than others, whether varying results relate to implementation, or if some require a longer implementation period before effect is registered (Knivsberg et al. 2002). Furthermore, it is important to note that individuals with autism are as different from each other as are individuals who do not have a developmental disorder. Therefore dietary intervention is not a cure that can remove all autistic traits in all individuals with autism (Knivsberg et al. 2001).

### Is it safe?

It is essential that any decision on whether to take up such a diet should be made in consultation with a doctor and preferably with a dietitian or nutritionist. Lewis (1994) reports that initially individuals may experience side effects including stomach upset, anxiety, and slight ill temper. Further research is required to establish a recommended trial period (Lewis [1994] reports suggested trial periods of between three months and a year).

## Yeast-Free Diet

### Who could benefit?

It has been argued that most children with autism, pervasive developmental disorder (PDD), and attention deficit hyperactivity disorder

(ADHD) have excessive amounts of intestinal yeast, known as Candida. Therefore, it is possible that a large number of these children could benefit from a diet free of yeast. Rimland has mentioned what he considers to be the two major factors for this problem: Overuse of antibiotics and too much sugar in the diet.

### How successful has this diet proved? Have any tests been done?

It is known that in a healthy intestinal tract bacteria, yeasts, and fungi work together to digest food. Antibiotics destroy both harmful and beneficial bacteria, while allowing the amount of yeast to increase, which means that the yeast can thrive by taking up all the food that the person eats. Candida produces enzymes that aid digestion and these can attack the intestinal wall, allowing undigested food to be absorbed into the bloodstream. This is called leaky gut. This causes an increase in peptides, which are opiates. Thus, as with the gluten- and casein-free diet, the parts of the brain that control speech and behavior are affected detrimentally. Treatment involving a low-sugar diet and anti-fungal compounds has shown benefits in reducing the symptoms of autism and PDD. In particular, an increase in concentration, better sleep patterns, less aggressive and self-destructive behavior, greater use of speech, and improved sociability have been noted. Also, a reduction in, or complete removal of, yeast from the diet could be helpful.

### Is it safe?

Clearly, such a radical step as removing yeast, which is in such a large number of different foods, is difficult. It is an extremely restrictive diet and success depends completely on the compliance of the child and the understanding of his or her school and relatives. Any form of treatment, including a yeast-free diet, should be done only following tests of the person's urine and close consultation with a doctor and a dietitian to ensure that a well-balanced diet is maintained.

## Vitamin A

Megson has suggested that natural vitamin A may help people with autism, especially those with vision, sensory perception, language processing, and attention problems. Vitamin A can be found in cold-water fish such as salmon and cod, as well as liver, kidney, and milk fat. A useful supplement to take may be cod liver oil.

At present, it is not possible to verify this completely.

## Serotonin

Serotonin is a neurotransmitter that acts on the brain to influence motivation and mood. The observation that levels of 5-HT (serotonin) were sometimes raised in children with autism was first made in 1961 in a study by Richard J. Schain and Daniel X. Freedman. Their research found that in approximately 30 percent of children with autism, blood serotonin levels are significantly raised (a condition known as hyperserotonemia). This finding has been validated by many subsequent studies but the reasons for it and the ways in which it can be treated have yet to be identified. Further, the relationship between secretion of neurotransmitters and mood is more subtle than had been previously supposed.

Several drugs have been tried to redress this problem, none of which have been proven to be very successful, although some have reported some improvement. However, one of these drugs, fenfluramine, has been withdrawn due to side effects.

With regard to diets that may be able to improve the levels of serotonin in people on the autistic spectrum, there are a number of foods that contain high levels. The most common foods are tomatoes, bananas, plums, pecan nuts (among others), and pineapples. Alternatively, if the levels of serotonin need to be reduced then these foods could be avoided. Knivsberg (1990) reported that some parents found that autistic episodes increased when children ate certain foods (for example, bananas), which lends support to the hyperserotonemia case. It is not clear what the effects of reducing serotonin in the diet would be, but if parents wish to experiment with this then we recommend that a dietitian or nutritionist is consulted to ensure that a balanced diet is maintained.

## Fatty Acids

Omega-3 and omega-6 fatty acids play key roles in brain development and function (Richardson 2001; Richardson 2003a; Richardson 2003b; Richardson and Ross 2003). Research suggests that imbalances or deficiencies in highly unsaturated fatty acids (HUFA) of the omega-3 and omega-6 series may contribute to a range of behavioral and learning difficulties, including autistic spectrum disorders (Bell et al. 2000; Richardson and Ross 2000; Richardson 2001; Vancassel et al. 2001; Richardson 2003a; Richardson and Ross 2003; Richardson 2004).

In a small ninety-day trial Patrick and Salik (2005) reported that eighteen of twenty-two children with autism or Asperger syndrome taking a supplement of essential fatty acids displayed significant increases

338

in their language and learning skills based upon a criterion-referenced measure. The authors conclude that information obtained from future studies utilizing large sample sizes and placebo-controlled formats would be of great benefit to individuals with autism and Asperger syndrome.

Richardson (2004) states that definitive evidence of a causal contribution can come from only intervention studies, specifically in the form of randomized, double-blind, placebo-controlled trials. No randomized, controlled trials of fatty acid treatment for autism have yet been reported (Richardson and Montgomery 2005).

Richardson and Montgomery (2005) conducted a randomized, controlled trial of dietary supplementation with omega-3 and omega-6 fatty acids, compared with placebo, among 117 children with developmental coordination disorder (DCD). Significant improvements for active treatment versus placebo were found in reading, spelling, and behavior. Though the study focused on DCD specifically, the authors suggest that the results may be more widely generalizable.

Further research, particularly with specific reference to autism, is required to add to our knowledge in this area. Richardson (2003b) and Richardson (2004) provide a review of key findings prior to 2003–4.

HUFA is present in fish and seafood, nuts and seeds, and green leafy vegetables. However these nutrients can be lacking in modern diets. It is possible to increase dietary supply of HUFA via supplementation. Supplements generally contain fish oils, however alternatives are available such as flax or hemp seed oil. Products may be single oils or blends and will offer varying levels of omega 3 and 6. Please check the label. Both fish- and non-fish-oil-based supplements can be found in health shops, pharmacies, and supermarkets and on the internet.

Richardson and Montgomery (2005) state that the optimal dosage and combination of fatty acids are at present unknown and call for further studies to establish both the optimal composition and dose-response relationships.

It is important to note that fatty acids should not be expected to help all individuals with a particular diagnostic label, and nutritional approaches are to be viewed as complementary to other methods of management (Richardson 2003b). Specific advice concerning HUFA supplementation should be sought from a doctor or dietitian.

## *Bibliography and Further Reading*

Adams, C. and Conn, S. Nutrition and its relationship to autism. *Focus on Autism and Other Developmental Disabilities*, 1997, 12(1): 53–58.

Adams, J. B. and Holloway, C. Pilot study of a moderate dose multi-vitamin/mineral supplement for children with autistic spectrum disorder. *Journal of Alternative and Complementary Medicine*, 2004, 10(6): 1033–39.

Bell, J. G. et al. Red blood cell fatty acid compositions in a patient with autistic spectrum disorder: a characteristic abnormality in neurodevelopmental disorders? *Prostaglandins Leukotrienes and Essential Fatty Acids*, 2000, 63(1–2): 21–25.

British Medical Association and the Royal Pharmaceutical Society of Great Britain. *British National Formulary (49)*. London: British Medical Association and the Royal Pharmaceutical Society of Great Britain, 2005.

Converse, J. Diets and supplements—are they any value to autistic children? *Autism File*, 2003, 12: 12–17.

Dolske, M. C. et al. A preliminary trial of ascorbic acid as a supplement therapy for autism. *Progress in Neuro-Psychopharmacology and Biological Psychiatry*, 1993, 17: 765–74.

Equazen. Fatty acids and learning conditions. Equazen, 2003.

Equazen. *Fatty acids and the autistic spectrum*. Equazen, 2003.

Gardner, M. Assembling the jigsaw puzzle. *Looking Up*, 1999, 1(8): 33–34.

Gardner, M. et al. The role of diet in the cause and treatment of the autistic syndromes. In: *Autism on the agenda: papers from a NAS conference*, 1996, 208–11.

Garvey, J. Diet in autism and associated disorders. *Journal of Family Health Care*, 2002, 12(2): 34–38.

Gold, K. Will he or won't he eat it? *Autism File*, 1999, 1: 21–23.

Haas, E. M. Vitamin $B_{15}$: pangamic acid. 1998. Available to download at www.healthy.net/scr/article.asp?PageType=article&ID=1925.

Holford, P. *Optimum nutrition for the mind*. London: Piatkus, 2003.

Jackson, L. *A user guide to the GF/CF diet for autism, Asperger syndrome and AD/HD*. London: Jessica Kingsley, 2002.

Kessick, R. C. T. Autism à la carte. Available to download at www.autismconnect.com.

Knivsberg, A. M. Dietary interventions in autistic syndromes. *Brain Dysfunction*, 1990, 3: 315–27.

Knivsberg, A. M. Autistic traits in a diet and a control group in a single blind controlled study on dietary intervention in autism. In: *Building bridges: a collection of papers from the conference held at Van Mildert College, University of Durham, April 10th–12th 2002*. Sunderland: Autism Research Unit, 2003, 59–68.

Knivsberg, A. M. and Reichelt, K. L. Autistic symptoms and diet: a single blind study. In: *Focus on autism research*, 2004, 213–45.

Knivsberg, A. M. et al. A survey of dietary intervention in autism. In: *Research into therapy: a collection of papers from the conference held at Van Mildert College, University of Durham*, 1999, 117–28.

Knivsberg, A. M. et al. Reports on dietary intervention in autistic disorders. *Nutritional Neuroscience*, 2001, 4: 25–37.

Knivsberg, A. M. et al. A randomised, controlled study of dietary intervention in autistic syndromes. *Nutritional Neuroscience*, 2002, 5(4): 251–61.

Knivsberg, A. M. et al. Effect of a dietary intervention on autistic behaviour. *Focus on Autism and Other Developmental Disabilities*, 2003, 18(4): 247–56.

Knivsberg, A. M. et al. A case study of dietary intervention in autism. In: *In this together: a collection of papers from the Durham International Research Conference on Autism, 2003*. Sunderland: Autism Research Unit, 2004, 63–72.

Le Breton, M. Diet intervention and autism. *Implementing the gluten free and casein free diet for autistic children and adults a practical guide for parents*. London: Jessica Kingsley, 2001.

Lee, T. Allergy-induced autism. *Communication*, 1996, Spring, 12.

Lewis, L. S. *An experimental intervention for autism: understanding and implementing a gluten and casein free diet*. San Diego, California: The Autism Research Institute, 1994.

Lewis, L. *Special diets for special kids: understanding and implementing a gluten and casein free diet to aid in the treatment of autism and related developmental disorders*. Arlington, Texas: Future Horizons, 1998.

Lewis, L. S. What's for dinner? *Autism-Asperger's Digest*, 2000, 1: 28–32.

Martineau, J. et al. An open middle-term study of combined vitamin $B_6$-magnesium in a subgroup of children selected on their sensitivity to this treatment. *Journal of Autism and Developmental Disorders,* 1988, 18(3): 435–46.

McGinnis, W. Fatty acids and autism: some researchers believe boosting fatty acid intake helps reduce symptoms of autism. *Advocate,* 2001, 34(4): 26–27.

McKelvey, V. Diet: A personal view. *Communication,* 1997, Spring, 12–13.

Millward, C. et al. Gluten and casein-free diets for autistic spectrum disorder. *Cochrane Database of Systematic Reviews,* 2004, 2.

Nye, C. and Brice, A. Combined vitamin $B_6$-magnesium treatment in autism spectrum disorder. *Cochrane Database of Systematic Reviews,* 2002, 4.

Patrick, L. and Salik, R. The effect of essential fatty acid supplementation on language development and learning skills in autism and Asperger's syndrome. *Autism Asperger's Digest,* 2005, January–February, 36–37.

Pfeiffer, S. I. et al. Effects of vitamin $B_6$ and magnesium in the treatment of autism: a methodology review and summary of outcomes. *Journal of Autism and Developmental Disorders,* 1995, 25(5): 481–93.

Raiten, D. J. Nutrition and developmental disabilities. In: Schopler, E. and Mesibov, G. *Neurobiological issues in autism.* Washington, D.C.: Plenum Press, 1987.

Raiten, D. J. and Massaro, T. F. Nutrition and developmental disabilities: an examination of the orthomolecular hypothesis. In: Cohen, D. and Donnellan, A. *Handbook of Autism and Pervasive Developmental Disorders.* Washington, D.C.: Wiley, 1987, 566–83.

Reichelt, K. L. et al. Biologically active peptide: containing fractions in schizophrenia and implementing a gluten and casein free diet. *Advances in Biochemical Psychopharmacology,* 1981, 28: 627–43.

Reichelt, K. L. et al. Diet and autism: a four year follow up. Probable reasons and observations relevant to a dietary and genetic aetiology. In: *Therapeutic intervention in autism: perspectives from research and practice. Collected papers from the conference organised by the Autism Research Unit and supported by the National Autistic Society and the*

*University of Sunderland. (The College of St. Hild and St. Bede, University of Durham, April 1st–3rd, 1996).* Sunderland: Autism Research Unit, 1996, 281–308.

Richardson, A. Fatty acids in dyslexia, dyspraxia, ADHD and the autistic spectrum. *The Nutrition Practitioner*, 2001, 3(3): 18–24, 66.

Richardson, A. (2003a). Fatty acids in dyslexia, dyspraxia, ADHD, and the autistic spectrum. *Food and Behaviour Research*, 2003. Available to download at www.fabresearch.org.

Richardson, A. J. (2003b). The role of omega 3 fatty acids in behaviour, cognition and mood. *Scandinavian Journal of Nutrition*, 2003, 47(2): 92–98.

Richardson, A. J. Clinical trials of fatty acid treatment in ADHD, dyslexia, dyspraxia and the autistic spectrum. *Prostaglandins Leukotrienes and Essential Fatty Acids*, 2004, 70(4): 383–90.

Richardson, A. J. and Montgomery P. The Oxford-Durham study: a randomized, controlled trial of dietary supplementation with fatty acids in children with developmental coordination disorder. *Pediatrics*, 2005, 115(5): 1360–66.

Richardson, A. J. and Ross, M. A. Fatty acid metabolism in neurodevelopmental disorder: a new perspective on associations between attention-deficit/hyperactivity disorder, dyslexia, dyspraxia and the autistic spectrum. *Prostaglandins Leukotrienes and Essential Fatty Acids*, 2000, 63(1–2): 1–9.

Richardson, A. and Ross, M. Physical signs of fatty acid deficiency. *Food and Behaviour Research*, 2003. Available to download at www .fabresearch.org.

Rimland, B. Dimethylglycine (DMG), a nontoxic metabolite, and autism. *Autism Research Review International*, 1990, 4(2): 3.

Rimland, B. Vitamin $B_6$ in autism: the safety issue. *Autism Research Review International*, 1996, 10(3): 3.

Rimland, B. $B_6$: breaking through autism. *What Doctors Don't Tell You*, 1998, 8(10): 12.

Rimland, B. What is the right "dosage" for vitamin $B_6$, DMG, and other nutrients useful in autism? *Autism Research Review International*, 1998, 11(4): 3.

Rimland, B. Vitamin C in the prevention and treatment of autism. *Autism Research Review International*, 1998, 12(2): 3.

Rimland, B. High dose vitamin $B_6$ and magnesium in treating autism: response to Findling et al. *Journal of Autism and Developmental Disorders*, 1998, 28(6): 580–81.

Schain, R. J. and Freedman, D. X. Studies on 5-Hydroxyindole metabolism in autistic and other mentally retarded persons. In: Donnellan, A., ed., *Classic readings in autism*. New York: Teacher's College Press, 1985, 74–83. (First published in *Journal of Pediatrics,* 1961, 58: 315–20.)

Schaumburg, H. et al. Sensory neuropathy for pyroxidine abuse: a new megavitamin syndrome. *New England Journal of Medicine*, 1983, 309: 445–48.

Shattock, P. Diet. *Communication*, 1998, Summer, 22–25.

Shattock, P. and Whiteley, P. Dietary interventions for the treatment of autism *and related syndromes. Paper presented at the internet conference* (www.autism99.org), 1999.

Shattock, P. et al. *Autism as a metabolic disorder: guidelines for the implementation of a gluten and / or casein free diet with people with autism or associated spectrum disorders.* Sunderland: Autism Research Unit, 2004.

Tommey, J. 5th annual Defeat Autism Now (DAN) conference. *Autism File*, 2000, 2: 21–25.

Tommey, J. The guts—the problem: the first step in combating autism is to get the gut functioning properly. *Autism File*, 2003, 12: 31–33.

Vancassel, S. Plasma fatty acid levels in autistic children. *Prostaglandins Leukotrienes and Essential Fatty Acids*, 2001, 65(1): 1–7.

Waring, R. The sulphation connection. *Looking Up*, 1999, 1(8): 30–33.

Waring, R. H. and Ngong, J. M. Sulphate metabolism in allergy-induced autism: relevance to the disease aetiology. In: *Biological perspectives in autism. Collected papers from the conference organised by the Autism Research Unit*. Sunderland: Autism Research Unit, 1993.

Whiteley, P. et al. Preliminary findings from the implementation of a gluten free diet with children with autism and associated spectrum disorders. In: *Living and learning with autism: perspectives from the individual, the family and the professional: a collection of papers.* Sunderland: Autism Research Unit, 1997, 189–97.

Whiteley, P. et al. A gluten-free diet as an intervention for autism and associated spectrum disorders: preliminary findings. *Autism*, 1999, 3(1): 45–65.

## Section 27.2

# *Secretin for Autism: Hope and Disappointment*

By David A. Cooke, M.D. © 2007 Omnigraphics, Inc.

Secretin, a widely used treatment for autism, has proven to be a major disappointment. Multiple well-designed clinical trials have shown it to be completely ineffective for treatment of autistic symptoms.

Secretin is a hormone produced in the gastrointestinal tract. Traditionally, its only medical use has been administration during certain tests to diagnose intestinal ailments.

Interest in the hormone as a possible treatment for autism arose in the late 1990s, after a single author published a report of three children with autism whose symptoms seemed to improve after receiving a single dose. In 1998, NBC *Dateline* ran a story reporting on one of these children, sparking a near-frenzy of interest among families of autistic children. Secretin began being widely used for autism, to the point that national shortages of the hormone occurred. A black market in secretin sprung up, which sold it at very high prices and often provided counterfeit medication. Despite this dramatic and widespread interest, there had been almost no scientific study of its use in autism at the time.

As a result, a number of double-blind, placebo-controlled studies of this therapy were performed. These were studies where volunteers with autism were randomly assigned to receive either secretin or an identical-appearing substance containing no medication (placebo).

Neither the patients nor the researchers knew who was receiving the medication or the placebo until the end of the study. This allowed objective assessment of the effects of the medication, without bias from expectations.

To date, there have been at least fifteen published double-blind, placebo-controlled studies of secretin use in autism. All but one have found no improvements with secretin therapy. Several of these studies are summarized here.

A large 2001 study, published by Owley et al. in the *Journal of the American Academy of Child and Adolescent Psychiatry*, was funded by the National Institutes of Health. This studied children at multiple geographic locations who received either a pig-derived form of secretin (the form most often used in diagnostic testing) or a placebo. Each child received two doses of intravenous medication four weeks apart. One dose contained secretin and one contained placebo. However, neither the treating physicians nor the families knew whether they were receiving secretin or placebo. A battery of behavioral and symptom-measurement tests were performed before, after, and eight weeks after each of the treatments. No significant differences on any of the measures were seen between the secretin infusions and the placebo infusions. The authors concluded that single doses of secretin have no effect on autistic symptoms or behaviors.

A 2001 study by Roberts et al. studied the effects of multiple doses of porcine secretin and looked at behavior ratings by physicians and caregivers. Like the Owley study, no significant differences in symptoms or behaviors were seen in patients who received multiple doses of secretin, versus those who received placebos.

A group of researchers at the Children's Hospital of Philadelphia published the results of a comparison between synthetic human secretin and a placebo in 2003. There were no significant differences in behavioral measurements between children who received secretin and those who received placebo. In addition, families could not tell from their children's behavior whether they received a placebo or secretin. A second study by the same group of researchers, published in 2007, also failed to find improvement with secretin therapy.

A study published in 2005 looked at secretin or placebo, given as an ointment absorbed transdermally (through the skin). This was done to determine whether prior studies had not treated the children for long enough periods. In this study, children were treated for four weeks at a time, and received courses of secretin or placebo at various times. The study did not find significant changes that related to when the children were receiving secretin.

Several studies have tried to determine whether there may be a subgroup of autistic patients who might respond to secretin. The only double-blind study that has reported an effect of secretin was published by Kern. et al in 2002. This study used porcine (pig-derived) secretin, which is the form most often used in medical testing. This study found some improvements with secretin, but only in a subgroup of children who had significant problems with diarrhea and gastrointestinal symptoms. Other studies with similar methods have failed to reproduce these results. To date, there is no subgroup that has been consistently shown to benefit from secretin therapy.

It now appears quite clear that secretin does not work for autism. Studies of single doses, multiple doses, and continuous transdermal dosing have shown no differences compared to placebos. Studies of porcine secretin, synthetic human secretin, and even a homeopathic secretin formulation have yielded consistently negative results.

How did well-meaning parents and researchers initially conclude that secretin might be helpful? The symptoms of autism are difficult to measure consistently without the use of detailed rating scales, so personal impressions of behavioral changes may not always be accurate. Some of the controlled studies noted that parents' assessments and teachers' assessments of their children's behavior were often quite different.

Other studies noted that even children who received placebo tended to have periods of significant improvement and worsening of their symptoms over time. This seemed to occur unrelated to any therapy or lack of therapy. It may be that some children had some spontaneous improvement around the time they happened to receive a dose of secretin. It is easy to see how this could lead to an incorrect conclusion that the secretin was responsible for the improvement. In addition, when a caregiver knows a patient is receiving therapy, his or her impressions may be unconsciously altered by the hope that the medication will help, and this may lead people to see improvements where none really exist.

The search for effective treatment for autism continues.

## Section 27.3

# *Is Eliminating Casein and Gluten from a Child's Diet a Viable Treatment for Autism?*

"Is Eliminating Casein and Gluten from a Child's Diet a Viable Treatment for Autism?" William H. Ahearn, Ph.D. © Cambridge Center for Behavioral Studies (www.behavior.org). Reprinted with permission.

Dietary interventions for developmental and learning disabilities have been controversial for decades. When a child presents with a metabolic disorder, it often follows that diet may be a critically important variable. Certain metabolic disorders, like phenylketonuria, are effectively managed by diet. Feingold (1975) first proposed that eliminating certain substances like preservatives would result in a child with attentional problems becoming more focused and less hyperactive. These claims did not turn out to be valid for 95 percent of the children treated with diet (NIH, 1996), and those who were helped tended to have identifiable food allergies. Evidence suggests that attention deficit hyperactivity disorder (ADHD) is a neurological condition but it is a complex disorder with little solid information about its cause. We do know that ADHD is unlikely to be caused by food allergies, excessive sugar intake, or other variables that do not affect an individual's neurological makeup (NIH, 1996).

Although there was no solid evidence that Feingold's approach was effective, this strategy has also been applied to autism. Additionally, other diets have been developed with a variety of hypotheses that also lack scientific confirmation. These diets have been applied as treatments for autism as well as for various other disabilities. However, unless a child has a food allergy/intolerance or metabolic condition it is unlikely that dietary changes will affect his or her disability. Given that a child with an autistic spectrum disorder (ASD) may also have a food allergy and that gastrointestinal difficulties have been suggested as more prevalent in people with autism, it may be useful to determine whether there is any good reason to think that the gastrointestinal system causes autism.

The "gut theory" of autism has been most popularly promoted by Andrew Wakefield. Wakefield and his colleagues (1998) have suggested an association between chronic gastrointestinal difficulties and autism caused by an insult to the gut that occurs as an adverse reaction to the measles, mumps, and rubella (MMR) vaccine. Wakefield's research was somewhat suspect in the soundness of the methods used, especially in how cases were identified for inclusion. It has recently come to light that Wakefield was paid a substantial amount of money by the Legal Aid Board to study whether children were harmed by the MMR before conducting his research (Lyall, 2004). The editor who approved the study's publication stated that he would not have published it had this conflict of interest been disclosed (Lyall). Furthermore, this conflict of interest led ten of the study's co-authors to retract the suggestion of a link between MMR and autism (Mayor, 2004).

Prior to the recent revelation of unacceptable scientific practice, many investigated Wakefield's claims. Fombonne and Chakrabarti (2001) did an extensive survey of the potential relation between autism and the MMR vaccine and found that there was no evidence for a relation between the vaccine and autism. The most definitive study to date was conducted by Danish researchers (Hviid et al., 2003) who studied well over two million children that received either a vaccine containing thimerosal or the same vaccine without this preservative and found that the rates of autism were not higher in the group that received vaccines with thimerosal. Some have said that thimerosal damages the gut, however, Taylor and his colleagues (2002) in a study with nearly five hundred children with an autistic spectrum disorder (ASD) found no relation between the MMR and bowel problems. Looking specifically at gut problems in persons with autism, Black, Kaye, and Jick (2002) found that children with ASD were no more likely to have a gastrointestinal problem than their age-matched peers. These studies strongly indicate that there is no link between the gut and autism.

Autism is thought by the scientific community to be of genetic origin (e.g., Folstein and Rosen-Sheidly, 2001; IMGSAC, 2001; Muhle, Trentacoste, and Rapin, 2004). It has also come to be well accepted that ASDs are the manifestation of a neurological condition. Acosta and Pearl (2003) posit that the best scientific evidence indicates that autism likely results from "genetically determined prenatal alterations in brain development." Although we are hopeful that empirically validated biological interventions can be developed to treat or perhaps prevent ASDs, it is more likely that the nature of successful therapy will not target the gastrointestinal system.

Nonetheless, it is still unknown whether a dietary intervention could treat autism. Currently, the most popular diet promoted as a cure for autism involves restricting casein and gluten from the child's diet. The unfounded assumption behind recommending that casein and gluten be restricted is that the processing of these substances causes many of the symptoms of autism. Beside the fact that most of the evidence provided as support for the casein/gluten theory of autism comes from individuals involved in selling these products or diet-related advice, the lack of scientific acceptance of casein and gluten processing difficulties as a cause of autism is one good reason to be wary of this approach.

Though children with ASD seem no more likely to have gastrointestinal difficulties, including food allergies, than typically developing children, the fact is that both children with ASD and those who are typically developing can have this problem. It is also the case that children are more likely to have food allergies than adults. So food allergies are clearly an appropriate concern. In fact, at times they can involve severe reactions that are life threatening. Food allergies occur because the body develops antibodies specific to the allergen in the offending food. The next time that this substance is ingested, the antibodies then trigger the release of histamine and an allergic reaction occurs. Most children with a significant food allergy appear sickly. They have symptoms that are typical of an allergic reaction, may vomit frequently, and often have abnormal bowel movements. Shortly after the food the child has an allergy to is ingested, symptoms (e.g., diarrhea, tingling/swelling in the mouth area, difficulty breathing, pronounced rashes especially on the face or torso) appear. Most children outgrow their allergies although it is thought that allergies to nuts (and peanuts), fish, and shellfish are likely lifelong allergies.

For over a decade I have worked with children with feeding difficulties with and without ASDs and one frequently encountered cause of a child's feeding problem is food allergy. If a child has a documented food allergy then removing the allergen(s) from the child's diet is one necessary component of resolving the problem. However, determining that the child has a food allergy is a critical first step. If a child is suspected of having an allergy because of symptoms, then there are two tests commonly accepted as valid means of diagnosing food allergy. These are the skin prick and RAST (radioallergosorbent) tests. So long as the allergic reaction is not severe, these tests can then be combined with information gathered by alternately exposing or restricting access to the suspected allergen and determining whether symptoms respectively appear and dissipate to confirm test results. For the child with a food allergy, the benefit of removing the allergen will be apparent in that the overt symptoms caused by ingestion of the offending substance will dissipate, but if the child has a disability as well, the disability will persist. The child who is no longer in discomfort will also likely be more receptive to instruction and have a more positive affect.

So, why not restrict access to casein and gluten just to make sure you are doing everything you can for your child? First, the lack of scientific evidence that casein and gluten cause autism is concerning. This combined with the evidence that gastrointestinal (GI) difficulties and autism are not linked, should cause you to question the plausibility of dietary intervention for this disorder. Then again, most significant in my mind is the fact that children with ASD are prone to selective eating (Ahearn et al., 2001). During our study of the eating habits of children with an ASD, my colleagues and I provided children with a variety of foods across six meals spread out over at least two weeks. Over half of the children we observed presented with some form of selective eating. Though we saw selectivity for various food groups, the food group that our selective eaters were most likely to prefer was starch. Gluten is a constituent of many starches, and restricting access to this substance can lead to eliminating the only foods that a child regularly eats.

The course of action that I have followed as a clinician treating selective eating has been to attempt to expand the variety of foods a child eats. I've worked with children who ate only one food and would not eat unless that food was prepared in a specific manner (e.g., macaroni and cheese made with whole milk and butter served straight out of the pan). Going from such selective acceptance of food to eating other foods often takes quite a long time. The only situations in which I would recommend restricting access to food would be if the child had a documented food allergy or excessively consumed food. Several parents have reported to me that they have tried the casein/gluten-free diet and their children would not eat any of the foods presented to them. To be fair, I've also had a number of parents swear to me that this diet was very helpful, but none of them answered yes when I asked them if the diet cured their child of autism. It is my opinion that children with an ASD will not benefit from dietary restrictions of any kind unless they also have a food allergy or intolerance. Furthermore, children who are selective eaters are likely to become more selective and may stop eating when their diet is radically restricted. Because children with ASDs are prone to selective eating it is probably a good idea to attempt to expand their diets rather than restrict them.

## References

Acosta, M.T. and Pearl, P.L. (2003). The neurobiology of autism: New pieces of the puzzle. *Current Neurology and Neuroscience Reports*, 3:149–56.

Ahearn, W.H., Castine, T., Nault, K., and Green, G. (2001). An assessment of food acceptance in children with autism or pervasive developmental disorder-not otherwise specified. *Journal of Autism and Developmental Disorders*, 31:505–12.

Black, C., Kaye, J., and Jick, H. (2002). Relation of childhood GI disorders to autism: Nested case-control study using data from the UK General Practice Research Database. *British Medical Journal*, 325:419–21.

Feingold, B.F. (1975). *Why your child is hyperactive*. New York: Random House.

Folstein, S.E., and Rosen-Sheidley, B. (2001). Genetics of autism: Complex aetiology for a heterogeneous disorder. *Nature Reviews: Genetics*, 2(12): 943–55.

Fombonne, E. (1999). The epidemiology of autism: A review. *Psychological Medicine*, 29:769–86.

Fombonne, E. and Chakrabarti, S. (2001). No evidence for a new variant of measles-mumps-rubella-induced autism. *Pediatrics*, 108:E58.

Hviid, A., Stellfeld, M., Wohlfahrt, J., and Melbye, M. (2003). Association between thimerosal-containing vaccine and autism. *Journal of the American Medical Association*, 290:1763–66.

International Molecular Genetic Study of Autism Consortium (2001). A genome-wide screen for autism: Strong evidence for linkage to chromosomes 2q, 7q, and 16p. *American Journal of Human Genetics*, 69:570–81.

Lightdale, J.R., Hayer, C., Duer, A., Lind-White, C., Jenkins, S., Siegel, B., Elliot, G.R., and Heyman, M.B. (2001). Effects of intravenous secretin on language and behavior of children with autism and gastrointestinal symptoms: A single-blinded, open-label pilot study. *Pediatrics*, 108(5). URL: http://www.pediatrics.org/cgi/content/full/108/5/e90.

Lyall, J. (2004). Editor in the eye of the storm. *British Medical Journal*, 328:528 (28 Feb). doi:10.1136/bmj.328.7438.528.

Mayor, S. (2003). Authors reject interpretation linking autism and MMR vaccine. *British Medical Journal*, 328:602 (13 Mar). doi:10.1136/bmj.328.7440.602-c.

Muhle, R., Trentacoste, S.V., and Rapin, I. (2004). The genetics of autism. *Pediatrics*, 113:472–86.

National Institutes of Health. (1996). NIH Publication No. 96-3572, printed 1994, reprinted 1996. Booklet. 44p. Retrieved September, 1997 from http://www.nimh.nih.gov/publicat/adhd.cfm#adhd6.

Roberts, W., Weaver, L., Brian, J., Bryson, S., Emelianova, S., Griffiths, A., MacKinnon, B., Yim, C., Wolpin, J., and Koren, G. (2001). Repeated doses of porcine secretin in the Treatment of autism: A randomized, placebo-controlled trial. *Pediatrics*, 107(5). URL: http://www.pediatrics.org/cgi/content/full/107/5/e71.

Ritvo, E.M., and Freeman, B.J. (1978). National society for autistic children definition of the syndrome of autism. *Journal of Autism and Childhood Schizophrenia*, 8:162–70.

Taylor, B. et al. (2002). MMR vaccination and bowel problems or developmental regression in children with autism: Population study. *British Medical Journal*, 324:393–96.

Wakefield et al. (1998). Ileal-lymphoid-nodular hyperplasia, nonspecific colitis, and pervasive developmental disorder in children: An early report. *Lancet*, 351:637–41.

# Chapter 28

# *Pharmacological Interventions*

## *Chapter Contents*

Section 28.1—Medications Used in the Treatment of
Autism .................................................................. 356
Section 28.2—Risperdal Approved to Treat Irritability
Associated with Autism ...................................... 359
Section 28.3—Oxytocin in the Treatment of Repetitive
Behaviors and Social Cognition Difficulties
in Adults with Autistic Disorders ..................... 360

## Section 28.1

# *Medications Used in the Treatment of Autism*

Excerpted from "Autism Spectrum Disorders (Pervasive
Developmental Disorders)," National Institute of Mental Health,
National Institutes of Health, July 11, 2006.

Medications are often used to treat behavioral problems, such as
aggression, self-injurious behavior, and severe tantrums, that keep the
person with an autism spectrum disorder (ASD) from functioning
more effectively at home or school. The medications used are those
that have been developed to treat similar symptoms in other disorders. Many of these medications are prescribed "off-label." This means
they have not been officially approved by the U.S. Food and Drug
Administration (FDA) for use in children, but the doctor prescribes
the medications if he or she feels they are appropriate for your child.
Further research needs to be done to ensure not only the efficacy but
also the safety of psychotropic agents used in the treatment of children and adolescents.

A child with ASD may not respond in the same way to medications
as typically developing children. It is important that parents work
with a doctor who has experience with children with autism. A child
should be monitored closely while taking a medication. The doctor will
prescribe the lowest dose possible to be effective. Ask the doctor about
any side effects the medication may have and keep a record of how
your child responds to the medication. It will be helpful to read the
"patient insert" that comes with your child's medication. Some people
keep the patient inserts in a small notebook to be used as a reference.
This is most useful when several medications are prescribed.

**Anxiety and depression:** The selective serotonin reuptake inhibitors (SSRIs) are the medications most often prescribed for symptoms
of anxiety, depression, or obsessive-compulsive disorder (OCD). Only
one of the SSRIs, fluoxetine (Prozac®), has been approved by the FDA
for both OCD and depression in children age seven and older. Three
that have been approved for OCD are fluvoxamine (Luvox®), age eight
and older; sertraline (Zoloft®), age six and older; and clomipramine

356

(Anafranil®), age ten and older.[1] Treatment with these medications can be associated with decreased frequency of repetitive, ritualistic behavior and improvements in eye contact and social contacts. The FDA is studying and analyzing data to better understand how to use the SSRIs safely, effectively, and at the lowest dose possible.

**Behavioral problems:** Antipsychotic medications have been used to treat severe behavioral problems. These medications work by reducing the activity in the brain of the neurotransmitter dopamine. Among the older, typical antipsychotics, such as haloperidol (Haldol®), thioridazine, fluphenazine, and chlorpromazine, haloperidol was found in more than one study to be more effective than a placebo in treating serious behavioral problems.[2] However, haloperidol, while helpful for reducing symptoms of aggression, can also have adverse side effects, such as sedation, muscle stiffness, and abnormal movements.

Placebo-controlled studies of the newer "atypical" antipsychotics are being conducted on children with autism. The first such study, conducted by the National Institute of Mental Health (NIMH)-supported Research Units on Pediatric Psychopharmacology (RUPP) Autism Network, was on risperidone (Risperdal®).[3] Results of the eight-week study were reported in 2002 and showed that risperidone was effective and well tolerated for the treatment of severe behavioral problems in children with autism. The most common side effects were increased appetite, weight gain, and sedation. Further long-term studies are needed to determine any long-term side effects. Other atypical antipsychotics that have been studied recently with encouraging results are olanzapine (Zyprexa®) and ziprasidone (Geodon®). Ziprasidone has not been associated with significant weight gain.

**Seizures:** Seizures are found in one in four persons with ASD, most often in those who have low IQ or are mute. They are treated with one or more of the anticonvulsants. These include such medications as carbamazepine (Tegretol®), lamotrigine (Lamictal®), topiramate (Topamax®), and valproic acid (Depakote®). The level of the medication in the blood should be monitored carefully and adjusted so that the least amount possible is used to be effective. Although medication usually reduces the number of seizures, it cannot always eliminate them.

**Inattention and hyperactivity:** Stimulant medications such as methylphenidate (Ritalin®), used safely and effectively in persons with attention deficit hyperactivity disorder, have also been prescribed for

357

children with autism. These medications may decrease impulsivity and hyperactivity in some children, especially those higher-functioning children.

Several other medications have been used to treat ASD symptoms; among them are other antidepressants, naltrexone, lithium, and some of the benzodiazepines such as diazepam (Valium®) and lorazepam (Ativan®). The safety and efficacy of these medications in children with autism has not been proven. Since people may respond differently to different medications, your child's unique history and behavior will help your doctor decide which medication might be most beneficial.

## References

1.  Newschaffer CJ (Johns Hopkins Bloomberg School of Public Health). Autism Among Us: *Rising Concerns and the Public Health Response* [Video on the Internet]. Public Health Training Network, 2003 June 20. Available from: http://www .publichealthgrandrounds.unc.edu/autism/webcast.htm.

2.  McDougle CJ, Stigler KA, Posey DJ. Treatment of aggression in children and adolescents with autism and conduct disorder. *Journal of Clinical Psychiatry*, 2003; 64 (supplement 4): 16–25.

3.  Research Units on Pediatric Psychopharmacology Network. Risperidone in children with autism and serious behavioral problems. *New England Journal of Medicine*, 2002; 347(5): 314–21.

## Section 28.2

## *Risperdal Approved to Treat Irritability Associated with Autism*

Reprinted from "FDA Approves the First Drug to Treat Irritability Associated with Autism, Risperdal," U.S. Food and Drug Administration, October 6, 2006.

On October 6, 2006, the U.S. Food and Drug Administration (FDA) approved Risperdal (risperidone) orally disintegrating tablets, an adult antipsychotic drug, for the symptomatic treatment of irritability in autistic children and adolescents. The approval is the first for the use of a drug to treat behaviors associated with autism in children. These behaviors are included under the general heading of irritability, and include aggression, deliberate self-injury, and temper tantrums.

"This approval should benefit many autistic children as well as their parents and other care givers," said Steven Galson, M.D., director of FDA's Center for Drug Evaluation and Research. "Our agency strongly encourages the development of appropriate pediatric labeling for adult drugs, and Risperdal is a welcome addition to the growing number of such products that have been shown to have an appropriate risk-benefit profile when tested in children."

Risperdal has been approved since 1993 for the short-term treatment of adults with schizophrenia, and since 2003 for the short-term treatment of adults with acute manic or mixed episodes associated with extreme mood swings.

The product's effectiveness in the symptomatic treatment of irritability associated with pediatric autistic disorders was established in two eight-week, placebo-controlled trials in 156 patients aged five to sixteen years, 90 percent of whom were five to twelve years old. The results, which were evaluated using two assessment scales, showed that children on Risperdal achieved significantly improved scores for certain behavioral symptoms of autism compared to children on placebo. The most common side effects of the use of Risperdal included drowsiness, constipation, fatigue, and weight gain.

## Section 28.3

# Oxytocin in the Treatment of Repetitive Behaviors and Social Cognition Difficulties in Adults with Autistic Disorders

Reprinted with permission from the American College of Neuropsychopharmacology (ACNP), from "New Research Suggests Oxytocin's Potential for Treatment of Two Core Autism Symptom Domains," Press Release, December 4, 2006.

Preliminary new research discussed on December 4, 2006, at the American College of Neuropsychopharmacology's Annual Meeting finds that oxytocin, when administered using intravenous fluid and nasal technology, may have significant positive effects on adult autism patients. The study, funded by the Seaver Foundation, examined the effects of oxytocin on repetitive behaviors and aspects of social cognition in adults with autism.

Investigators Eric Hollander, M.D., and Jennifer Bartz, Ph.D., presented results of both intravenous and intranasal administration of oxytocin in high-functioning adult autism patients and discussed the implications of this research for the treatment of autism. Dr. Hollander is chairman of psychiatry and at the Mt. Sinai School of Medicine in New York, New York, and director of the Seaver and New York Autism Center of Excellence, one of eight NIH-funded Studies to Advance Autism Research and Treatment (STAART) centers devoted to the study of autism. Dr. Bartz is a postdoctoral fellow at the Seaver Center at the Mt. Sinai School of Medicine.

"Studies with animals have found that oxytocin plays a role in a variety of behaviors, including parent-child and adult-to-adult pair bonding, social memory, social cognition, anxiety reduction, and repetitive behaviors," explained Dr. Bartz. "However," adds Dr. Hollander, "we have only recently considered that administration of oxytocin can have behavioral effects. Autism is a particularly ripe neuropsychiatric disorder for studying this approach because it presents with the types of symptoms that have been found to be associated with the oxytocin system."

High-functioning adults with autism or Asperger disorder received an intravenous infusion of Pitocin (synthetic oxytocin) or placebo (saline solution) over a four-hour period. During that time, participants were monitored for repetitive behaviors that are hallmarks of autism spectrum disorders, including need to tell/ask, touching, and repeating. These behaviors were assessed at a baseline and throughout the course of the infusion.

"Repetitive behaviors are often overlooked as symptoms of autism in favor of more dramatic symptoms like disrupted social functioning," noted Hollander. "However, early repetitive behavior is often the best predictor of a later autism diagnosis."

The infusion produced results that were both clinically and statistically significant. Hollander noted a rapid reduction of repetitive behaviors over the course of the oxytocin infusion, whereas no such reduction occurred following the placebo infusion, suggesting that oxytocin does indeed address these symptoms.

Researchers also looked at the effects of oxytocin on social cognition. Autism patients are often unable to detect or read emotion in others through facial and voice cues, resulting in the decreased ability to have meaningful interactions with others that characterizes individuals with this disease.

To test participants' ability to assign affective significance to speech, participants listened to prerecorded sentences with neutral semantic content that were presented with different intonations such as anger, sadness, or happiness. Participants were asked to identify the emotion. Participants received intravenous infusions of Pitocin (synthetic oxytocin) or placebo (saline solution) over a four-hour period; participants then returned approximately two weeks later, receiving the alternate compound. Comprehension of affective speech was assessed throughout the four-hour infusion on both occasions, that is, once with intravenous infusion of oxytocin and once without.

Most interestingly, participants who received oxytocin on the first testing day retained the ability to assign affective significance to speech, performing above expectations when they returned approximately two weeks later. This effect was not found among participants who received the placebo on the first testing day.

Hollander and his colleagues are now using nasal technology to study the treatment implications of oxytocin in a controlled six-week trial. "The intranasal administration of oxytocin is important because it may allow for better penetration of the blood-brain barrier, and is easier to administer," explained Hollander. "When administered orally, oxytocin is metabolized and only a small amount reaches the brain.

This is important because the behavioral effects of oxytocin are thought to result from its action on the brain."

Hollander and his colleagues are among the first group to have used intravenous fluid technology and nasal technology to study the behavioral effects of oxytocin in autism spectrum disorders. Though the findings are promising, Hollander cautions that this research is still very preliminary.

"Our findings will need to be replicated in large-scale, placebo-controlled trials to fully explore treatment potential," said Hollander. "And, though both intravenous and intranasal approaches have been well tolerated, we need to understand more about the safety of these potential treatments, particularly before these effects are explored in autistic children."

# Chapter 29

# *Social Intervention Strategies*

## Chapter Contents

Section 29.1—Son-Rise Program: Encouraging Love and
        Acceptance of Children ...................................... 364
Section 29.2—Daily Life Therapy (Higashi): Educating
        Children with Autism through Physical
        Activity, Academic Activity, and Vocational
        Training ............................................................. 376

Section 29.1

## *Son-Rise Program: Encouraging Love and Acceptance of Children*

### How the Program Began

It is said by the Option Institute that after Raun Kaufman was diagnosed with autism at eighteen months, professionals suggested to his parents that he be institutionalized. They say that after looking for programs to help their son and finding nothing they felt was suitable, the Kaufmans instead decided to develop their own home-based program. They worked with him seven days a week, twelve hours a day, and after three years it is reported that he was able to attend a mainstream school (Kaufman, B. 1981). After writing the book *Son Rise* and the showing of the subsequent film, the family was inundated with requests for help. As a result, they set up the Option Institute in Sheffield, Massachusetts, and launched the Son-Rise Program in 1983 (Kaufman, S. 1998). Raun Kaufman now works with parents and children in the program.

### The Theory of the Program

There are five underlying principles that the Institute teaches and believes in as part of its program:

- **The importance of a loving and accepting attitude:** The institute believes that the attitudes of love and acceptance are what all interactions and programs are built on. This is particularly important with regard to the child, who is often viewed negatively. It claims that as a result, parents learn to accept both themselves and their child first, including all their behaviors and "isms" (the description given to a child's repetitive behavior, positively)

(Kaufman, S. 1998). It believes that adults who are accepting, sincere, enthusiastic, and exciting are appealing to the child and as a result will encourage interactions (Horler et al. 1998) and that the child works better and is more interactive if the adult is completely comfortable (Kaufman, R. 2002).

- **The gift of a special child:** This is closely linked to the first attitude. Parents are taught to see their child as a gift, to whom parents can respond with "energy and dedication" (Kaufman, S. 1998).

- **The parents as the child's best resource:** Parents are seen by the institute as the people who understand their child the best. The institute feels that other programs and professionals often ignore this fundamental point.

- **The question of hope and false hope:** The claim made by the institute that "autism doesn't have to be a life sentence" is seen by some as misleading in its claim of recovery from autism. Conversely, the institute also states that doing the Son-Rise Program is no longer a guarantee of results. However, they believe that this should not stop you from trying (Kaufman, S. 1998).

- **The child as teacher:** Rather than teaching a preset standard of skills, the program is run by the child, at a pace set by the child. He or she can then explore and develop in his or her own time. This entails others joining the child in his or her world by mimicking his or her "isms"—the activities he or she often repeats. The aim of the activity is not simply to copy the child's actions but to gain his or her trust. As trust is gained the child will lead the adult into his or her world. Accordingly, it is then believed that it is possible to use the child's motivation as a teaching tool, simplifying every activity and event, breaking them down into digestible parts. Interaction can then become a pleasurable activity and make people more attractive to the child than the objects and obsessions (MacDonald and MacDonald 1991).

The institute believes that joining the child in his or her "isms" also indicates acceptance of the child's behavior and gives "social meaning" to the task so that retreating into the "ism" will no longer block out the world (Jordan and Powell 1993). Although the Son-Rise Program has never carried out any formal assessments, Dawson and Adams (1994) found that children with autism were more socially responsive and showed more eye contact when the experimenter imitated their behavior (Dawson and Adams in Escalona et. al. 2002).

Alongside these principles are a number of other approaches taught by the program. It teaches that parents need to become "happy detectives," observing the child first to watch for clues and cues to help them learn the child's behavior and routines. It also teaches that they need to learn to take into account sensitivities to things such as sound (Kaufman, B. 1981) and to try out different pitches and levels of noise to see which the child is more responsive to. Another recommendation is to limit language so the child knows what to focus on. For example, instead of saying, "Do you want some dinner?" say, "Dinner?"

Eye contact is also particularly emphasized in the Son-Rise Program. The institute believes that the more a child looks, the more he or she learns. As a result eye contact is encouraged at every opportunity (i.e., mimicking the "ism" at eye level, feeding food at eye level, raising objects to eye level). Often the program will introduce eye contact through the use of a mirror, as some children can at first find it uncomfortable to give direct eye contact.

Dietary intervention is also focused upon. The institute strongly recommends looking into a gluten- and casein-free diet, eliminating caffeine, reducing sugar intake, and exploring the possibility of Candida yeast overgrowth (Kaufman, R. 2004). Investigation of any other intolerance the child may have is also recommended.

## The Playroom

A calm, safe, and distraction-free playroom is one of the key elements of the Son-Rise Program. The institute highlights this as the place where it believes children will find it easiest to process information and relate to the people around them. The idea developed from the fact that the Kaufmans found their bathroom to be the best environment in which to work with their son, as it was the most calm and distraction-free environment in the house. Sensory processing is often an area that people with autistic spectrum disorders find difficult, often finding it difficult to concentrate while competing with background noises, visual stimuli, and the like. Parents are strongly encouraged to create such a playroom at home.

The institute has a number of recommendations to make the playroom as "distraction-free" as possible. These include putting filters on the windows to prevent the outside world from becoming distracting as well as making the room as soundproof as possible. The playroom walls should be a fairly neutral color, with few displays on them and with equipment kept high out of reach on shelves. It recommends vinyl flooring without a pattern, as it is durable, easily cleaned, and not distracting for the child. Many children are hypersensitive to light, so lights that do not flicker are recommended, with a particular note not to use fluorescent lighting. The institute also recommends removing any electronic equipment such as televisions and videos, as this is a passive form of entertainment and also often hypnotic and absorbing for children (Kaufman 2004).

Wooden shelves should be built about four feet off the floor, high enough that the child cannot reach, and food and toys should be kept on these. As a result the room is not only distraction-free but also requires the child to learn to request toys and food.

Most playrooms also have an observation window, so that volunteers and parents can observe sessions as part of ongoing training, as well as having an intercom system. A baby-monitoring device is a relatively inexpensive solution.

Other objects suggested for the room are exercise balls, a wooden slide with detachable steps, a low wooden table, a bench, and a small trampoline. The idea is to use the large items to help the child use his or her body but not have so many objects as to form a distraction.

Another key aspect of the room is that there is only one other person in the room with the child at a time. As a result the whole playroom is centered on the child and the environment is very predictable. The Options Institute believes that one of the reasons that children with autism retreat into their "isms" is because they, unlike the outside world, are predictable and therefore comforting. By making the environment similarly predictable, the child is less likely to retreat into his or her "isms" and will learn to trust his or her environment (Horler et. al. 1998). The volunteer is encouraged "to go in with a bang," showing the child how exciting life can be (Macey 1994). "Excitement, enthusiasm, and energy are the order of the day in the Option playroom" (Macey 1994). It is a room where the word "no" does not exist, the idea being that the child has full control and the ability to control the room.

## Who Is the Program Aimed At?

Although the program is mostly marketed toward people with autism, the Kaufmans see the Son-Rise Program as being a global program for people with a variety of difficulties, including autism, pervasive developmental disorders (PDD), and Down syndrome at a variety of ages (Kaufman, R. 2002). Early intervention is emphasized, with the recommendation that the approach be used from the earliest possible age. However, they also claim that older children can carry out the program and make significant progress (Kaufman, R. 2002).

# The Different Son-Rise Programs Offered by the Institute

## The Start-Up Program

This is an introductory five-day program designed to give people the tools to design and implement their own home program. The institute's website recommends the program to parents who are already running a home program they are not happy with or who are contemplating running either a full- or part-time program, family members and volunteers interested in supporting a family, or professionals who are working with children with special needs. A number of teachers use a wide range of program topics including speech and language development, handling behavior, and leading a program, among many others. This is all done through slides, videos, lectures, activities, and question-and-answer sessions. Creating a playroom and recruiting and training volunteers are also covered, as well as providing attitudinal training. At the end, everyone is given a manual to refer to at home. This program is run a number of times a year in both the United States and the United Kingdom.

## The Intensive Program

This program is the most individual and intensive program offered and is held only at the Options Institute in Massachusetts. Parents and their children live and work in the Son-Rise house for a week. The house includes a playroom with a two-way mirror so the child can be observed at all times. An individual program is designed. The child is kept locked in a playroom from 8:30 to 5:30, with lunch being left at the door for a volunteer to collect. The child, as a result, interacts with only one other person during this time. Parents also work the same hours, either with the child or in one-to-one dialogue. One-to-one dialogue is one of the key teaching tools at the institute. Parents have one-to-one sessions with members of staff, a questioning process to find out parental areas of stress to help maintain an attitude of acceptance and enthusiasm with the child.

As a result, at the end of the program, the child will have received thirty-five hours of intensive interaction and parents will have received forty-five hours. Before attending the program parents talk to a member of staff to provide personal history, and to share concerns and what they would like to get out of the program. Teaching is done in a number of ways, including observing staff with your child to learn the skills, hands-on practice working with the child, and confidence-building to manage a program at home. A video of you working with your child is also produced for you and for training for others. A team meeting of all staff and parents is also held to create clear baselines and directions to establish the child's motivations and also to use data, observations, techniques, and experience.

### The Maximum Impact Program

This is a more advanced version of Start-Up for parents who have done Start-Up and perhaps the Intensive Course as well. It is a similar course to Start-Up in teaching style and includes presentations by Barry Neil and Samahria Lyte Kaufman. Individualized sessions with them can also be scheduled. They focus more on question and answers than in the other program. Again, this program is run a couple of times a year in both the United States and the United Kingdom.

After parents have been trained, they then can get further support by telephone or they can send a video to get feedback (Kaufman, S. 1998). It is also possible for families to have a free twenty-five-minute consultation with a family counselor before attending a program.

### New Frontiers: The Son-Rise Advanced Training Program

This is a new program recently launched by the Options Institute. It is offered to parents who have completed at least one of the other programs: Start-Up, Maximum Impact, or the Intensive Program. This program is set to a curriculum. Its purpose is to assess a child's social development and determine how to develop these skills further. Goals include developing eye contact, communication, physical interaction, and friendship skills.

### In-Home Outreach Service

This is a service for parents who have attended one of the above programs and are now running a Son-Rise Program at home. One of the institute's certified teachers will come to the home and work with your family and any volunteers or professionals that are working with your child.

### Costs

It is very difficult to find out the costs of the different programs, as this is not something readily advertised on their website. However, estimates of the costs for the courses are as follows:

- $1,995 for the Start-Up Program in the United States
- $2,385 for the Start-Up Program in the United Kingdom
- $11,500 for the Intensive Program
- $1,995 for the Maximum Impact Program in the United States
- $2,385 for the Maximum Impact Program in the United Kingdom
- Phone consultation $550 (50 minutes), though this can vary greatly depending on the professional to whom you talk

The institute can also provide information and possibly help to families in regard to financial assistance and fund-raising (Kaufman, S. 1998).

It is worth bearing in mind that you will need ongoing financial assistance to maintain the program.

## *Volunteers*

Running and maintaining such an intensive program does rely on having a team of dedicated and reliable volunteers to help maintain it. The institute produces guidelines and tips on recruiting volunteers, including providing examples of posters and fliers to advertise for volunteers as well as covering letters, interview techniques, and possibly training. It recommends recruiting from a large number of places such as colleges, sports centers, churches, and social clubs, as well as asking friends, colleagues, and acquaintances. It also suggests writing an interest story for the local paper.

Many parents advertise in the psychology and nursing departments of their local universities, as students are often looking for experience in the field of special needs. There is also a section on the Son-Rise Program website where parents can advertise for volunteers and in turn volunteers can advertise for placements.

It is important that volunteers are made aware of the number of hours and the length of time they are required to commit to the program. The program recommends asking for at least four to eight hours a week as well as attending a bi-weekly team meeting with all other volunteers. They should be expected to keep a formal journal of behavior, changes, and the like so that these changes can be discussed at the team meetings and used to decide what the goals should be for forthcoming sessions.

# Pros and Cons of the Program

## *Pros*

One of the biggest advantages reported by parents doing the program is the amount of productive and positive time they can spend with their child (Jordan and Powell 1993). Williams (2004) carried out a survey of parents doing the program, and many noted that the family generally felt more positive and interaction among the whole family had improved since doing the program (Williams 2004). The program shares a number of features with other autism-specific programs, particularly the environmental and sensory impact and the need to develop empathy for the way the child sees the world. However, possibly the most striking feature of the program is the huge amount of one-to-one intervention the child can receive on a daily basis. There is research to support that such huge levels of intensive interaction can encourage development in the child, though this is not specifically in regard to Son-Rise (Jordan and Powell 1993).

## *Cons*

Apart from the costs of the program, a major criticism of Son-Rise is that the Options Institute has never allowed or carried out any formal research on the effectiveness of it. It argues that it does not have the resources to carry out any large-scale evaluation of the success rate (Kaufman, R. 2002), but it is said to have turned down external researchers' requests as well. Jordan (1993) points out that the informal, successful reports there have been of the program have been with young children and there are no reports on older children (Jordan 1993). It is possible that the program works better for some children than others, with Jordan suggesting that it may depend on a "certain level of intellectual potential" (Jordan 1993 and Williams and Wishart 1999).

Another difficulty that parents commonly face is recruiting and retaining enough volunteers for the program. This can be unreliable, especially around the holidays, when many students go home, resulting in the parents having to cover many hours of the program themselves (Macey 1994). Williams (2004) found in her survey that the most common obstacle was the lack of, or high turnover of, volunteers. Parents worked for an average of eleven hours a week out of a possible nineteen, and as a result other problems arise, such as not spending enough time with the rest of the family. Howlin (1997) emphasizes that any benefits to a child from an intensive program must be weighed against the disruption to family life and relationships (Williams and Wishart 1999).

The emphasis on gaining eye contact is also questioned by some professionals. For some people on the autistic spectrum, eye contact can be distressing and uncomfortable. Luke Jackson, a teenager with Asperger syndrome, describes giving someone eye contact as feeling "as if their eyes are burning me" (Jackson 2002, 70). He also finds it difficult to listen to someone at the same time that he is looking at him or her (Jackson 2002). This again emphasizes how the intervention may be more effective for some children than others.

## Alternatives to the Son-Rise Program

There are now a number of interventions designed for people on the autistic spectrum. Son-Rise sees the program in direct contrast to other programs such as Lovaas. While both are home-based, intensive, and one-on-one, there are a number of differences (Lynch 1996). While the Son-Rise Program is child-led, Lovaas is therapist-led; Son-Rise is a more flexible program, whereas Lovaas is more structured (Lynch 1996).

The Growing Minds Institute also provides an alternative to the Son-Rise Program. It is a program directed and taught by Steven Wertz, who has been both a Son-Rise and an applied behavioral analysis (ABA) teacher in the past. This institute provides individual education plans based on a number of different teaching methods, including Son-Rise, Lovaas, TEACCH, and floor-time, to develop your own teaching style for the child. Steven Wertz is certified in ABA and Son-Rise.

It is reported that some parents have found that the Son-Rise Program has given them a good launch pad for other programs. One set of parents found that it was good at getting their child to establish rapport and confidence with a large number of people and increasing listening and understanding skills. However, it did not allow the child to fulfill his or her potential academically but gave the child good skills for other programs (Horler et. al. 1998).

As all of these programs require such a large amount of commitment from the family, it is always useful to do as much research on them as possible.

## Recommended Reading and References

Adams, A. (1993) Coaxed Away from a Shut-Away Existence. *The Independent*, 28 September 1993.

Archer, M. (1997) Welcome to My World. *Special Children*, November–December 1997, 21–23.

Bennie, M. (2 February 2005) It's All in How You Look at It. *Autism Today*, www.autismtoday.com/articles/How_You_Look_At_It.htm.

Escalona, A., Field, T., Nadel, J., and Lundy, B. (2002) Brief Report: Imitation Effects on Children with Autism. *Journal of Autism and Developmental Disorders*, 32: 141–44.

Gaunt, M. and Howard Taylor G. (1997) *QED: Challenging Children: I Want My Little Boy Back.* This BBC television program followed the Broadrick family to the Options Institute to see the help they got for their son.

Hamilton-Ely (1990) The Option Method. *Communication*, 24(1): 7–8.

Heggessey, L. (ed.) (1997) *QED: Challenging Children* London: BBC Learning Support.

Horler, M., Jobson, R., and Grayson, A. (1998) *Combining a Home-Based Intervention with a Young Autistic Boy. Psychobiology of Autism: Current Research and Practice. Collected papers from a conference organised by the Autism Research Unit*, 231–38.

Jackson, L. (2002) *Freaks, Geeks and Asperger Syndrome*. London: Jessica Kingsley Publishers.

Jones, G. (ed.) (2002) Autism Early Intervention. A Special Supplement. *Good Autism Practice Journal*. BILD Publications.

Jordan, R. (1999) Making Relationships with Individuals with Autism: Rationale and Practical Approaches. www.autismconnect.org/autism99.

Jordan, R. (1990) *The Option Approach to Autism: Observer Project Report*.

Jordan, R. and Powell (1993) Reflections of the Option Method as a Treatment for Autism. *Journal of Autism and Developmental Disorders*, 23: 682–85.

Kaufman (1994) *Son-Rise—The Miracle Continues*. Tiburon, Calif.: H. J. Kramer Inc.

Kaufman, B. (1984) *Autism Can Be Cured: Loving Children Back to Life. An Option Presentation*. Sheffield, Mass.: Option Indigo Press.

Kaufman, B. N. (1981) *A Miracle to Believe In*. USA: Ballantine Books.

Kaufman, R. (7 February 2005) Moving the Mountain: Autism, Recovery and the Answer "Yes." *Autism Today*, www.autismtoday.com/articles/moving_the_mountain.htm.

Kaufman, R. (7 February 2005) The Journey out of Autism. *Autism Today*, www.autismtoday.com/articles/Journey_Out_of_Autism.htm.

Kaufman, R. (7 February 2005) Autism and the Myth of False Hope. *Autism Today*, www.autismtoday.com/articles/Autism_and_the_Myth_of_False_Hope.htm.

Kaufman, R. (2002) Building the Bridges: Strategies for Reaching Our Children. *Good Autism Practice*, 3: 10, 16.

Kaufman, R. (2002) Raun Kaufman and Son-Rise Program. *Communication*, Spring 2002, 26–28.

Kaufman, S. (1998) The Son-Rise Program at the Option Institute. *Communication*, Spring 1998, 19–23.

Kaufman, S. L. (1989) *Special Children / Special Solutions: A Journey of Love*. Sheffield Mass.: Option Indigo Press.

Knott, F. (1996) *Approaches to Autism in the USA*. London: Winston Churchill Memorial Trust.

Levy (1999) Teaching Critical Social Skills: Utilizing Attitude, Environment, Joining, and Motivation in the Son-Rise Program. www.autismconnect.org/autism99.

Levy, J. (1998) The Son-Rise Program: Letters. *Communication*, Winter 1998, 2.

Lynch, S. (1996) Intensive Behavioural Intervention with a Seven Year Old Girl with Autism. *Therapeutic Intervention in Autism: Perspectives from Research and Practice. Collected papers from the conference organised by the Autism Research Unit*, 343–60.

MacDonald and MacDonald (1991) Option Method—Part 2. *Communication*, 25: 5–6.

Macey, E. (1996) Using the Option Approach in Schools. *Autism on the Agenda. A collection of papers from a National Autistic Society Conference*, 203–5.

Rimland, B. and Edelson, S. (1999) The Autism Treatment Evaluation Checklist www.autism.com/atec/atec.jpg or *Autism Review International*, 13: 2.

Roberts, Y. (1996) John's Story. *Daily Express*, 13 April 1996

Romanczyk, R. and Gillis, J. (2005) Chapter 14: Treatment Approaches for Autism: Evaluating Options and Making Informed Choices. In *Autism Spectrum Disorders. Identification, Education and Treatment*, 3rd ed., ed. Dianne Zager, New York: Lawerence Erlbaum Assoc. Inc., 515–35.

Shakeshaft, L. (1998) They Said Our Son Was Autistic and That Was That. *Daily Mail*, 10 February 1998.

Spinks, A. The Option Institute's Son-Rise Program—A Parent's View, www.nas.org.uk/nas/jsp/polopoly.jsp?d=297&a=3729&view=print.

Stehli, A. (1995) *Dancing in the Rain: Stories of Exceptional Progress by Parents of Children with Special Needs*. Westport, Conn.: Georgiana Organisation.

Tissot, C. (1999) Decisions after Diagnosis: A Practical Path for Parents, www.autismconnect.org/autism99.

Walters, T. (1994) Kieran's World. *Nursery World*, 17 November, 10–11.

Williams, K. (2006) The Son-Rise Program Intervention for Autism: An Investigation into Prerequisites for Evaluation and Family Experiences. PhD diss., University of Edinburgh.

Williams, K. and Wishard, J. (2003) The Son-Rise Program Intervention for Autism: An Investigation into Family Experiences. *Journal of Intellectual Disability Research*, 47: 291–99.

Williams, K. and Wishart, J. (2001) Combining School Attendance with Home-Based Interventions for Autism, *NASEN Journal for Research in SEN*, vol. 1.

Williams, K. and Wishart, J. (1999) The Experience of Families Implementing the Son-Rise Program Intervention for Autism. From *Research into Therapy: Collected papers from the conference organised by the Autism Research Unit*, 91–102.

## Section 29.2

# Daily Life Therapy (Higashi): Educating Children with Autism through Physical Activity, Academic Activity, and Vocational Training

"Daily Life Therapy: Higashi," © 2007 The National Autistic Society (www .autism.org.uk). All rights reserved. Adapted and reprinted with permission. Information from The National Autistic Society is regularly updated. For the most current information, visit www.autism.org.uk.

### History and Philosophy

Boston Higashi School, Inc. is an international program serving individuals, aged three to twenty-two, with autism. The philosophy is based upon the acclaimed tenets of daily life therapy developed by the late Dr. Kiyo Kitahara of Tokyo, Japan. The holistic approach captures the essence of humanity and reflects the sensibilities and sensitivities, the intellect and the aesthetics of humankind, attaining harmony in all aspects of life.

Dr. Kiyo Kitahara's method provides children with systematic education through group dynamics, modeling, and physical activity. The goal of this educational approach is for the children to develop as closely to normal physically, emotionally, and intellectually as possible, and to achieve social independence and dignity.

### Programs and Services

Daily life therapy is an educational methodology framed within normal development based upon group dynamics, physical education, art, music, academic activity, and vocational training. Whole language and a socio-communicative approach are utilized with language acquisition and the development of communication skills. The computer center, with state-of-the-art software, enhances language and literacy. Academic activities designed for individual capabilities are emphasized. Physical education and vigorous exercise reduce anxiety, increase stamina, and establish rhythm and routines. Exercises founded upon principles of sensory integration and vestibular stimulation develop coordination and cooperative group interaction.

Academic activities, in the areas of language, arts, mathematics, social studies, and science, are compatible with typical school curricula to prepare each student for inclusion opportunities. Art and music provide opportunities to gain mastery and appreciation of aesthetics.

The residential program is a related educational service designed to teach daily living and social skills and support the day program in order that students can maintain and derive educational progress. The residential program is an educational component to optimize life-long inclusion in the community and not a place to provide long-term living arrangements. Family support services offer parent training and involvement through regularly scheduled parent study meetings.

The day program operates 217 days a year and the residential program operates 304 days a year.

- Age range served: Three to twenty-two
- Age at admission: Three to twelve and up to sixteen
- Staff to pupil ratio: Day 1:6, Residential 5:16
- Current enrollment: 102

## Publications

Collins, M. et al. *Common Ground: Report on a Visit by the National Autistic Society to the Boston Higashi School, 5th–9th November 1995.* London: The National Autistic Society.

Edwards, D. The efficacy of Daily Life Therapy at the Boston Higashi School. In: Therapeutic Approaches to Autism: Research and Practice. Collected papers from a Conference. Sunderland: Autism Research Unit, 1995, 115–27.

Elgar, S. Report of my visit to Dr. Kiyo Kithara's Boston Higashi School, Boston, USA. *Communication*, 1989, 23 (1): 5–6.

Evans, J. Boston Higashi: a parent's eye view. *Stop Press!* (Newsletter of the West Midlands Autistic Society), February 1995.

Kitahara, K. Daily life therapy: a method of educating autistic children. *Record of Actual Education at Musashino Higashi Gakuen School*, Japan. Volume 1. Boston, Mass.: Nimrod Press, 1984.

Kitahara, K. Daily life therapy: a method of educating autistic children. *Record of Actual Education at Musashino Higashi Gakuen School*, Japan. Volume 2. Boston, Mass.: Nimrod Press, 1984.

Kitahara, K. Daily life therapy: a method of educating autistic children. *Record of Actual Education at Musashino Higashi Gakuen School*, Japan. Volume 3. Boston, Mass.: Nimrod Press, 1984.

Larkin, A. S. and Gurry, S. Brief report: progress reported in three children with autism using Daily Life Therapy. *Journal of Autism and Developmental Disorders*, 1998, 28 (4): 339–42.

Martell, R. Vision need not be a miracle. *Therapy Weekly*, 22 August 1996, 4. Reports on a visit to Boston Higashi school which has been criticized for its emphasis on physical exercise.

Peacock, G. Higashi: implementing Daily Life Therapy in Japan. *A visit to the Musashino Higashi Gakuen School in Tokyo*. London: The National Autistic Society, 1994.

Quill, K. Daily Life Therapy: a Japanese model of educating children with autism. *Journal of Autism and Developmental Disorders*, 1989, 19 (4): 625–35.

Upton, G. Two hours in the Musashino Higashi Gakuen. *Communication*, 1992, 26 (1): 9–12.

# Chapter 30

# *Occupational Therapy in the Treatment of Autism*

Occupational therapists and occupational therapy assistants help people with autism find ways to adjust tasks and conditions that match their needs and abilities. Such help may include adapting the environment to minimize external distractions, finding specially designed computer software that facilitates word processing to ease communication, or identifying skills that build capabilities.

## Where do occupational therapists and occupational therapy assistants work with individuals with autism?

Occupational therapists and occupational therapy assistants provide interventions to clients in the environments where they typically engage in their occupations, such as a child care center or preschool, school, home, worksite, adult day care, residential setting, or any range of community settings.

## What information do occupational therapy practitioners offer to families and to teams?

Occupational therapy assistants and occupational therapists help families and other people learn how to adapt the environment to increase the comfort and performance of individuals with autism spectrum disorders (ASD). Occupational therapy assistants and occupational therapists also can provide information about other services that may support the individual or family.

## What occupational therapy services are available for people with autism?

Occupational therapy intervention helps individuals with autism develop or improve appropriate social, play, learning, community mobility, and vocational skills. The occupational therapy practitioner aids the individual in achieving and maintaining normal daily tasks such as getting dressed, engaging in social interactions, completing school activities, and working or playing.

## What can occupational therapists do?

- Evaluate an individual to determine whether he or she has accomplished developmentally appropriate skills needed in such areas as grooming and play or leisure skills.

- Provide interventions to help a child appropriately respond to information coming through the senses. Intervention may include developmental activities, sensory integration or sensory processing, and play activities.

- Facilitate play activities that instruct as well as aid a child in interacting and communicating with others.

- Devise strategies to help the individual transition from one setting to another, from one person to another, and from one life phase to another.

- Collaborate with the individual and family to identify safe methods of community mobility.

- Identify, develop, or adapt work or engagement in meaningful activities that enhance the individual's quality of life.

## How can I find occupational therapy services?

Pediatricians can help parents identify early intervention programs available through a state's Department of Social Services or Department of Health. These programs can refer young children and their families to occupational therapy and other needed services. Services also may be available through local health centers, hospitals, private clinics, and home health agencies. Additionally, adults with ASD who need occupational therapy services may find resources through developmental disability programs or social services agencies.

### *Who pays for occupational therapy services?*

Occupational therapy is a skilled service covered by private insurance, Medicare, Medicaid, worker's compensation, vocational programs, behavioral health programs, early intervention, and school programs. Services also may be covered through Social Security, state mental health or mental retardation agencies, health and human services agencies, private foundations, and grants. Many providers accept private payments.

Chapter 31

# Music Therapy and Individuals with Autism Spectrum Disorders

## What is music therapy?

Music therapy is a well-established allied health profession similar to occupational and physical therapy. It consists of using music therapeutically to address behavioral, social, psychological, communicative, physical, sensory-motor, and/or cognitive functioning. Because music therapy is a powerful and nonthreatening medium, unique outcomes are possible. For individuals with diagnoses on the autism spectrum, music therapy provides a unique variety of music experiences in an intentional and developmentally appropriate manner to effect changes in behavior and facilitate development of skills.

Music therapy may include the use of behavioral, biomedical, developmental, educational, humanistic, adaptive music instruction, and/or other models. Music therapy enhances one's quality of life, involving relationships between a qualified music therapist and individual; between one individual and another; between the individual and his or her family; and between the music and the participants. These relationships are structured and adapted through the elements of music to create a positive environment and set the occasion for successful growth.

### Why music therapy for individuals with diagnoses on the autism spectrum?

- The literature reports that most individuals with autism respond positively to music (DeMyer, 1974; Edgerton, 1994; Euper, 1968; Snell, 1996; Thaut, 1992).

- People with diagnoses on the autism spectrum often show a heightened interest and response to music, making it an excellent therapeutic tool to work with them.

- Music is a very basic human response, spanning all degrees of ability/disability. Music therapists are able to meet clients at their own levels and allow them to grow from there. The malleability of music makes it a medium that can be adapted to meet the needs of each individual.

- Music is motivating and enjoyable.

- Music can promote relatedness, relaxation, learning, and self-expression.

- Music therapy addresses multiple developmental issues simultaneously.

- Music therapy can provide success-oriented opportunities for achievement and mastery.

- The structure and sensory input inherent in music help to establish response and role expectations, positive interactions, and organization.

### How does music therapy make a difference for individuals with diagnoses on the autism spectrum?

Individuals with diagnoses on the autism spectrum may display "qualitative impairments in social interaction and communication" and often manifest "restricted repetitive and stereotyped patterns of behavior, interests and activities." Delays and/or abnormal functioning usually occur before age three and may be marked by a lack of symbolic or imaginative play as well. (*Diagnostic Statistical Manual-IV*, pp. 70–71).

Music therapy can be effective in addressing the typical characteristics of autism listed above in the following ways:

- Music is considered a "universal language" which provides bridges in a nonthreatening setting between people and/or between individuals and their environment, facilitating relationships, learning, self-expression, and communication.

• Music captures and helps maintain attention. It is highly motivating and engaging and may be used as a natural "reinforcer" for desired responses. Music therapy can stimulate clients to reduce negative and/or self-stimulatory responses and increase participation in more appropriate and socially acceptable ways.

• Music therapy can enable those without language to communicate, participate, and express themselves nonverbally. Very often music therapy also assists in the development of verbal communication, speech, and language skills. The interpersonal timing and reciprocity in shared play, turn-taking, listening, and responding to another person are augmented in music therapy with children and adults with autism to accommodate and address their styles of communication.

• Music therapy allows individuals with diagnoses on the autism spectrum the opportunity to develop identification and appropriate expression of their emotions.

• Because music is processed in both hemispheres of the brain, music can stimulate cognitive functioning and may be used for remediation of some speech and language skills.

• Music provides concrete, multisensory stimulation (auditory, visual, and tactile). The rhythmic component of music is very organizing for the sensory systems of individuals diagnosed with autism. As a result, auditory processing and other sensory-motor, perceptual/motor, gross and fine motor skills can be enhanced through music therapy.

• Musical elements and structures provide a sense of security and familiarity in the music therapy setting, encouraging clients to attempt new tasks within this predictable but malleable framework.

• Many people with diagnoses on the autism spectrum have innate musical talents; thus, music therapy provides an opportunity for successful experiences. Emphasis is placed on strengths, which in turn may be utilized to address each individual's areas of need.

### What do music therapists do?

Music therapists provide direct or consultative services. They work individually or in small groups, using a variety of music and techniques to engage children and adults with diagnoses on the autism spectrum. They involve clients in singing, listening, moving, playing instruments, and creative activities in a systematic, prescribed manner to influence change in targeted responses or behaviors and help clients meet individual goals and objectives. They create a musical, familiar environment that encourages positive interpersonal interaction and allows clients freedom to explore and express themselves. They utilize music that is preferred by and reinforcing to clients and is appropriate for ages, cultures, and environments in which the clients interact.

Music therapists are trained professionals who accept referrals, observe clients' behavior and interactions, and assess their behavioral/psychosocial/emotional, communication/language, perceptual and sensory-motor, cognitive/academic, and musical skills. After designing realistic goals and target objectives to address identified needs, music therapists plan and implement individualized music therapy treatment programs with strategies, procedures, and interventions to develop skills necessary to achieve an optimum level of success or quality of life for individuals with diagnoses on the autism spectrum. Music therapists document client responses, conduct ongoing evaluations of progress and performance, and make recommendations for future consideration. They often work as team members in conjunction with families and professionals to best address each individual's needs. Music therapists may also make recommendations to team members and families regarding ways to include successful music therapy techniques in other aspects of clients' lives.

### What can one expect from a music therapist?

A music therapist is:

- Professionally trained to utilize clinical musical interventions to address behavioral/psychosocial/emotional, communication/language, sensory-motor, and cognitive needs of individuals;

- A competent musician who is both creative and resourceful;

- An understanding, caring, ethical therapist, with a broad range of skills;

- Well-versed in a variety of music therapy applications and pertinent research;

- Informed regarding individuals with diagnoses on the autism spectrum and able to provide adaptations to address unique processing styles;

- Able to create a therapeutic environment and engage in the therapeutic process;

- An effective communicator, with clients, other team members, and the public.

## *Who is a qualified music therapist?*

Graduates of colleges or universities from one of approximately seventy approved music therapy degree programs are eligible to take a certification examination in music therapy. Those who pass the exam become board certified (MT-BC), demonstrating entry-level skills in the profession. In addition to the MT-BC credential, other recognized professional designations are registered music therapist (RMT), certified music therapist (CMT), and advanced certified music therapist (ACMT) listed with the National Music Therapy Registry. Any individual who does not have proper training and credentials is not qualified to provide music therapy services.

## *Where do music therapists work?*

Music therapists may work in public school systems, where, in accordance with the Individuals with Disabilities Education Act (IDEA), music therapy is recognized as a related service that provides a "significant motivation and/or assist" in the achievement of Individual Education Plan (IEP) goals and objectives.

In addition, music therapists may provide service in the following settings: early intervention centers, Head Start programs, day care centers, preschools through high schools, day treatment centers, hospitals, hospices, clinics, rehabilitation centers, substance abuse facilities, mental health centers, group homes, sheltered workshops, long-term care facilities, correctional institutions, private homes, camps, community schools of the arts, music retailers, wellness centers, holistic treatment centers, private practice, and more.

## *How does music therapy help families of individuals with diagnoses on the autism spectrum?*

Families of those with diagnoses on the autism spectrum may reap many benefits from music therapy:

- An individual's growth through music therapy may improve the quality of life for the whole family. If the client's behavior is improved, there may be less stress or strain on other family members. In addition, with an increase in skills, the client may become more independent and aware and more able to interact and communicate with others.

• Music therapy can provide additional opportunities for positive interaction and building relationships among family members and the client. New music-related leisure options among family members may be explored, while providing an acceptable emotional outlet.

• Greater family cohesiveness, support, and coping skills may be achieved through shared, equal music making during sessions or in the home environment.

• Music therapy interventions can teach family members alternative ways to interact, socialize, and communicate with their loved ones.

• Music therapy can help promote generalization and transfer of skills in sessions to the home environment.

• Participation in music therapy often allows family members to see their loved one in a "different light," to witness their relative's areas of strength and aptitude, perhaps seeing or hearing novel responses in this setting that they have not noted elsewhere. Music therapy may provide hope for the future and belief in the individual's abilities.

### *Is there research to support music therapy for individuals with diagnoses on the autism spectrum?*

Through peer-reviewed journals inside the profession such as *Music Therapy, the Journal of Music Therapy, Music Therapy Perspectives*, and extensive articles in journals outside the profession, the American Music Therapy Association (AMTA) has promoted much research exploring the benefits of music therapy with individuals with diagnoses on the autism spectrum. A research bibliography of select articles and publications is available from AMTA for those interested in specific research examples.

# Part Six

# Family and Lifestyle Issues for People with Autism

Chapter 32

# Autism's Effect on Family Relationships

## Chapter Contents

Section 32.1—Stress on Families of Autistic Children ........... 392
Section 32.2—Helping Siblings Understand Autism and
            Encouraging Positive Relationships ................. 397

# Section 32.1

# *Stress on Families of Autistic Children*

Stress—something parents in general are all too familiar with. There is the physical stress from carpools, preparing meals, bathing, homework, shopping, and so on. This is compounded by such psychological stressors as parent-child conflicts, not having enough time to complete responsibilities and concern regarding a child's well-being. When a family has a child on the autism spectrum, unique stressors are added.

## *Sources of Stress for Parents*

**Deficits and behaviors of autism:** Research indicates that parents of children with autism experience greater stress than parents of children with intellectual disabilities and Down Syndrome (Holroyd & McArthur, 1976; Donovan, 1988). This may be a result of the distinct characteristics that individuals with autism exhibit. An individual with autism may not express his or her basic wants or needs in a manner that we would expect. Therefore, parents are left playing a guessing game. Is the child crying because he or she is thirsty, hungry, or sick? When a parent cannot determine his or her child's needs, both are left feeling frustrated. The child's frustration can lead to aggressive or self-injurious behaviors that threaten his or her safety and the safety of other family members (e.g. siblings). Stereotypic and compulsive behaviors concern parents since they appear peculiar and interfere with functioning and learning. If a child has deficits in social skills, such as the lack of appropriate play, stress may be increased for families; individuals lacking appropriate leisure skills often require constant structure of their time, a task not feasible to accomplish in the home environment.

Finally, many families struggle with the additional challenges of getting their child to sleep through the night or eat a wider variety of foods. All of these issues and behaviors are physically exhausting for families and emotionally draining. For families of children on the autism spectrum this can be a particular challenge. Scheduled dinner times may not be successful due to the child's inability to sit appropriately for extended periods of time. Bedtime routines can be interrupted by difficulties sleeping. Maladaptive behaviors may prevent families from attending events together. For example, Mom might have to stay home while Dad takes the sibling to the soccer game. Not being able to do things as a family can impact the marital relationship. In addition, spouses often cannot spend time alone due to their extreme parenting demands and the lack of qualified staff to watch a child with autism in their absence.

**Reactions from society and feelings of isolation:** Taking an individual with autism out into the community can be a source of stress for parents. People may stare, make comments, or fail to understand any mishaps or behaviors that may occur. For example, individuals with autism have been seen taking a stranger's food right off their plate. As a result of these potential experiences, families often feel uncomfortable taking their child to the homes of friends or relatives. This makes holidays an especially difficult time for these families. Feeling like they cannot socialize or relate to others, parents of children on the autism spectrum may experience a sense of isolation from their friends, relatives, and community.

**Concerns over future caregiving:** One of the most significant sources of stress is the concern regarding future caregiving. Parents know that they provide their child with exceptional care. They fear that no one will take care of their child like they do. There may also be no other family members willing or capable of accomplishing this task. Even though parents try to fight off thinking about the future, these thoughts and worries are still continually present.

**Finances:** Having a child on the autism spectrum can drain a family's resources due to expenses such as evaluations, home programs, and various therapies. The caregiving demands of raising a child with autism may lead one parent to give up his or her job, yet financial strains may be exacerbated by having only one income to support all of the families' needs.

**Feelings of grief:** Parents of children with autism spectrum disorder are grieving the loss of the "typical" child that they expected to have. In addition, parents are grieving the loss of lifestyle that they expected for themselves and their family. The grief that parents experience can be an additional source of stress due its ongoing nature. Current theories of grief suggest that parents of children with developmental disabilities experience episodes of grief throughout the life cycle as different events (e.g., birthdays, holidays, unending caregiving) trigger grief reactions (Worthington, 1994). Experiencing "chronic sorrow" is a psychological stressor that can be frustrating, confusing and depressing.

## Sources of Stress for Siblings

There are also potential sources of stress for siblings. Not all siblings will experience these issues, but here are some to be aware of:

- Embarrassment around peers; jealousy regarding amount of time parents spend with their brother or sister
- Frustration over not being able to engage or get a response from their brother or sister
- Being the target of aggressive behaviors
- Trying to make up for the deficits of their brother or sister
- Concern regarding their parents' stress and grief
- Concern over their role in future caregiving

## Sources of Stress for Grandparents

Like parents, grandparents can grieve over the loss of the "typical" grandchild they expected to have. In addition, grandparents are concerned about the stress and difficult situations they see their children experiencing.

Many grandparents want to help but they often face two obstacles. First, most of them do not have the training in behavior management that is required to handle behavioral episodes. They may offer advice related to their experiences, but these may not be successful for individuals with autism. This can cause parents to become frustrated when they perceive the grandparents as not understanding their situations. Second, grandparents may not be physically able to manage the behaviors of individuals with autism. Grandparents just want to play with their grandchildren and "spoil" them. Unfortunately, at times it may seem that a diagnosis of an autism spectrum disorder gets in the way of these desires. In reality, through understanding, experience, and acceptance many learn to relate to the child, understand the child's differences, celebrate his or her strengths and gifts, and gain insight into the unique situations involved with parenting a child with autism and find that children on the autism spectrum are just as easy to love and "spoil" as any other grandchild.

## What Can Be Done to Address Family Stress

Luckily, family members can take action to address the stress that they experience. Accessing services or doing any additional tasks can be overwhelming, considering what parents are already dealing with on a daily basis. However, remember that it is only by taking action that challenges can be tackled and progress toward solutions made. Following are some suggestions to get started with in enhancing family functioning.

### *Take Time For Yourself and Other Family Members*

In order to avoid burnout, parents must make time for themselves. Parents often respond to this suggestion by saying that they don't have any time to do that. However, you must keep in mind that even a few minutes a day can make a big difference. Some parents do such simple things for themselves as taking the time to apply hand lotion or cook their favorite dinners to make themselves feel better. Parents, just like individuals with autism, need rewards in order to be motivated. Parents who have children on the autism spectrum have even more of a need to reward themselves, because parenting their child can be frustrating and stressful.

In addition to rewarding themselves, family members need to reward one another. Spouses need to acknowledge the hard work that each is achieving. Also remember to thank siblings for watching or helping out their brothers and sisters. It is also important that spouses try to spend some time alone. Again, the quantity of time is not as important as the quality. This may include watching television together when the children are asleep, going out to dinner, or meeting for lunch when the children are in school.

Families may also want to occasionally engage in activities without the individual with autism. This may include mom, dad, and the siblings attending an amusement park together. Often families feel guilty not including the individual with autism, but everyone deserves to enjoy time together that is not threatened by the challenges of autism.

## Network with Other Families Affected by Autism or Another Disability

It gives us comfort to know that we are not the only ones experiencing a particularly stressful situation. In addition, one can get the most useful advice from others facing similar challenges and using similar services and supports. Support groups for parents, siblings, and grandparents are available through educational programs, parent resource centers, local chapters of the Autism Society of America (ASA), and developmental disabilities offices. In addition, there are now online supports available for family members. You can locate these sources of support and many other services in your area by using ASA's online referral database, Autism Source, at www.autismsource.org.

### Other Strategies to Address Stress

When it comes to reducing stress, be creative. You may want to consider one or more of the following approaches:

- Prayer
- Exercise/yoga
- Deep breathing/relaxation exercises/meditation
- Writing in a journal
- Keeping a daily schedule of things to accomplish
- Joining others in advocacy efforts at the local, state, or federal level
- Individual, marital, or family counseling

If you or a family member is exhibiting signs of stress, you need to take action. Even if it takes the last bit of energy you have left, getting assistance can only make things better. Yes, waiting lists, burdensome paperwork, and bureaucracy can make accessing supports stressful, but in the long run it will be worth it.

Note: This section was contributed by Adrianne Horowitz, CSW, director of family services for the Eden II Programs for Autistic Children.

Section 32.2

# *Helping Siblings Understand Autism and Encouraging Positive Relationships*

## *Understanding My Sibling's Disability*

### *"Telling" Does Not Guarantee Understanding*

The process of sharing information has two components, telling and understanding. As a child's ability to understand changes significantly as he or she grows and matures, the "telling" process must involve determining the child's level of understanding at his or her particular stage of development and re-presenting the same information in different ways over time.

### *Misconceptions and Misinformation*

Research indicates that siblings often do not understand or have misinformation regarding the definition and cause of their brother or sister's disorder. Additionally, it has been indicated that parents often overestimate siblings' understanding of the implications of their brother or sister's disorder.

## *My Perspective as a Sibling*

### *Things to Know*

Siblings are likely to spend more time with the child in their family who has special needs than anyone else, other than the mother or primary caregiver. In addition, because the sibling relationship is the longest-lasting relationship in the family, sibling issues are lifelong issues and change throughout the lifespan.

## *Of Concern or to Be Expected?*

Many situations that arise around sibling relationships can be attributed to typical sibling concerns. However, having a sibling with a disability or disorder impacts a child in many ways. Sibling concerns can be compounded by their level of understanding of their brother or sister's disorder and its implications, as well as the coping abilities and strategies exhibited by parents (so be sure to take care of not only your children but yourself and your other significant relationships!!). It is also important to remember that factual understanding and emotional acceptance are different processes.

## *Other Impacting Factors*

- Type and severity of the child's disorder
- Number of children in the family
- Age differences between siblings
- Family's child-rearing practices
- Family's lifestyle
- Other stress-producing conditions existing in the family
- Parental/family coping styles and interaction patterns
- The resources, support services and networks available to the family

## Developmental Stages

Depending on the siblings' developmental stage or level of understanding, their concerns are likely to focus on the cause of their brother or sister's disorder, their brother or sister's thoughts and feelings, whether or not he or she will get better, what is expected of them as a sibling, treatment and supports, and what the future holds for everyone involved.

## *Early Childhood*

**Understanding autism:** Autism is understood in terms of isolated behaviors that are specific, observable, and concrete (i.e., understanding is based on what the sibling sees rather than on logic).

The sibling may believe "illness" or disability can be almost magically transmitted.

The sibling has not yet devised logical strategies to relate observations and does not yet have the capacity to reason or understand on an abstract level what "autism" means or what the related implications may be.

Focus on concrete strategies and simple explanations that are specific, factual, and concrete (e.g., if the child is scared by tantrum behaviors, remove him or her from the immediate area and provide reassurance and comfort; explain that brother Billy waves his hands because he is excited).

**Sibling's perspective:** The sibling will notice differences between self and brother or sister but expects typical sibling interactions and relationships.

The sibling may be fearful of unpredictable behaviors (e.g., fearful for own safety, fear possessions will be taken or destroyed).

The sibling may take on caregiver or teacher role.

The sibling may believe something is wrong with him or her since he or she receives less parental/adult attention; the sibling may attempt to become the "perfect" child.

The sibling is unable to articulate his or her feelings and may do so using behavior.

The sibling may regress or mimic his or her brother or sister's behaviors in order to gain the same attention.

The sibling may develop jealousy and resentment toward parent for giving more attention to brother or sister, leading to feelings of rejection.

### *Middle Childhood*

**Understanding autism:** Autism is understood in terms of physical events; the concept of "contamination" results in the sibling understanding "illness" or disorder as being transmitted through physical contact.

The sibling is developing the ability to draw meaningful connections between current and past experiences and consider the connection between multiple symptoms, behaviors and/or events; develops understanding that the disorder is enduring.

However, understanding may be based on mistaken assumptions and "magical thinking" (e.g., the sibling might believe that Billy's autism came from getting sick, because he once heard the disorder described as an illness).

The sibling is not yet able to consider "possibilities" or implications of his brother or sister's disorder (e.g., parents may assume the sibling understands that the family can not attend the parade due to the sister or brother's inability to sit and attend, but the sibling may not yet have the cognitive abilities to relate the two).

The sibling is able to understand concrete definitions of his or her brother or sister's disorder and explanations of related needs described in familiar terms he or she understands; understands and becomes a "storehouse" of "facts."

**Sibling's perspective:** The sibling may worry that his or her brother or sister's "illness" or disorder is contagious or can be "caught"; may believe that his or her "bad" behavior or thoughts resulted in the brother or sister's "illness" or disorder.

The sibling may feel guilt for having negative feelings toward sister or brother; may feel "survivor's guilt."

The sibling may feel hurt or take brother or sister's behaviors personally.

The sibling may develop awareness of parents as "flawed" and may be critical of their efforts in addressing both their and their brother or sister's needs

The sibling is becoming aware of differences among people in the "outside" world; may develop feelings of isolation and embarrassment or shame.

The sibling may attempt to take on parental responsibilities and become overprotective of sister or brother, leading to conflicts with peers.

The sibling may continue to demonstrate own needs through behavior (e.g., demonstrating noncompliance, being overly well behaved).

### *Adolescence/Young Adulthood*

**Understanding autism:** Autism is understood in terms of "physiology"; the sibling has developed an abstract concept of "illness" or disorder and views this in terms of a malfunctioning body part or system.

The sibling can reason logically about past and future events and use knowledge rather than perception to reason.

The sibling can evaluate the impact of his or her brother or sister's disorder on situations that have not yet occurred.

The sibling understands and desires more detailed information and explanations regarding his or her brother or sister's specific disorder.

**Sibling's perspective:** The sibling may worry that brother or sister's disorder is hereditary.

The sibling wants to conform to peer group; may be embarrassed by brother or sister.

The sibling feels conflicted between desire for independence and for maintaining their special relationship.

The sibling may resent the degree of responsibility taken on by or imposed on them; may feel anger toward parents, professionals, sister or brother, and self.

The sibling may begin to worry about his or her and the brother or sister's future, even to the point of "what if . . . " and may question his or her possible role in the sister or brother's future.

The sibling may have concerns regarding how others will treat and accept his or her brother or sister (e.g., social groups, dating, marriage).

The sibling may sacrifice his or her own life, dreams, and goals to fulfill family responsibilities.

The sibling may grieve the loss or absence of independence and the development of relationships (e.g., typical sibling relationships, friendships).

## Talking to Mom and Dad

**When to "tell":** In your eagerness to inform your child, don't make the mistake of giving too much information at one time. You have an entire childhood to help your child understand what he or she needs to know to feel confident of his or her factual information, to become accepting of him- or herself and the brother or sister, and to handle the curiosity and ignorance (whether intentional or accidental) that he or she is likely to encounter on the journey through childhood. However, open the door by mentioning the topic of autism from time to time and act on the following opportunities when they arise:

- Transitional periods (e.g., when brother or sister enters a treatment program or new school)

- When a brother or sister's report card or program report is sent home

- Following an incident that has possibly upset the sibling

- When the sibling first comes into contact with other children the same age as his or her brother or sister

- During developmental and social transitions experienced by the sibling (e.g., reaching puberty, entering junior high school, developing a new peer group)

- When issues arise resulting with the sibling wanting specific information (e.g., brother or sister begins medication)

Watch for and respect signals indicating that the sibling has the information he or she needs at that time (e.g., changing the subject, asking if you are "done").

## Strategies for Developing Positive Relationships

### Ways to Divide Your Time

Do things as a family and separately:

- If the sibling without autism has a school concert and you know the sibling with autism will be a disruption, do not bring the sibling with autism. The sibling without autism needs a chance shine.

- Go camping as a family.

Give each child separate time with mom and dad:

- Dad takes his daughter to the hardware store to pick up a tool.

- Both parents take turns putting a different child to bed each night.

Allow for private time. Time alone is also important for the sibling without autism. He or she should have time to take part in his or her own interests, daydream, and be a kid.

### Sharing the Load and Special Moments

Divide up the household workload. Give each member of the household chores and this includes the child with autism. Remember that chores should be divided up according to developmental ages.

Use resources to give yourself a break:

- Close friends and extended family members
- Other families who have children with autism
- Formal support networks (e.g., respite, counseling)

Let everyone know they are special. Take time to tell each member of the family what they've done well, praise them, give hugs and kisses. This should include all members of the family, including yourself, so let family members know when you need a hug.

Laugh together. Autism is a serious disorder and can be very trying on a family. The family will come to a place where they gain some perspective and when that happens it is important to regain a sense of humor and laugh about those embarrassing moments that autism bring. Remember, laughter relieves tension and it allows you all to have fun together.

## Activities to Encourage Communication

**Feelings box:** Find a box with a lid and cut a hole in the top. Leave a pad and pencil nearby. On the pad siblings and parents can write unspoken anger, sadness, confusion, or happy moments they would like to share about their sibling or child with autism. Make time when the notes can be shared and discussed.

**Scrapbooking:** With help a child can create a book by cutting pictures out of a magazine and dictating a text, which summarizes his or her feelings about the autistic sibling.

**Puppet plays:** Using puppets, dolls, or other toys children can learn about autism or deal with their emotions around their sibling with autism through role-play. For example a child who is upset by his or her sibling who throws tantrums may find it helpful to act out the scenario and see how the situation is resolved by the parent puppet.

**Journaling:** An older child can use a journal to express all of his or her feelings (e.g., positive, negative, angry and confused). The journal allows the sibling to engage in self-reflection and gain strength and wisdom. (You can provide your child with a book but never insist that he or she write in it!)

**Favorite things:** Take time to share your favorite things about your child with autism with siblings and have them share with you as well.

**Together time:** Brainstorm activities together that the sibling can enjoy with his or her brother or sister who has autism (e.g., shopping, snack, bowling).

## Super Parent—Exit Stage Left

No one knows all the answers and it is not essential that your child view you as "all knowing." Siblings need a realistic perspective in which they see Mom and Dad as people who are able to cope with problems in spite of difficulties they may face. This provides the sibling with a role model to refer to as he or she develops, rather than a superhero he or she could never live up to!

## References

Barrett, K. (1993); Brill, M. T. (2001); Cunningham, Alexis (2001); Harris, Sandra (1994); Glasberg, Beth A. (2000); LaPorte, Jennie (2002); Meyer, Donald (1994); Powell, Thomas H. & Ahrenhold Ogle, Peggy (1985); Powers, Michael D. (1989); Siegel, Bryna (1996).

# Chapter 33

# *Ensuring Safety at Home for People with Autism*

## *How Do I Make My Home Safe for a Child with Autism?*

Most parents and caregivers are familiar with basic home safety precautions for young children such as stairwell gates, electrical outlet covers, and childproof locks on cupboards. Modifying your home environment may be even more necessary (sometimes well past the toddler stage) for children with autism spectrum disorders (ASDs). Many children with autism have serious behavioral problems that can put them and other family members at risk. Also, they may not be able to understand and remember the dangers of certain actions without consistent training and intervention. Here are some guidelines to make the home safer:

- **Arrange the furniture** to prevent throwing or sweeping of objects off surfaces, climbing up onto high shelves, or knocking over chairs and tables. Bookcases, dressers, china cabinets and freestanding shelves, laundry baskets, and other taller furniture objects can be screwed directly to walls to prevent them from tipping over when the child does climb on them. Seat child in chair with arms or a wrap-around style desk when doing work or eating meals. Seat against the wall or in a corner to prevent continual escape from the table.

---

- **Locks, gates, and barriers** can help prevent child falling down steps, escaping from the house, or climbing out a window and can limit access to dangerous areas. Safety locks can be placed on interior doors and bathroom and kitchen cabinets. Before putting locks on windows or bedroom doors, families must find out if this is legal in their location. In some places it is against fire regulations. Contact your local fire department for a consultation on home safety for your child and recommendations on the kinds of locks to be used. Travel intruder alarms may be very helpful to alert caregivers to an escaping child or a child going into a room that is off limits.

- **Some parents have tried using Plexiglas in windows** to protect children who pound on or push at glass but it should be noted that Plexiglas can also break and become very sharp when shattered.

- **Do not leave curtain and blind cords hanging.** Keep cords out of your child's reach whether the blind is up or down. Cut the cords short. Do not put a crib, bed, high chair, or playpen near a window or a patio door where a child can reach the curtain or blind cord and strangle. Sofas, chairs, tables, shelves, or bookcases should not be near windows where children could climb up to reach the curtain or blind cord.

- **Secure all potentially dangerous items.** Children with autism may be very curious and interested in how things work. Safety locks can be placed on every cabinet door in the house as well as on the stove, refrigerator, microwave, VCR, washer, dryer, and toilet (most baby sections of department stores and toddler catalogs sell these). Use safety covers for stove burners. Wiring for appliances and electronics should be hidden. Lock up household drugs and chemicals, lighters, matches, sharp knives, and small items that might be swallowed. Use child safety scissors for crafts or projects with supervision. Pad all hard objects in a child's room with foam if he or she engages in any self-injurious actions. Never leave toiletries or glue bottles where they can be reached.

- **Order and structure in the child's environment** can reduce frustration levels. Some people put visual labels (symbols, photos, words, textures) on everyday items, rooms, cabinets, drawers, bins, and closets. A child's things can be organized in see-through plastic bins with visual labels.

- **Visual warning prompts** can help to set boundaries. "Stop" signs, signs saying "No," or pieces of colored tape can be used to help children understand what is off-limits.

- **At mealtime,** eating utensils may need to be tied to string and attached to the chair or table so that if thrown, they remain attached, preventing unintentional injuries. If the child regularly throws things, plates and bowls can be attached to the table with adhesive Velcro on a placemat secured to the table. Use plastic or rubber plates, bowls, and cups to prevent breakage.

- **In the bathroom,** use an inflatable or foam cover on the faucet. Turn down the hot water tank to prevent accidental scalding. Use rubberized bath mats in the bath and remove soap and shampoo after washing so the child will not empty or ingest them. Water taps may have to be kept turned off under the sink to be safe. Keep sink plugs hidden so a child cannot plug a sink and fill it to overflowing.

- **Fire safety.** Try to teach the child the rules to follow for fire safety. Have regular fire drills. Some parents use social stories (with photographs, pictures, words) about smoke detectors, fire drills, fire alarms, touching fire, and so on.

- **Car safety.** A child may need to wear soft footwear so a shoe or boot will not hurt the driver if kicked off or thrown. Child locks may be installed on back doors and you may need to be creative about more involved seatbelts that can't be undone easily while driving. It may be necessary to talk to police and safety professionals in your region. Make certain the driver has hair up or secured so it can't be easily pulled while driving and a driver should not wear necklaces or other jewelry that can be pulled on. If an upset occurs while driving, it is often safest to pull over until calm is regained.

## Wandering/Running Away

Children and adults who are at risk and who run away or wander off from parents and caregivers are a concern. Some children with ASDs just like to be outside and on the go and might head off at any opportunity. Others with autism may be very attracted to water such as ponds, rivers, or swimming pools, which can be very dangerous. If running away is an issue:

- Outside doors can be locked, but this presents safety issues in emergency situations. Contact your local fire department for a consultation on home safety, as well as a professional locksmith or security company.

- Some parents find it helpful to use a Velcro wrist strap and coiled cord to attach their child to them when out shopping or walking. This may prevent children from dashing into traffic, falling into water, running away at shopping malls, and the like.

- Your child should always carry identification in case he or she gets lost and is unable to ask for help. Some children wear a medical ID bracelet or necklace. If the child won't wear or carry ID and doesn't speak, some parents label clothing with iron-on labels.

- Contact local police, fire, and ambulance services and ask your local 911 call center to keep identifying information about your child on record. Dispatchers can alert officers about your concerns.

- Get to know your neighbors and let those neighbors you trust know in advance that your child with an ASD might wander off. Explain any unusual behaviors or characteristics that might be confusing. Neighbors can be given a handout with a photo of your child and emergency contact information for you.

- Some municipalities will reduce the speed limit on a street where a child with autism is living if the child is prone to dashing out into the street without looking. There are signs available to warn drivers of deaf children and blind children but not yet children with autism, so reducing speed may be a useful option.

# Chapter 34

# *Understanding Self-Injurious Behavior in People with Autism*

## *How Science Is Delivering Answers*

Five to 17 percent of persons with mental retardation and autism do serious harm to themselves by biting, pulling out hair, banging their head, or gouging their eyes—on a regular basis. Unlike psychiatric disorders, this kind of self-destruction is not a suicide attempt. It is a repetitive ritual that causes mutilation, and in the past, was generally stopped with restraints. Because it is so disturbing to the family and difficult to control, a person with self-injurious behavior (SIB) would often have no choice but to live in an institution. Today, most people experiencing SIB live in the community.

Since the 1960s, scientists in medicine, neuroscience, psychology, and education have been documenting the reasons for SIB and developing effective treatments. The National Institutes of Health and the Office of Special Education and Rehabilitation Services have been instrumental in funding research at many universities across the United States. Today, we have some significant answers and a few approaches that bring relief.

Here is a sampling of facts from various research fields:

---

"Self-Injurious Behavior" by Joy Simpson was based on interviews with Stephen Schroeder, Director Emeritus of the Life Span Institute at the University of Kansas. Reprinted with permission from the University of Kansas–Merrill Advanced Studies Center. © 2002 University of Kansas–Merrill Advanced Studies Center. All rights reserved. For additional information, visit http://www.merrill.ku.edu.

- For some people with intellectual deficits, SIB is a way of communicating that something is wrong or they want to be left alone. Therefore, teaching new strategies for expressing needs and relating to other people is critical—a behaviorist approach.

- Chronic health problems increase the tendency to engage in SIB. It is important to diagnose and treat health conditions that are a constant aggravation, such as difficulty sleeping, inner ear imbalance, and digestive ailments.

- Persons with certain kinds of mental retardation are likely to have chemical imbalances in the brain. Their treatment must include medication.

"To be effective, we must treat the person's medical condition and make changes in the living environment as well," says Stephen Schroeder, retired director of the Life Span Institute at the University of Kansas. Schroeder believes that researchers from the behaviorist camp and from the disciplines of biomedicine must work together even though their approaches are vastly different. For this very reason, he directed the 1999 Merrill Center conference that brought together leading experts on SIB in the United States. Fifty scholars contributed to the book Schroeder edited with colleagues Travis Thompson and Mary Lou Oster-Granite. *Self-Injurious Behavior: Gene-Brain-Behavior Relationships* is the most comprehensive book on SIB to be released since 1992.

### Breakthroughs in Drug Treatment

No drug to date has been created specifically for self-injurious behavior (SIB). To find a medicinal treatment, scientists are testing drugs approved for psychiatric disorders. Risperidone originally came on the market for persons with schizophrenia. A group of researchers at the University of Kansas obtained permission to run clinical trials on risperidone for the treatment of SIB. Stephen Schroeder, Ph.D., headed the team that included Jessica Hellings, M.D., a professor of psychiatry at the Medical School, and Jennifer Zarcone, Ph.D., a research scientist at the Schiefelbusch Institute for Life Span Studies. Their clinical studies showed that half of the persons who took risperidone experienced a 50 percent reduction of SIB episodes. In all the patients but one, the drug reduced incidents by 25 percent.

Risperidone acts as a modulator adjusting the amount of serotonin and dopamine in the brain. Serotonin and dopamine regulate learning, reward, and emotions. Schroeder decided to pursue risperidone as a remedy because data from animal models showed a link between self-injury and an imbalance of the brain chemistry. His hypothesis is that SIB may be caused by a depletion of dopamine and an excess of serotonin in the basal ganglia region of the brain.

Approximately one-quarter of the persons with SIB do not show long-term benefits from "behavioral" interventions—changes made in the environment, or new learned patterns of behavior. In this instance, medicine plays an especially important role in treatment. Schroeder's study is noteworthy because he restricted participation to those persons who experience repeated, severe bouts of SIB and have not found relief elsewhere. With risperidone, he was able to show a significant reduction in the number of SIB incidents.

A complementary approach has been put forward by Curt Sandman, University of California at Irvine. His research involves the opioid system, which regulates the sensation of pain. He has also been successful in treating the most difficult cases of SIB—with drugs called opiate blockers. Naltrexone changes the brain chemistry in persons with an elevated pain threshold. The inability to feel normal pain is another compelling explanation for SIB.

"It is interesting," says Schroeder, "the opioid receptors for pain are located in the same area of the brain as the dopamine receptors that also influence SIB. It is likely these two systems interact and are part of a larger circuitry of neurons." Some patients may react well to the drug risperidone and others to naltrexone. This may be evidence that persons experiencing SIB don't all have the same diagnosis, according to Schroeder. The success of various treatments may depend on the person's unique brain chemistry.

## Genetics and the Environment—Two Heads of the Coin

"There are many possible genetic causes of SIB. The severe cases may very well be instances where genetics plays a significant role," says Stephen Schroeder. When looking at brain functions and behavior, genetic origins are certainly important. The role of the environment cannot be overlooked either. The circumstances of life ultimately affect the expression of any chemical imbalance in the brain. "Traumatic life events, eating, stress, even learning are all factors that can bring out—or control—a genetic condition like SIB," reports Schroeder.

Many forms of mental retardation are genetic. In certain kinds, SIB is so predictable that it is considered part of the disorder. In fact, scientists learn about SIB just from studying the origins of mental retardation. Mental retardation and SIB are linked in these genetic conditions: Lesch-Nyhan, Prader-Willi, Smith-Magenis, de Lange, and fragile X.

For example, researchers have pinpointed the origin of the Lesch-Nyhan syndrome. The gene is on the X chromosome and the molecular location is an enzyme called HPRT. The genetic defect causes an overproduction of purine 5, and leads to large amounts of uric acid being stored in body fluids. Scientists also know that a deficiency of HPRT changes the structure and function of the brain, resulting in cognitive and neurological deficits—and perhaps triggering SIB. However, SIB cannot be fully explained by the chemical process; scientists are also looking at the role of neurotransmitters with Lesch-Nyhan syndrome.

Genetic conditions do not destine a person to unrelenting self-abuse. "Treatment is possible and important," says Schroeder. Just as diabetes can never be cured, so too with SIB, the condition persists. But, people with diabetes can live out full lives by changing their eating patterns and taking insulin. With SIB also, education, behavioral supports, and sometimes medicine can change the way the behavior is expressed—says Schroeder—and significantly reduce the number of times it occurs. Because of advances in science, most individuals with SIB are no longer subject to repeated self-mutilation from biting, gouging, and head banging. Persons with SIB can often live in community housing or at home with their families.

## References

Hellings, J., Zarcone, J., Crandall, K, Wallace, D., and Schroeder, S. R. (2001). Weight gain in a controlled study of risperidone in children, adolescents and adults with mental retardation and autism. *Journal of Child and Adolescent Psychopharmacology*, 11, 229–38.

King, B.H. (1993). Self-injury by people with mental retardation: A compulsive behavior hypothesis. *American Journal on Mental Retardation*, 98, 93–112.

Lewis, M.H. and Baumeister, A.A. (1982). Stereotyped mannerisms in mentally retarded persons: Animal models and theoretical analyses. In N.R. Ellis (Editor), *International review of research in mental retardation* (volume 12). New York: Academic Press.

Luiselli, J., Singh, N.N., and Matson, J. (Editors) (1992). *Analysis, assessment, and treatment of self-injury*. New York: Springer-Verlag.

McAdam, D.B., Zarcone, J.R., Hellings, J., Napolitano, D.A., and Schroeder, S.R. (2002). Effects of risperidone on aberrant behavior in persons with developmental disabilities: II. Social validity measures. *American Journal on Mental Retardation*, 107, 261–69.

Sandman, C. and Touchette, P. (2002). Opioids and the maintenance of self-injurious behavior. In Schroeder, S. R., Oster-Granite, M.L., and Thompson, T. (Editors), *Self-injurious behavior: Gene-brain-behavior relationships*. Washington, D.C.: American Psychological Association.

Schroeder, S.R., et al. (2001). Self-injurious behavior: Gene-brain-behavior relationships. *Mental Retardation and Developmental Disabilities Research Reviews*, 7, 3–12.

Schroeder, S.R., Oster-Granite, M.L., and Thompson, T. (Editors) (2002). *Self-injurious behavior: Gene-brain-behavior relationships*. Washington, D.C.: American Psychological Association.

Thompson, T., and Gray, D.B. (Editors) (1994). *Destructive behavior in developmental disabilities: Diagnosis and treatment*. Thousand Oaks, California: Sage Publications.

Thompson, T., Symons, F., Delaney, D., and England, C. (1995). Self-injurious behavior as endogenous neurochemical self-administration. *Mental Retardation and Developmental Disabilities Research Reviews*, 1, 137–48.

Valdovinos, M., Napolitano, R., Hellings, J., Zarcone, J., Williams, D., and Schroeder, S.R. (2002). Multimodal assessment during a medication trial of risperidone for destructive behavior: Functional analysis, direct observations, checklists, and psychiatric impressions. *Journal of Experimental and Clinical Psychopharmacology*, 10, no. 3, 268–75.

Zarcone, J., Hellings, J., Crandall, K., Resse, R.M., Marquis, J., Fleming, K., Shores, R., Williams, D., and Schroeder, S.R. (2001). Effects of risperidone on aberrant behavior of persons with developmental disabilities: I. A double-blind crossover study using multiple measures. *American Journal on Mental Retardation*, 106, 525–38.

Chapter 35

# Personal Care and Grooming Issues

## Chapter Contents

Section 35.1—Handling Dressing and Bathing Issues
with the Autistic Child .......................................... 416

Section 35.2—Tips for Toilet Training the Autistic Child ....... 418

Section 35.3—Tips for Dealing with Sleeping Difficulties
in Autistic Children ............................................. 420

Section 35.4—Tips for Dealing with Eating Difficulties in
Autistic Children ................................................ 422

Section 35.5—Dental Care for Children with Autism ............. 424

# Section 35.1

# Handling Dressing and Bathing Issues with the Autistic Child

Excerpted from *The Autistic Spectrum Parents' Daily Helper* by Phillip Abrams and Leslie Henriques, Ulysses Press, © 2004. Reprinted with permission from Ulysses Press.

## Getting Dressed

Getting dressed independently is an important part of self-care. It seems simple enough to learn; children who are not impaired learn this skill primarily by imitation. Your child will probably have a more difficult time learning the process. Think about it. Not only do you have choices to make—what clothes to wear if it is cold or hot outside, which apparel is appropriate for the occasion—but you need to know how to put them on in the proper sequence. Then you need to figure out which is the front of the garment and whether it is inside out. Not so easy after all, is it?

Never fear, your child can learn to dress himself. His best chance to do this is through direct experience. One method of teaching this skill is called backward chaining. This method breaks a process down into small steps. Begin with the last step first, having your child master it before going on to the step that goes before it. For instance, perhaps you are teaching your child to put on socks. Begin by putting the sock almost all the way onto his foot, pulling it over toe and heel. Teach your child to pull the sock up the rest of the way. The next step is teaching him to pull the sock over his heel; then to put the toe into the sock, and so on. Be patient; it may take a long time for each step to be mastered.

Once your child has learned how to put on each article of clothing, it is time to teach her the proper order for dressing. Imagine if you put your pants on, then your underwear. How funny would that be? Use humor to help your child recognize the *incorrect* order for dressing. Next place the clothes in front of your child in the correct order so that she can learn how to do this.

Another method of teaching your child to dress is to manipulate her hands as you help dress her. For example, when buttoning a blouse, physically guide her through the movements necessary. (Try to select clothing with large buttons and other easy fasteners.) Her fingers may feel limp at first, but persevere—after a while she will be buttoning the garment herself. Be sure to give her positive feedback every time she does something right.

Sometimes, in this hectic world, you don't have time to wait for your child to dress himself. Still, try to remember that the more you do for your child the less he is interested in doing for himself. So give yourself plenty of time in the morning—and if putting on all the clothes is too daunting a task for your child, give yourself a break and pick one or two items that are your child's responsibility to put on while you do the rest. When you're in a hurry, reinforcers can also help speed up the process by motivating your child.

## Bathing

Learning self-care will obviously involve understanding proper hygiene. For younger children on the autistic spectrum, taking a bath can be an opportunity to develop imaginative play. On the other hand, when children hate the tub, bath time can be a nightmare for parents who want their child to be clean!

Bathing is an area where suggestions for typical children come in handy—even if they're not quite age appropriate for your child. Bathtubs can be safety hazards if you are not paying attention. Remember:

- Be aware of the water temperature—not to hot . . . and brrrr, not too cold;

- Place a rubber mat (or an old towel if your child doesn't like the feel of rubber) on the bottom of the tub to prevent slipping;

- Teach your child not to touch the taps so he won't burn himself;

- Keep the water shallow;

- Never leave your child unsupervised.

If your child really hates the bath, you might use a hand shower in an empty tub to rinse her off. Many kids really hate shampooing—this can be kept to a minimum if your child's hair is cut short. (Of course, then you have to deal with hair cutting. Decide which is more difficult!)

Bath toys inspire games. Ask questions that stimulate creative thinking and let your child initiate stories. For example, if your child pushes a toy boat under the water, point out that everyone on the boat must be getting wet. Ask whether they are enjoying swimming in the tub. Choose comments that invite a response.

Eventually you will want to teach your child the steps of soaping, rinsing, and drying off. This activity lends itself well to play. Have your child help wash the car, and talk about how you use soap to wash, the hose to rinse, and towels to dry the car. You can have your child practice washing a doll. Use your creativity to come up with playful learning opportunities.

## Section 35.2

# Tips for Toilet Training the Autistic Child

"Parent Skill Building Series: Toilet Training Difficulties," by Dr. Kimberley Ward, Chartered Psychologist, Associate Treatment Director, Autism Treatment Services of Canada/Association Canadienne pour L'Obtention de Services aux Personnes Autistiques. Reprinted with permission.

## Treatment Suggestions

Collect data regarding typical accident times (try to keep fluid intake consistent during the data collection period) to determine the most appropriate times to have the child sit on the toilet.

Initially focus on sitting on the toilet. It is often helpful to provide the child with a special "toilet toy" when he or she is sitting on the toilet (i.e., remove from the child's possession when he or she stands up). Gradually increase the length of time that the child is expected to sit on the toilet. For most children four to ten minutes is sufficient.

Some children respond positively to a picture script that outlines the routine associated with going to the toilet.

Some children develop toileting more quickly if they are provided with a visual model (e.g., sibling, peer, or parent). Kathleen Quill advocates the development of video scripts.

Provide the child with a foot rest to increase feelings of security and to reduce straining.

Try to encourage to a child to eat high-fiber foods and to drink plenty of water to ensure that stools are soft enough to avoid pain and straining. Salty foods such as crackers can increase fluid intake. Also, for children who resist drinking water, foods such as Jell-O, soup, and milkshakes can provide a "sneaky" source of liquid.

Whenever the child has a bowel movement in his or her pants or diaper, ensure that the stool is placed into the toilet. This can help the child learn where "poo" should be placed.

Ensure that the bathroom is perceived as a positive place. It should also be easily accessible to the child. On outings make sure that the child knows where the washroom is located.

Teach the child at least one word, sign, picture symbol, or gesture to indicate when he or she needs to use the toilet. Prompt the child to use the word/sign/gesture whenever you take him or her to the toilet (i.e., so the child will associate the word/sign/gesture with the act of going to the toilet).

Have the child take some responsibility for his or her accidents. For example, have the child take his or her soiled clothing to the laundry.

To help the child develop more awareness of his or her accidents, prompt the child to touch the wet pants, look at the wet pants, and so on. Tight-fitting clothing is often more uncomfortable when it is wet. Discomfort can be a big motivator for a child to use the toilet.

Toilet training often represents a good time to work on self-help skills such as pulling pants up and down, washing hands, and so on.

Consistency between home and school can often facilitate the toilet training process. One way to ensure consistency is to use the communication book to discuss the approaches that have been attempted and the effectiveness of each approach.

Remain as neutral as possible during clean-ups. Some children seem to find negative attention as reinforcing as positive attention.

Avoid warm baths after accidents. Some children inadvertently learn that the way to request a bath is to have an accident. As such, it is often a better idea to provide a sponge bath.

Some children engage in smearing to gain sensory feedback. Provide alternative sensory experience such as playing with dough, kneading dough, playing with shaving cream, and so on to satisfy their sensory craving.

# Section 35.3

# *Tips for Dealing with Sleeping Difficulties in Autistic Children*

"Parent Skill Building Series: Sleeping Difficulties," by Dr. Kimberley Ward, Chartered Psychologist, Associate Treatment Director, Autism Treatment Services of Canada/Association Canadienne pour L'Obtention de Services aux Personnes Autistiques. Reprinted with permission.

## *Treatment Suggestions*

Research indicates that approximately 56 percent of all developmentally delayed individuals present with sleep-related issues (e.g., difficulty falling asleep at night, early waking). It has also been demonstrated that children with autism do not tend to "grow out" of their sleeping difficulties.

Attempt to determine what is "causing" or maintaining your child's sleep difficulties (e.g., attention seeking, anxiety, medical issues). This will help you to decide which strategies to utilize.

Attempt to establish a consistent bedtime routine. The child's activity level should be gradually reduced over the course of the evening. It is also helpful to include "calming" activities such as warm baths, towel rubdowns, and lotion applications in the routine. Deep pressure and gentle rocking can also have a calming effect on children with autism. The routine can be outlined using words and/or picture symbols in a script or book.

Provide transition warnings before putting your child to bed.

Consider the role that diet may play in your child's sleep difficulties.

Increase the amount of physical activity that the child engages in during the day (e.g., community walks, swimming).

Avoid "sleeping in" and naps if your child has a tendency to get up during the night or has difficulty falling asleep. This may help your child to establish a more regular sleep pattern.

Allow your child to stay up until he or she is very sleepy/tired and then put him or her to bed. This may give your child experience falling asleep in his or her room without fussing. Over time the bedtime can be gradually adjusted to a more age-appropriate time.

420

For children who have difficulty lying still when they are put to bed it is often helpful to remain in their room and provide praise and concrete reinforcement for remaining still. For example, one could play music when the child is lying quietly and stop the music when he or she becomes restless.

Teach the child to imitate relaxation strategies (e.g., deep breathing, tensing/relaxing muscle groups, deep pressure) and engage in a relaxation session prior to bedtime.

If your child insists on sleeping in your room introduce a cot or air mattress on the floor. Inform the child that he or she must sleep on the cot if he or she wants to remain in the room. Over time the cot can be gradually moved toward the door, to the hallway, and so on. Some children choose to sleep in their bed when the cot is introduced, as they realize their bed is more comfortable.

Make your child's bedroom as safe as possible (e.g., remove cord from blinds, cover electrical outlets, remove breakable items). This may make it easier for parents to withdraw their attention when their child gets up in the night.

Some parents have found it effective to put a lock on their child's bedroom door. This makes it easy to withdraw attention after the child is put to bed.

Make an effort to reduce how much attention/reinforcement the child receives when he or she gets up. Try to limit physical contact, discussions, and eye contact. It is also important to remain as neutral and businesslike as possible.

Gradually reduce or phase out parental attention after your child has been put to bed. For example, gradually increase the length of time before you respond to crying or screaming.

Some children find it difficult to fall asleep in a dark environment. Night-lights can be comforting in this situation. Also, some parents have found that a fish aquarium provides a low-intensity light source as well as a calming stimulus.

Some children have difficulty falling asleep when it is light outside (or they wake up with the sun). In such situations black blinds can be very effective.

Some parents find it effective to provide their child with quiet toys to play with when or if the child wakes up. That is, the child is directed to remain in his or her room until it is time to get up.

Provide the child with a concrete cue about when it is time to get up (e.g., when daddy gets up, when the alarm goes off). Direct the child to return to bed until he or she hears or sees the cue.

Plan ahead—do not attempt to address bedtime issues the night before a big presentation at work. Plan to start on a weekend or during a holiday period. You may miss a few nights sleep, but most parents report the sacrifice is well worth it in the end.

Utilize respite or school hours to catch up on your sleep to ensure that you have the resources to effectively cope with sleep difficulties the next night.

Have a family meeting prior to implementing any bedtime strategies. It is critical that all caregivers are in agreement to ensure that issues are dealt with in a consistent manner.

## Section 35.4

# Tips for Dealing with Eating Difficulties in Autistic Children

"Parent Skill Building Series: Eating Difficulties," by Dr. Kimberley Ward, Chartered Psychologist, Associate Treatment Director, Autism Treatment Services of Canada/Association Canadienne pour L'Obtention de Services aux Personnes Autistiques. Reprinted with permission.

## Treatment Suggestions

Provide a "buffet" of choices and allow the child an opportunity to try the food on his or her own (i.e., avoid prompting and power struggles).

Set up an if-then contingency with preferred food items (i.e., if you try "x" then you can have the preferred item). If the child is not motivated by the preferred food item you may want to use a special toy as the reward for tasting a new food item.

Mix a small amount of new taste or texture into established/accepted foods (e.g., mixing a small amount of tuna into macaroni). However, this should be done cautiously, as it may turn a child "off" a previously preferred food item.

Have children engage in food-related activities (e.g., baking, pudding painting) and feeding activities (e.g., feeding dolls, feeding pets) to desensitize them to the notion of eating.

Limit between-meal snacks and the use of edible reinforcers. After all, a hungry child is more apt to try a new or less preferred food item than a child who is already full.

Keep in mind that different textures and temperatures can impact mood. Crunchy foods (e.g., popcorn, raw vegetables, crackers) tend to have an alerting influence, foods that must be sucked (e.g., hard candies, frozen treats) are thought to have a calming influence, and chewy foods (e.g., fruit leather, dried fruits, bagels) are thought to have an organizing influence on the nervous system.

Ensure that the child is positioned at the table in a manner that is conducive to eating. The child's feet should be flat on the floor (or a stool) and his or her elbows should be supported by the table.

Encourage appropriate utensil use during all meals and snacks.

Make an effort to include the child in the family mealtime routine (e.g., the preparation, the eating of the meal, clean up). This will allow the child to observe other family members eating. If the child's behavior is very disruptive, it may be a good idea to initially have him or her sit with the family during only the first or last portion of the meal.

Expect the child to remain seated whenever he or she is eating or drinking.

Strive for consistency between home and school with regard to mealtime rules and approaches.

Have the child engage in oral sensory play (e.g., blowing bubbles, blowing whistles, brushing teeth) approximately fifteen minutes before meals. This may help to warm up or sensitize the mouth region.

Expect children to sit to at least smell and/or touch new food items to their lips. Rejected food items should be left on the plate. That is, the child should be expected to cope with the presence of new food items and not be allowed to push them away or throw them into the garbage.

Consult your family physician, pediatrician, or dietitian if you are concerned about the quality of your child's diet. They can make suggestions regarding what food groups or elements are missing.

## Section 35.5

# Dental Care for Children with Autism

"Healthy Smiles for Children with Autism," made possible by the California State Council on Developmental Disabilities grant funds to the Anderson Center for Dental Care, Rady Children's Hospital and Health Center. © 2007 California State Council on Developmental Disabilities. All rights reserved. Reprinted by permission of Rady Children's Hospital and Health Center.

### Did You Know?

Cavities are the most common chronic disease of children.

The germs that cause cavities can be passed from parent to child so it's important to not share foods.

Children with cavities in their primary (baby) teeth are more likely to have cavities in adult teeth.

Primary (baby) teeth are very important for nutrition, speech, and your child's self esteem.

Children with autism/pervasive developmental disorders (PDD) may experience more dental problems due to oral sensitivities around the mouth, diet, difficulty accessing dental care, and difficulty brushing.

### Prevent Early Childhood Cavities

Don't share anything with your child that has been in your mouth, such as spoons, foods, or water bottles.

Put only formula, breast milk, or water in baby's bottle.

Don't put baby to bed with a bottle or sipper cup.

Don't let child walk around with a bottle or sipper cup with anything except water.

Brush baby's teeth as soon as they come in.

Take your child for a dental check-up by age one.

Ask the dentist or doctor about fluoride.

Start flossing when two teeth touch each other.

### Drinking from a Cup

Introduce the cup around six months and switch from bottle to cup by one year. Avoid using bottles and no-spill sipper cups. When children drink from them throughout the day, the sugar in the drink (anything but water) is in contact with the teeth longer and promotes cavities.

## Healthy Snacks

Snack on cut-up vegetables and fruits.

Avoid sticky or sugary foods like fruit-roll-ups or crackers because they increase the time sugar is on the teeth and can cause cavities.

Lift your child's lip and look for chalky white or brown spots. Check upper front teeth, on the inside and outside. This is where early childhood cavities often start.

If you see any spots, take your child to the dentist.

## Introducing New Textures

Puffed or crunchy chips or crackers may be used to introduce new textures. Brush after crackers when possible, since they stick to the teeth. Once your child readily accepts crunchy textures, use fruits, cheese, or other non-sticky snacks, when possible.

## Visiting the Dentist

Find a pediatric or general dentist who has experience with children with special needs.

Inform the dentist's office of your child's special needs. Explain any sensitivities to touch or lights.

Ask if the appointment can be made for the quietest time of the day.

Ask for a private exam room if possible.

Ask for any paperwork to be mailed so it can be completed ahead of time.

Ask the dentist if you can schedule an "orientation" visit before the first appointment to get used to the office and meet the staff.

Get a video or book on visiting the dentist and review several times with your child.

Practice looking in your child's mouth with a disposable mouth mirror available at drug stores.

Take your child's favorite music or toy.

Get dental check-ups every six months. Children with disabilities may need more frequent visits.

Ask your dentist about sealants and fluoride.

## Oral Sensitivities and Tooth Brushing

Children with Autism/PDD may have oral (mouth) sensitivity that makes tooth brushing difficult. When this occurs, it may be helpful to try the following steps:

- Stabilize your child's head. Sit child in a high chair or the corner of the couch. This will help stabilize child's head if he or she pulls away. Avoid brushing with the child standing at the sink.

- Start by touching the lips or just inside the mouth with the toothbrush for a few seconds morning and night if the child is very sensitive. Praise after each touch. After a week, start tooth brushing as outlined in the following text.

- Break the tooth brushing into six small steps. As early as age one, start using a tiny pea-size of fluoride toothpaste. If your child objects to toothpaste, dip the brush once in ACT fluoride rinse before brushing. Brush one area at a time as outlined in the following. Then take the brush out of the mouth. Reinforce each step by smiling, clapping, and saying, "Good brushing." You may try bubbles or other reinforcement that your child likes. Ignore any negative behavior! For additional help, ask your occupational or behavioral therapist.

  1. Brush the outside of the bottom back teeth. Wiggle-jiggle the brush back and forth where the teeth and gums come together for a few seconds, then move the brush to the chewing surfaces and wiggle-jiggle. Then move to the inside to brush the tongue side of the teeth. Try singing while brushing. You may not be able to sing all of the song in the beginning (to the tune of Row, Row, Row Your Boat). Brush, brush, brush your teeth. Brush them everyday. That's the way we will fight Mr. Tooth Decay.

  2. Brush the bottom front teeth outside and inside in the same manner while singing.

  3. Brush the bottom back teeth on the other side.

  4. Brush the top back teeth on one side.

  5. Brush the top front teeth outside and inside.

  6. Brush the top back teeth on the other side.

- Brush morning and night even if only for a few seconds. Some brushing is better than none. Don't give up. Once a routine is established, brushing will get easier. Use only a pea-sized amount of toothpaste.

- Try a two-sided toothbrush to reduce brushing time. Special brushes can brush the inside and the outside of the teeth at the same time. To use them, press the brush on the chewing surface of the teeth so that the bristles reach the gums and "hug" the sides of the teeth. Wiggle the brush back and forth. Brush in the six areas as described.

- Social stories may help. Take pictures of you and your child before, during, and after brushing (smiling) and put the pictures together with a brief story about brushing. Read the story every day. A social story can also be made about your child's trip to the dentist.

- Make tooth brushing a routine. If you are using picture schedules, add a picture of tooth brushing as part of the morning and bedtime routine.

- Supervise tooth brushing for children. A good rule is to brush your child's teeth until the child can tie his or her shoes. Some children with disabilities will continue to need partial or total assistance.

- Once two teeth touch and your child accepts brushing, start flossing. Use the same step-by-step approach as brushing. Try floss holders that are available at drug stores.

# Chapter 36

# *Encouraging Successful Play Dates for Autistic Children*

I am the mother of a nine-year-old boy with Asperger syndrome. I have very simple goals in life for my son—for him to be happy, have friends, and a job he enjoys. I believe that these goals can be attained only by his having adequate social skills. Unfortunately, our children have a deficit in this area. I frequently say to friends "social skills are my number-one priority for my son—the 'cognitive stuff' can always be taught. How often do we use calculus in our daily lives"? I have made this a top priority, and I have come to realize over the years that play dates have helped my son greatly improve his social skills and assisted him in making and keeping friends.

In the 1990s a social skills study was conducted at UCLA by Dr. Fred Frankel. The most important finding was that one-on-one play dates are the best way to build close friendships. A one-on-one play date is when your child invites only one guest over and plays with him or her in private. These play dates are the only time when children can get to know each other intimately without interruption. They also help your child maintain a continuing relationship with friends. One-on-one play dates have been shown to enhance self-esteem and make your child feel special. Your child is able to see that another child wants to play with him or her exclusively.

I have practiced this one-on-one play date theory over the past four years, and after much trial and error, I can provide the following tips from my experience:

"One-on-One Playdates," by Marsha Parrish, © ASPEN® (www.aspennj.org). Reprinted with permission.

- **Have lots of play dates.** I know it's time-consuming, but studies have shown if you are able to schedule, on average, one play date every week for your child, tremendous improvement in social skills will occur.

- **Make your house the "fun" house in the neighborhood.** Buy the best games, snacks, and toys. Is this bribery? Yes—but for a noble cause. I am on a mission to help my child have friends. I also tell myself that this is actually "behavioral." My son can be difficult to play with, he has difficulty losing, he usually wants to do very specific types of make-believe play, and sometimes he "melts down." If other children are being asked to put up with his behavior, external incentives are needed at my house. At a social skills seminar I recently attended, quite a few parents of children with social skills difficulties mentioned that they had purchased trampolines, and although they require a great deal of parental supervision, children love this activity. The parents reported that the trampoline worked to "lure" the neighborhood kids to their house. One parent even placed it in the front yard, where it became a "kid magnet" (this particular trampoline was apparently a slightly smaller one, which was only three feet off the ground).

- **"Scope out" the best children in your child's class for play dates.** Visit your child's classroom or volunteer for class parties in order to determine which children would make good playmates. There are always at least a couple of children in each class who have particularly tolerant personalities. Also choose children with the same interests as your child (i.e., dinosaurs, space, animals). There are a few children I consider my favorites, and I invite them over regularly, I have made my share of mistakes in choosing playmates, but keep trying: Invite a few new children every couple of months.

- **If possible, "ship" the siblings to a friend's house for a couple of hours.** I am very lucky in this regard, as my son is an only child. Your goal is to have a one-on-one play date, and that is possible only without interference from siblings. Also, many parents have told me that the playmate ends up playing with the sibling, even if the sibling is older or younger, because the sibling is much easier to play with. This will also allow you to better monitor the play date.

- **Start with a semi-structured activity and then let the children decide what to do.** One of my favorite activities with which to start a play date is Play Dough. We have a "center island" in our kitchen, and I have lots of colors of Play Dough set out and ready to go, and a couple of the Play Dough kits handy. My son and I practice greeting the guest at the door and inviting him or her to play the first activity. Most children like Play Dough (or some craft activity), and the initial transition is smoothed. Also, a table or a center island allows the children to stand up while still playing in one spot, and this provides a great opportunity for conversation. The children can also converse while working on their project, and they don't have to have much eye contact while talking. Eye contact is difficult for my son, especially with people who are not family members. This helps disguise his poor eye contact.

- **"Hover" in the background, and then step in when necessary.** Try to let your child do as much as possible by him- or herself in the way of conversation and play. When you detect a disagreement, stand back for a couple of seconds and see if they can resolve it themselves. If not, step in as unobtrusively as possible, whisper a quick cue to your child, and disappear into the background again as soon as possible. If you see a true "meltdown," discuss the consequences ahead of time with your child, and enforce it.

- **Rehearse the "rules of a play date" ahead of time.** These rules can be any reminders that are particularly applicable to your child, however, I use the rules outlined in *Good Friends are Hard to Find* just prior to the guest arriving:

  - *The guest is always right.* If there is an argument, such as the rules of a game, the guest is always right. This means that you will never have to get to the bottom of an argument, and that your child will learn that a good host bends over backward to make a guest feel welcome. A good host puts his guest's wishes ahead of his own. Remember, your child has been warned about this ahead of time! (Obviously an exception would be if the guest has physically hurt your child or the guest does not obey you).

  - *If your child is bored, he or she suggests a change in an activity.* Rehearse ahead of time ways to suggest an activity change. An example might be, "Can we play ____ when it's my turn again?" or, "Can we play this for five more minutes and then play ____?" If your child is able to say this, (and remember you heard it because you are hovering in the background), be ready with the timer to help your child with the latter suggestion.

- *Don't criticize the guest.* Explain that being polite will get your child what he or she wants without hurting the guest's feelings.

- *Don't leave the guest alone for more than a few minutes.* If the guest wants to see your child's room, make it clear that your child will go up to the room with him or her, even if it means stopping an activity your child is presently engaged in.

- **Try to get the guest's parent to drop off at your house, so you take the guest home.** This gives you control over a finite end to the play date. As we all know, things can deteriorate rapidly. I made the mistake once of having the other parent pick up the guest and they were twenty minutes late. Unfortunately this was twenty minutes too long, and during that time a great play date took a turn for the worse because of my son's "meltdown." If I had taken the guest home I could have foreseen that my son was getting tired and cranky and ended the play date on a positive note.

- **Get your child into a formal social skills group and keep him or her there.** I know this is not specific play date advice; however, this is where your child is going to learn many of the skills that can be practiced in your home during a play date. Social skills are very difficult to teach, so find an experienced social skills group teacher, and attend regularly. A seven-week social skills course is unfortunately not going to accomplish this. My son has been going to a social skills group almost weekly for 1.5 years, and the progress has been slow and steady. These are difficult skills for our children to learn and they take time. I envision that my son will need formal social skills training for years, and he may always need a professional with which to consult regarding these matters throughout his life.

Teaching my child to find and keep friends is the most important gift I can give him in life. I hope that he is able to live a life filled with friends.

Chapter 37

# Integrating the Autistic Child into the World outside the Home

## Chapter Contents

Section 37.1—Taking an Autistic Child to the Grocery
Store .................................................................... 434

Section 37.2—Making Medical Appointments Less
Challenging for Children with Autism .............. 436

Section 37.3—Autism and Airport Travel Safety Tips ............. 438

## Section 37.1

# *Taking an Autistic Child to the Grocery Store*

Going to the supermarket with a child with autism can be a stressful experience for parents concerned about serious behavior problems. They worry that their child might throw a tantrum, run away, talk to or touch other shoppers inappropriately, or open food items before they are purchased. A successful visit, on the other hand, can make this routine family chore much more pleasant, and presents the child with numerous opportunities for learning.

What can parents do to make these trips successful? First, bear in mind that success requires both the direct teaching of necessary skills and the consistent managing of behavior problems. Parents should employ a structured teaching and behavior management plan that includes proven procedures such as teaching in small steps, presenting frequent opportunities for practice, providing clear instructions and assistance, using positive rewards, and having a consistent response to any behavior problems if they occur.

Parents should work with their child's school to ensure that specific goals—such as learning supermarket skills—are included in their child's Individual Education Plan (IEP). Then, instruction can be individually designed for the child in a way that both parents and teachers can implement. It is very important to select and consistently implement a strong reward system, especially during the early stages of instruction.

For most children, instruction should begin in simulated practice settings at home or in school before moving on to a small grocery or convenience store. The child should be able to follow a number of basic instructions in a more controlled environment before visiting a larger supermarket.

Developing a plan to address problem behaviors is an important component in the training program. The plan should be the same for school and home. Immediately leaving the store and not providing a reward can be effective, unless the child's behavior problems occur because he or she wants to leave the store. "Giving in" and offering the child a toy or edible treat to avoid or stop a tantrum may be effective for the moment, but will likely make the problem worse in the future.

Shannon Kay, Ph.D., director of the May Center in West Springfield, Massachusetts, recommends teaching the child the following instructions:

- "Come here." Use two adults to teach so rewards and assistance can be provided immediately. Start with a small distance—about six feet—between child and adults.

- "Stop." Also use two adults so you do not have to chase the child if he or she does not comply.

- "Hold my hand." Give the child a reward for walking small distances (fifteen feet) while holding an adult's hand without pulling away or falling on the floor.

- "Stay with me." After holding hands is mastered, reward the child for walking small distances and staying next to the adult.

- "Wait in line with me." Start with very short lines.

Once the child masters the basic skills outlined here, the supermarket experience will be much more positive for both the parent and the child. Then, more advanced supermarket skills can be taught, such as making and using a shopping list, locating one or more items from the list, pushing the cart appropriately, asking for help from a store employee, and mastering counting and other money skills.

I would encourage parents to avoid stores that are too large or crowded, and to keep the initial visits brief. It is better to have multiple short successes and slowly build up to longer, successful outings.

435

## Section 37.2

## *Making Medical Appointments Less Challenging for Children with Autism*

"Medical Appointments Can Be Made Less Challenging for Children with Autism," by Alan Harchik, Ph.D., BCBA. © 2007 The May Institute, Inc. Reprinted with permission.

Even the most basic healthcare activities can become quite challenging for children with autism and their families. For example, medical and dental office visits, blood tests, haircuts, and even fingernail and toenail clipping can be extremely uncomfortable to a child with heightened sensitivities. Putting the child in these kinds of situations may sometimes result in severe behavior problems, including tantrums, aggression, and toilet accidents. As a result, parents may fear or avoid these situations, and may not know where to turn for help.

If an activity is discontinued because of the child's response, the child may learn to use problem behaviors to escape from these situations. Although physical holds and sedating medications may be recommended in some circumstances, most parents don't like these procedures. What else can be done?

Following are some methods that the professionals at May Institute have found helpful. They can be used individually or together, based upon the child's needs. Many physicians, dentists, and hairstylists are patient and willing to work with children and families once they understand that a child has special needs.

One method is called desensitization. It means gradually exposing the child to the situation that is feared. Michelle Pratt, director of May Institute's School Consultation Program in western Massachusetts, recommends that parents with a child who has difficulty with medical appointments start with short, frequent visits that end with a reward or preferred activity, such as a favorite toy or treat.

The appointment can be broken down into a sequence of steps. Have the child complete only the first step on the first visit. On the next visit, try to complete the first two steps, and so on. Recent research by Carole Conyers, a child development researcher from North Dakota State

University, showed success with this method when dividing a dental visit into eighteen steps. Steps included waiting, walking to the chair, opening mouth, and allowing a dental mirror to be placed.

A second method involves teaching the child about the situation in advance of the visit. One way this might be done is by creating a series of pictures that present appropriate behaviors in a story format. Ms. Pratt recommends making a book with photos of the child, or someone the child knows and likes, going through all of the steps of the activity in the actual setting, including receiving the treat at the end of the activity. A variation is to make a video for the child to watch.

Another teaching method is to create a simulated pretend situation. Research suggests that if the situation is made realistic, it can result in improved behavior in the real setting. Simulation allows for many more practice opportunities than what might be available if traveling to the actual location. Simulation also enables the child to practice with a variety of materials and instructors.

A third method involves modifying the environment to make it feel more comfortable or safe for the child. Examples include letting the child sit on a parent's lap or hold a favorite item or toy during the office visit, talking about a favorite topic, telling the child what will be happening next, and supervising his or her holding some special item, such as a stethoscope, prior to its use.

A fourth method is to provide specific positive rewards for participation. This is an important component of the desensitization and instructional procedures described previously. Examples include a coupon for a local ice cream store and access to a favorite video.

Researchers and practitioners are exploring a fifth method—providing the child with ten- to twenty-second "breaks" from the activity, whether or not he or she is cooperating. Initially, the breaks may occur every fifteen to thirty seconds. Over time, they can be spaced further apart.

At May Institute, we have found that concentrating on successful outcomes is more beneficial than focusing on the problem as an anxiety or sensory processing disorder. We need to treat each problem as a skill deficit that children with disabilities (and adults, too) can overcome with systematic use of effective teaching and reward procedures. Teaching a child to master each of these situations makes that child happier, more independent, and better able to function in the world. That is the ultimate goal for providers and parents alike.

Section 37.3

## Autism and Airport Travel Safety Tips

Excerpted from "Autism and Airport Travel Safety Tips," by Dennis Debbaudt. © 2001 Dennis Debbaudt. For additional information, visit www.autismriskmanagement.com. Reviewed by David A. Cooke, M.D., March 2007.

Traveling through airport security will never be the same. Every traveler passing through a security checkpoint will now encounter waiting in long lines, having to produce two forms of picture identification at multiple locations, mandatory questioning and inspections of personal belongings by strangers and the increasing likelihood of a light touch from a stranger holding a Geiger counter–like sound-producing wand. When you add to the mix the possibility of a complete physical frisk or pat down—and the presence and scrutiny of armed, uniformed paramilitary personnel and contraband-sniffing dogs—the accompanying sensory-enhancing gauntlet of sounds, lights, and touch can tax the system of any traveler, let alone one who has autism. This experience has quickly become standard operating procedure at U.S. airports.

People with autism, parents, and caregivers may want to consider taking some extra measures to make passing through a security checkpoint easier.

As daunting as a security checkpoint is for some children and adults with autism, we must consider the point-of-view of the security professional. The behavior or characteristics of the child or adult with autism may make the security professional extremely anxious. Consider the reliance on visual cues and innocent echolalia a person with autism may display, such as repeating a phrase observed on a close-by poster. At a security checkpoint that phrase might include words that cite the laws or warn against the use of the words "bomb threat" or "hijacking." Someone who repeats this phrase would quickly come under suspicion at a security checkpoint. Those that repeat a question, run from, or blanche at passing through a metal detector, or become overanxious at attempts to touch them would also merit extra scrutiny. Left unexplained, the behaviors and characteristics of some persons with autism may delay their trip and cause unnecessary anxiety. These encounters are the types of situations that can easily escalate into misinterpretations, verbal and physical confrontations, physical containment, and restraint.

As reported in my latest book, *Autism, Advocates and Law Enforcement Professionals*, "Those with autism, parents and caregivers may want to consider carrying autism handout information which would at least include a basic autism brochure, and a person-specific handout that at least includes their picture, description, information about behaviors that security may find suspicious and the best way a security professional can communicate with or interact with that person. Many parents find business card handouts that might contain a message such as 'Perhaps my son/daughter's behavior is surprising to you. This is because he/she has autism,' a brief definition of autism, and the phone number/website address of a local or national advocacy organization."

If possible, make travel plans well in advance. Call the airlines and security companies (soon to be mainly federalized) and ask what you can do to help the security experience go more smoothly for the person with autism and the security professionals with whom they will interact. If the trip has to be made suddenly, arrive extra early, bring plenty of handouts, and explain to the gate agent what your needs are. Those that have the time may want to inquire with their air carrier about assistance plans they may offer inexperienced travelers. Northwest Airlines, for example, offers the Adult Assistance Program for a fee ranging from $40.00 to $75.00. This may prove to be money well spent. The program offers personal assistance from check-in, through security and boarding, and through the destination airport. While the program does not assist with eating, personal hygiene, or medication issues, it does provide assistance through the crucial security checkpoints. Parents and caregivers of a passenger using travel assist can also pass through security with their loved one even if they are not traveling with him or her. Special security passes would be issued in lieu of tickets. A program like Northwest Airlines' Adult Assistance could be utilized by caregivers even if they are traveling with a loved one.

Anticipating the worst is never a pleasant proposition. But it's something we do all the time in our everyday lives when we put on seatbelts, lock our back doors, and pay the life insurance. The downside for not doing these things is extremely negative in each example. But do we shudder in fear every time we do these things? Of course not. They are commonsense options associated with everyday life.

Taking extra precautions is also an everyday consideration that those with autism, parents, and caregivers also can become accustomed to doing. When traveling through our communities, and airports, taking the precautions—alerting security, carrying identification and informational handouts, considering the needs of others, anticipating the possibilities—can help make our trips and travel a lot safer and a lot more relaxing. Give yourself at least two weeks to seek the best that our airlines and airport security can offer. But it's never too late to alert the airlines and security professionals to a special request for assistance.

Chapter 38

# *Handling Puberty in Children with Autism Spectrum Disorders*

For many of us growing up is an interesting journey and reaching puberty can be a time of great confusion, anxiety, and change. It can also be a very exciting time for teenagers and a *very* anxious time for parents and caregivers. For young people with intellectual disability this is no different.

It can be expected that teenagers will want to lock themselves in their bedrooms and say that you don't understand. They will want to choose their own clothes, friends, hairstyles, and types of music. They will get crushes and believe that this love is forever. This will be a time when they strive to be more independent and take bigger risks.

For families and caregivers it's a time of trying to instill boundaries and helping the teenager in your life understand about society—and all the enticements and risk that this brings. Attitudes within society toward sexuality have changed with each generation, so what may have guided you as a teenager will probably be quite different for the teenager in your life.

Below are some ideas and resources that may help you to communicate with your teenager.

## Public and Private Body Parts

Teaching young people about their bodies can be a complex business but below are some handy hints that may make this process easier for them and for you.

Public body parts are any body parts that its okay for others to see, such as arms, hands, necks, faces. But then there are some exceptions to the rule, like showing your whole leg to someone when you are at McDonald's may not be the thing to do. So coupled with body parts comes the need to talk to the person about *where* it is okay or not okay to show certain body parts.

Private body parts are any body parts that are not okay for just anyone to see and that are usually hidden by clothing (e.g., breasts, bottoms). Again it's useful to talk about the different situations and places where it may be okay to show private body parts (e.g., if you go to the doctor and they need to look at a person's body.)

## Explaining Body Parts

It is important for you as parents/caregivers to explain to your young person how different parts of his or her body function and what they are for. It will be up to you decide how much information your young person needs. Remember to keep it straightforward.

It's good practice to use the formal terms for body parts, even though you may have "family" names. It's good if your family member can learn both versions (e.g., "boobs" and "breasts").

It's especially important that any caregivers you have coming into your home follow the same guidelines.

## Identity and Body Changes

Puberty and adolescence can be a very challenging and confusing time not just for parents/caregivers but for the young people themselves. Again the more information you can give the young person the better without overwhelming them. Some families have said that they have found it hard to determine whether their family member's behavior is to do with their disability or because of their adolescence. There is no magic trick to sort this out—just breathe through it!

## Menstruation

Teaching teenage girls about menstruation (periods) is extremely important. Some parents/caregivers have had great success in doing this by starting to teach their daughters about periods when they are about eleven or twelve years old.

Actual situation: One parent whose daughter has autism and has behaviors that were quite challenging started introducing the idea of periods to her about a year before she actually started menstruating. She did the following things that proved to be quite successful:

- She gave her daughter good information about her genitals and where the menstrual blood would be coming from. This was done by having her daughter stand over a mirror and look at her genitals.

- She encouraged her daughter to wear pads one day each month.

- Wearing a pad before she actually had her period meant that she got used to the sensation and when she would (at times) pull them out it was less embarrassing for her and the people she was showing.

- The days for wearing pads were gradually increased and marked on the calendar.

- Fake blood (from a magic shop) was put on the pads so that she became used to seeing it.

The above strategies meant that this young girl was less traumatized by having her period.

Following are other strategies that can work:

- Menstruation kits—this involves making up a fun bag for the young girl that is her special bag. Inside will be underwear that already has pads attached. This means that when she goes to the toilet she doesn't have to make a judgment about when to change her pad. She just takes everything off and puts a fresh pair on.

- It's good to have a paper bag that she can place the soiled pad and underwear into.

- For young girls with autism, or without, it works well for her to have the same colored underwear for the whole time that she has her period. Red is a good color to use. When other colored underwear arrives she will then know that her period has finished.

Not many young girls seem to use tampons—again young women with autism have stated that this can be quite uncomfortable for them. Of course it is all about personal choice and where possible those choices are supported.

## Pain Relief

For premenstrual pain the following can be effective:

- Evening primrose oil (capsules or liquid form)
- Vitamin B$_6$ pills

For menstrual pain, try the following:

- Naproxen (Aleve)
- Ponstel (mefenamic acid)

It's always best to consult with a pharmacist or a medical professional before using any medications.

## Masturbation

For many young adolescents masturbation is a natural time of self-discovery but like many facets of sexuality it can be confusing and for some people quite frightening. Boys and young men with autism can find masturbation both appealing and scary. This can be to do with not understanding what is happening to their body.

Some strategies that work well are as follows:

- Describing to the boy or young man what happens to his body physically when he masturbates

- Explaining the difference between urine and semen—some boys with autism have thought that they were going to wet themselves when they ejaculate

- Explaining that the penis gets hard from blood pumping around the body—and that there is *no* bone in there

- Talking about the fact that their bodies might get hot and they might feel slightly out of control but that it will be okay

- Having lubrication such as KY jelly can mean that there is no friction on the skin—this applies to both boys and girls

- For some adolescents, having a soft fabric to lie on works well

- Teaching about public and private places—making sure that if the young person has his or her own bedroom that he or she knows that this is the *most* private room in the house, as bathrooms and toilets are usually shared rooms

The questions below might be helpful if you are uncertain as to whether the young person is masturbating:

- Is there any physical discomfort due to trousers, underpants, or pads?

- Is there a hygiene problem?

- Is there a medical reason—for example, a rash or infection, or is the person taking medication with a side effect of delaying or preventing orgasm?

- Has the person developed an allergy to a new soap or fabric?

- Is the person unoccupied or bored?

- Is the person using the behavior to get attention?

- Is the person using this behavior to avoid tasks or things the person does not want to do?

- Is the person masturbating for sexual pleasure?

- Is the person trying to masturbate, but unable to reach orgasm because of his or her technique?

- Is there a possibility the person has been sexually abused?

## Keeping Safe

For some young people with disability, vulnerability to abuse is a very real and unfortunate fact. Teaching young people about their bodies can help combat this, as they will be more aware of their public and private body parts. If they have difficulty understanding that concept, then teaching their peer group about body safety can mean that they can look out for their disabled friends.

The Circles Program is used around the world. It involves teaching the young person about who the different people in their lives are and the rules about touching those people and them touching you. It's important that young people know that *they* are in charge of their bodies and also that they know who to talk to if something happens that they don't like.

With the circles program people's names and/or photos can be placed in each circle. These can be put on Velcro dots and can then be moved about. For example, a young person may move the picture of their taxi driver from their red stranger circle into their hug circle. This may mean that there was a near accident on the way home and the taxi driver comforted the young person or it may mean there has been a situation of abuse. Either way it gives you an opportunity to ask more questions.

Each circle denotes a different activity (e.g., orange could be a wave circle, yellow a handshake circle, and so on). You can add as many circles as required and it's good to have a symbol for each activity attached to each color.

Another strategy that can work is to give everyone in that young person's network a picture (e.g., a flower or an animal) and if that young person is approached by someone in a car and they do *not* have that picture then the young person should *not* take a ride with them.

# Part Seven


# Education and Independence Issues for People with Autism

# Chapter 39

# *A Guide to the Individualized Education Program*

## *Basic Information about the Individualized Education Program*

Each public school child who receives special education and related services must have an Individualized Education Program (IEP). Each IEP must be designed for one student and must be a truly individualized document. The IEP creates an opportunity for teachers, parents, school administrators, related services personnel, and students (when appropriate) to work together to improve educational results for children with disabilities. The IEP is the cornerstone of a quality education for each child with a disability.

To create an effective IEP, parents, teachers, other school staff— and often the student—must come together to look closely at the student's unique needs. These individuals pool knowledge, experience, and commitment to design an educational program that will help the student be involved in, and progress in, the general curriculum. The IEP guides the delivery of special education supports and services for

"Basic Information about the Individualized Education Program" is reprinted from "A Guide to the Individualized Education Program," U.S. Department of Education, July 2000. "Updates in the Individualized Education Program with IDEA 2004" is reprinted from "IDEA 2004 Roadmap to the IEP: IEP Meetings, Content, Review and Revision, Placements, Transition, and Transfers," © 2007 Peter W. D. Wright and Pamela Darr Wright. All rights reserved. Reprinted with permission. For additional information, visit www.wrightslaw.com.

the student with a disability. Without a doubt, writing—and implementing—an effective IEP requires teamwork.

This chapter explains the IEP process, which we consider to be one of the most critical elements to ensure effective teaching, learning, and better results for all children with disabilities. The chapter is designed to help teachers, parents, and anyone involved in the education of a child with a disability develop and carry out an IEP. The information in this chapter is based on what is required by our nation's special education law—the Individuals with Disabilities Education Act, or IDEA.

The IDEA requires certain information to be included in each child's IEP. It is useful to know, however, that states and local school systems often include additional information in IEPs in order to document that they have met certain aspects of federal or state law. The flexibility that states and school systems have to design their own IEP forms is one reason why IEP forms may look different from school system to school system or state to state. Yet each IEP is critical in the education of a child with a disability.

## The Basic Special Education Process under IDEA

The writing of each student's IEP takes place within the larger picture of the special education process under IDEA. Before taking a detailed look at the IEP, it may be helpful to look briefly at how a student is identified as having a disability and needing special education and related services and, thus, an IEP.

**Step 1—Child is identified as possibly needing special education and related services:** The state must identify, locate, and evaluate all children with disabilities in the state who need special education and related services. To do so, states conduct "Child Find" activities. A child may be identified by "Child Find," and parents may be asked if the "Child Find" system can evaluate their child. Parents can also call the "Child Find" system and ask that their child be evaluated.

Alternatively, a school professional may ask that a child be evaluated to see if he or she has a disability. Parents may also contact the child's teacher or other school professional to ask that their child be evaluated. This request may be verbal or in writing. Parental consent is needed before the child may be evaluated. Evaluation needs to be completed within a reasonable time after the parent gives consent.

**Step 2—Child is evaluated:** The evaluation must assess the child in all areas related to the child's suspected disability. The evaluation results will be used to determine the child's eligibility for special education and related services and to make decisions about an appropriate educational program for the child. If the parents disagree with the evaluation, they have the right to take their child for an independent educational evaluation (IEE). They can ask that the school system pay for this IEE.

**Step 3—Eligibility is decided:** A group of qualified professionals and the parents look at the child's evaluation results. Together, they decide if the child is a "child with a disability," as defined by IDEA. Parents may ask for a hearing to challenge the eligibility decision.

**Step 4—Child is found eligible for services:** If the child is found to be a "child with a disability," as defined by IDEA, he or she is eligible for special education and related services. Within thirty calendar days after a child is determined eligible, the IEP team must meet to write an IEP for the child.

**Step 5—IEP meeting is scheduled:** The school system schedules and conducts the IEP meeting. School staff must do the following:

- Contact the participants, including the parents

- Notify parents early enough to make sure they have an opportunity to attend

- Schedule the meeting at a time and place agreeable to parents and the school

- Tell the parents the purpose, time, and location of the meeting

- Tell the parents who will be attending

- Tell the parents that they may invite people to the meeting who have knowledge or special expertise about the child

**Step 6—IEP meeting is held and IEP is written:** The IEP team gathers to talk about the child's needs and write the student's IEP. Parents and the student (when appropriate) are part of the team. If the child's placement is decided by a different group, the parents must be part of that group as well.

Before the school system may provide special education and related services to the child for the first time, the parents must give consent. The child begins to receive services as soon as possible after the meeting.

If the parents do not agree with the IEP and placement, they may discuss their concerns with other members of the IEP team and try to work out an agreement. If they still disagree, parents can ask for mediation, or the school may offer mediation. Parents may file a complaint with the state education agency and may request a due process hearing, at which time mediation must be available.

**Step 7—Services are provided:** The school makes sure that the child's IEP is being carried out as it was written. Parents are given a copy of the IEP. Each of the child's teachers and service providers has access to the IEP and knows his or her specific responsibilities for carrying out the IEP. This includes the accommodations, modifications, and supports that must be provided to the child, in keeping with the IEP.

**Step 8—Progress is measured and reported to parents:** The child's progress toward the annual goals is measured, as stated in the IEP. His or her parents are regularly informed of their child's progress and whether that progress is enough for the child to achieve the goals by the end of the year. These progress reports must be given to parents at least as often as parents are informed of their nondisabled children's progress.

**Step 9—IEP is reviewed:** The child's IEP is reviewed by the IEP team at least once a year, or more often if the parents or school ask for a review. If necessary, the IEP is revised. Parents, as team members, must be invited to attend these meetings. Parents can make suggestions for changes, can agree or disagree with the IEP goals, and can agree or disagree with the placement.

If parents do not agree with the IEP and placement, they may discuss their concerns with other members of the IEP team and try to work out an agreement. There are several options, including additional testing, an independent evaluation, or asking for mediation (if available) or a due process hearing. They may also file a complaint with the state education agency.

**Step 10—Child is reevaluated:** At least every three years the child must be reevaluated. This evaluation is often called a "triennial." Its purpose is to find out if the child continues to be a "child with a disability," as defined by IDEA, and what the child's educational needs are. However, the child must be reevaluated more often if conditions warrant or if the child's parent or teacher asks for a new evaluation.

## A Closer Look at the IEP

Clearly, the IEP is a very important document for children with disabilities and for those who are involved in educating them. Done correctly, the IEP should improve teaching, learning, and results. Each child's IEP describes, among other things, the educational program that has been designed to meet that child's unique needs. This part of the chapter looks closely at how the IEP is written and by whom, and what information it must, at a minimum, contain.

## Contents of the IEP

By law, the IEP must include certain information about the child and the educational program designed to meet his or her unique needs. In a nutshell, this information is as follows.

**Current performance:** The IEP must state how the child is currently doing in school (known as present levels of educational performance). This information usually comes from the evaluation results such as classroom tests and assignments, individual tests given to decide eligibility for services or during reevaluation, and observations made by parents, teachers, related service providers, and other school staff. The statement about "current performance" includes how the child's disability affects his or her involvement and progress in the general curriculum.

**Annual goals:** These are goals that the child can reasonably accomplish in a year. The goals are broken down into short-term objectives or benchmarks. Goals may be academic, address social or behavioral needs, relate to physical needs, or address other educational needs. The goals must be measurable—meaning that it must be possible to measure whether the student has achieved the goals.

**Special education and related services:** The IEP must list the special education and related services to be provided to the child or on behalf of the child. This includes supplementary aids and services that the child needs. It also includes modifications (changes) to the program or supports for school personnel—such as training or professional development—that will be provided to assist the child.

**Participation with nondisabled children:** The IEP must explain the extent (if any) to which the child will not participate with nondisabled children in the regular class and other school activities.

453

**Participation in state and district-wide tests:** Most states and districts give achievement tests to children in certain grades or age groups. The IEP must state what modifications in the administration of these tests the child will need. If a test is not appropriate for the child, the IEP must state why the test is not appropriate and how the child will be tested instead.

**Dates and places:** The IEP must state when services will begin, how often they will be provided, where they will be provided, and how long they will last.

**Transition service needs:** Beginning when the child is age fourteen (or younger, if appropriate), the IEP must address (within the applicable parts of the IEP) the courses he or she needs to take to reach his or her post-school goals. A statement of transition services needs must also be included in each of the child's subsequent IEPs.

**Needed transition services:** Beginning when the child is age sixteen (or younger, if appropriate), the IEP must state what transition services are needed to help the child prepare for leaving school.

**Age of majority:** Beginning at least one year before the child reaches the age of majority, the IEP must include a statement that the student has been told of any rights that will transfer to him or her at the age of majority. (This statement would be needed only in states that transfer rights at the age of majority.)

**Measuring progress:** The IEP must state how the child's progress will be measured and how parents will be informed of that progress.

### Additional State and School-System Content

States and school systems have a great deal of flexibility about the information they require in an IEP. Some states and school systems have chosen to include in the IEP additional information to document their compliance with other state and federal requirements. (Federal law requires that school districts maintain documentation to demonstrate their compliance with federal requirements.) Generally speaking, extra elements in IEPs may be included to document that the state or school district has met certain aspects of federal or state law, such as the following:

- Holding the meeting to write, review, and, if necessary, revise a child's IEP in a timely manner

- Providing parents with a copy of the procedural safeguards they have under the law

- Placing the child in the least restrictive environment

- Obtaining the parents' consent

## *IEP Forms in Different Places*

While the law tells us what information must be included in the IEP, it does not specify what the IEP should look like. No one form or approach or appearance is required or even suggested. Each state may decide what its IEPs will look like. In some states individual school systems design their own IEP forms.

Thus, across the United States, many different IEP forms are used. What is important is that each form be as clear and as useful as possible, so that parents, educators, related service providers, administrators, and others can easily use the form to write and implement effective IEPs for their students with disabilities.

## *The IEP Team Members*

By law, certain individuals must be involved in writing a child's Individualized Education Program. Note that an IEP team member may fill more than one of the team positions if properly qualified and designated. For example, the school system representative may also be the person who can interpret the child's evaluation results.

These people must work together as a team to write the child's IEP. A meeting to write the IEP must be held within thirty calendar days of deciding that the child is eligible for special education and related services.

Each team member brings important information to the IEP meeting. Members share their information and work together to write the child's Individualized Education Program. Each person's information adds to the team's understanding of the child and what services the child needs.

Parents are key members of the IEP team. They know their child very well and can talk about their child's strengths and needs as well as their ideas for enhancing their child's education. They can offer insight into how their child learns, what his or her interests are, and other aspects of the child that only a parent can know. They can listen to what the other team members think their child needs to work on at school and share their suggestions. They can also report on whether the skills the child is learning at school are being used at home.

Teachers are vital participants in the IEP meeting as well. At least one of the child's regular education teachers must be on the IEP team if the child is (or may be) participating in the regular education environment. The regular education teacher has a great deal to share with the team. For example, he or she might talk about any of the following:

- The general curriculum in the regular classroom

- The aids, services, or changes to the educational program that would help the child learn and achieve

- Strategies to help the child with behavior, if behavior is an issue

The regular education teacher may also discuss with the IEP team the supports for school staff that are needed so that the child can do the following:

- Advance toward his or her annual goals

- Be involved and progress in the general curriculum

- Participate in extracurricular and other activities

- Be educated with other children, both with and without disabilities

Supports for school staff may include professional development or more training. Professional development and training are important for teachers, administrators, bus drivers, cafeteria workers, and others who provide services for children with disabilities.

The child's special education teacher contributes important information and experience about how to educate children with disabilities. Because of his or her training in special education, this teacher can talk about the following issues:

- How to modify the general curriculum to help the child learn

- The supplementary aids and services that the child may need to be successful in the regular classroom and elsewhere

- How to modify testing so that the student can show what he or she has learned

- Other aspects of individualizing instruction to meet the student's unique needs

Beyond helping to write the IEP, the special educator has responsibility for working with the student to carry out the IEP. He or she may do any of the following:

- Work with the student in a resource room or special class devoted to students receiving special education services

- Team teach with the regular education teacher

- Work with other school staff, particularly the regular education teacher, to provide expertise about addressing the child's unique needs

Another important member of the IEP team is the individual who can interpret what the child's evaluation results mean in terms of designing appropriate instruction. The evaluation results are very useful in determining how the child is currently doing in school and what areas of need the child has. This IEP team member must be able to talk about the instructional implications of the child's evaluation results, which will help the team plan appropriate instruction to address the child's needs.

The individual representing the school system is also a valuable team member. This person knows a great deal about special education services and educating children with disabilities. He or she can talk about the necessary school resources. It is important that this individual have the authority to commit resources and be able to ensure that whatever services are set out in the IEP will actually be provided.

The IEP team may also include additional individuals with knowledge or special expertise about the child. The parent or the school system can invite these individuals to participate on the team. Parents, for example, may invite an advocate who knows the child, a professional with special expertise about the child and his or her disability, or others (such as a vocational educator who has been working with the child) who can talk about the child's strengths or needs. The school system may invite one or more individuals who can offer special expertise or knowledge about the child, such as a paraprofessional or related services professional. Because an important part of developing an IEP is considering a child's need for related services, related service professionals are often involved as IEP team members or participants. They share their special expertise about the child's needs and how their own professional services can address those needs. Depending on the child's individual needs, some related service professionals attending the IEP meeting or otherwise helping to develop the IEP might include occupational or physical therapists, adaptive physical education providers, psychologists, or speech-language pathologists.

When an IEP is being developed for a student of transition age, representatives from transition service agencies can be important participants. Whenever a purpose of meeting is to consider needed transition services, the school must invite a representative of any other agency that is likely to be responsible for providing or paying for transition services. This individual can help the team plan any transition services the student needs. He or she can also commit the resources of the agency to pay for or provide needed transition services. If he or she does not attend the meeting, then the school must take alternative steps to obtain the agency's participation in the planning of the student's transition services.

Last but not least, the student may also be a member of the IEP team. If transition service needs or transition services are going to be discussed at the meeting, the student must be invited to attend. More and more students are participating in and even leading their own IEP meetings. This allows them to have a strong voice in their own education and can teach them a great deal about self-advocacy and self-determination.

### The Regular Education Teacher as Part of the IEP Team

Appendix A of the federal regulations for Part B of IDEA answers many questions about the IEP. Question 24 addresses the role of the regular education teacher on the IEP team. Here's an excerpt from the answer:

> While a regular education teacher must be a member of the IEP team if the child is, or may be, participating in the regular education environment, the teacher need not (depending upon the child's needs and the purpose of the specific IEP team meeting) be required to participate in all decisions made as part of the meeting or to be present throughout the entire meeting or attend every meeting. For example, the regular education teacher who is a member of the IEP team must participate in discussions and decisions about how to modify the general curriculum in the regular classroom to ensure the child's involvement and progress in the general curriculum and participation in the regular education environment.
>
> Depending upon the specific circumstances, however, it may not be necessary for the regular education teacher to participate

in discussions and decisions regarding, for example, the physical therapy needs of the child, if the teacher is not responsible for implementing that portion of the child's IEP.

In determining the extent of the regular education teacher's participation at IEP meetings, public agencies and parents should discuss and try to reach agreement on whether the child's regular education teacher that is a member of the IEP team should be present at a particular IEP meeting and, if so, for what period of time. The extent to which it would be appropriate for the regular education teacher member of the IEP team to participate in IEP meetings must be decided on a case-by-case basis.

## *Related Services*

A child may require any of the following related services in order to benefit from special education. Related services, as listed under IDEA, include (but are not limited to) the following:

- Audiology services
- Counseling services
- Early identification and assessment of disabilities in children
- Medical services
- Occupational therapy
- Orientation and mobility services
- Parent counseling and training
- Physical therapy
- Psychological services
- Recreation
- Rehabilitation counseling services
- School health services
- Social work services in schools
- Speech-language pathology services
- Transportation

If a child needs a particular related service in order to benefit from special education, the related service professional should be involved in developing the IEP. He or she may be invited by the school or parent to join the IEP team as a person "with knowledge or special expertise about the child."

### Transition Services

Transition refers to activities meant to prepare students with disabilities for adult life. This can include developing postsecondary education and career goals, getting work experience while still in school, setting up linkages with adult service providers such as the vocational rehabilitation agency—whatever is appropriate for the student, given his or her interests, preferences, skills, and needs. Statements about the student's transition needs must be included in the IEP after the student reaches a certain age.

**Transition planning:** This is for students beginning at age fourteen (and sometimes younger) and involves helping the student plan his or her courses of study (such as advanced placement or vocational education) so that the classes the student takes will lead to his or her post-school goals.

**Transition services:** This is for students beginning at age sixteen (and sometimes younger) and involves providing the student with a coordinated set of services to help the student move from school to adult life. Services focus upon the student's needs or interests in such areas as higher education or training, employment, adult services, independent living, or taking part in the community.

### Writing the IEP

To help decide what special education and related services the student needs, generally the IEP team will begin by looking at the child's evaluation results, such as classroom tests, individual tests given to establish the student's eligibility, and observations by teachers, parents, paraprofessionals, related service providers, administrators, and others. This information will help the team describe the student's "present levels of educational performance"—in other words, how the student is currently doing in school. Knowing how the student is currently performing in school will help the team develop annual goals to address those areas where the student has an identified educational need.

The IEP team must also discuss specific information about the child. This includes the following:

- The child's strengths
- The parents' ideas for enhancing their child's education
- The results of recent evaluations or reevaluations
- How the child has done on state and district-wide tests

In addition, the IEP team must consider the "special factors" described in the following text.

It is important that the discussion of what the child needs be framed around how to help the child do the following:

- Advance toward the annual goals
- Be involved in and progress in the general curriculum
- Participate in extracurricular and nonacademic activities
- Be educated with and participate with other children with disabilities and nondisabled children

Based on the preceding discussion, the IEP team will then write the child's IEP. This includes the services and supports the school will provide for the child. If the IEP team decides that a child needs a particular device or service (including an intervention, accommodation, or other program modification), the IEP team must write this information in the IEP. As an example, consider a child whose behavior interferes with learning. The IEP team would need to consider positive and effective ways to address that behavior. The team would discuss the positive behavioral interventions, strategies, and supports that the child needs in order to learn how to control or manage his or her behavior. If the team decides that the child needs a particular service (including an intervention, accommodation, or other program modification), they must include a statement to that effect in the child's IEP.

### Special Factors to Consider

Depending on the needs of the child, the IEP team needs to consider what the law calls special factors. These include the following:

- If the child's behavior interferes with his or her learning or the learning of others, the IEP team will consider strategies and supports to address the child's behavior.
- If the child has limited proficiency in English, the IEP team will consider the child's language needs as these needs relate to his or her IEP.

- If the child is blind or visually impaired, the IEP team must provide for instruction in Braille or the use of Braille, unless it determines after an appropriate evaluation that the child does not need this instruction.

- If the child has communication needs, the IEP team must consider those needs.

- If the child is deaf or hard of hearing, the IEP team will consider his or her language and communication needs. This includes the child's opportunities to communicate directly with classmates and school staff in his or her usual method of communication (for example, sign language).

- The IEP team must always consider the child's need for assistive technology devices or services.

### Will Parents Need an Interpreter in Order to Participate Fully?

If the parents have a limited proficiency in English or are deaf, they may need an interpreter in order to understand and be understood. In this case, the school must make reasonable efforts to arrange for an interpreter during meetings pertaining to the child's educational placement. For meetings regarding the development or review of the IEP, the school must take whatever steps are necessary to ensure that parents understand the meetings—including arranging for an interpreter. This provision should help to ensure that parents are not limited in their ability to participate in their child's education because of language or communication barriers.

Therefore, if parents need an interpreter for a meeting to discuss their child's evaluation, eligibility for special education, or IEP, they should let the school know ahead of time. Telling the school in advance allows the school to make arrangements for an interpreter so that parents can participate fully in the meeting.

### Deciding Placement

In addition, the child's placement (where the IEP will be carried out) must be decided. The placement decision is made by a group of people, including the parents and others who know about the child, what the evaluation results mean, and what types of placements are appropriate. In some states, the IEP team serves as the group making the placement decision. In other states, this decision may be made by another group of people. In all cases, the parents have the right to be members of the group that decides the educational placement of the child.

Placement decisions must be made according to IDEA's least restrictive environment requirements, commonly known as LRE. These requirements state that, to the maximum extent appropriate, children with disabilities must be educated with children who do not have disabilities.

The law also clearly states that special classes, separate schools, or other removal of children with disabilities from the regular educational environment may occur only if the nature or severity of the child's disability is such that education in regular classes with the use of supplementary aids and services cannot be achieved satisfactorily.

What type of placements are there? Depending on the needs of the child, his or her IEP may be carried out in the regular class (with supplementary aids and services, as needed), in a special class (where every student in the class is receiving special education services for some or all of the day), in a special school, at home, in a hospital and institution, or in another setting. A school system may meet its obligation to ensure that the child has an appropriate placement available by doing the following:

- Providing an appropriate program for the child on its own

- Contracting with another agency to provide an appropriate program

- Utilizing some other mechanism or arrangement that is consistent with IDEA for providing or paying for an appropriate program for the child

The placement group will base its decision on the IEP and which placement option is appropriate for the child.

Can the child be educated in the regular classroom, with proper aids and supports? If the child cannot be educated in the regular classroom, even with appropriate aids and supports, then the placement group will talk about other placements for the child.

### After the IEP Is Written

When the IEP has been written, parents must receive a copy at no cost to themselves. The IDEA also stresses that everyone who will be involved in implementing the IEP must have access to the document. This includes all of the following people:

- The child's regular education teacher(s)

- The child's special education teacher(s)

- The child's related service provider(s) (for example, a speech therapist)

- Any other service provider (such as a paraprofessional) who will be responsible for a part of the child's education

Each of these individuals needs to know what his or her specific responsibilities are for carrying out the child's IEP. This includes the specific accommodations, modifications, and supports that the child must receive, according to the IEP.

### Parents' Permission

Before the school can provide a child with special education and related services for the first time, the child's parents must give their written permission.

### Implementing the IEP

Once the IEP is written, it is time to carry it out—in other words, to provide the student with the special education and related services as listed in the IEP. This includes all supplementary aids and services and program modifications that the IEP team has identified as necessary for the student to advance appropriately toward his or her IEP goals, to be involved in and progress in the general curriculum, and to participate in other school activities. While it is beyond the scope of this chapter to discuss in detail the many issues involved in implementing a student's IEP, certain suggestions can be offered.

- Every individual involved in providing services to the student should know and understand his or her responsibilities for carrying out the IEP. This will help ensure that the student receives the services that have been planned, including the specific modifications and accommodations the IEP team has identified as necessary.

- Teamwork plays an important part in carrying out the IEP. Many professionals are likely to be involved in providing services and supports to the student. Sharing expertise and insights can help make everyone's job a lot easier and can certainly improve results for students with disabilities. Schools can encourage teamwork by giving teachers, support staff, and paraprofessionals time to plan or work together on such matters as adapting the general curriculum to address the student's unique needs. Teachers, support staff, and others providing services for children with disabilities may request training and staff development.

- Communication between home and school is also important. Parents can share information about what is happening at home and build upon what the child is learning at school. If the child is having difficulty at school, parents may be able to offer insight or help the school explore possible reasons as well as possible solutions.

- It is helpful to have someone in charge of coordinating and monitoring the services the student receives. In addition to special education, the student may be receiving any number of related services. Many people may be involved in delivering those services. Having a person in charge of overseeing that services are being delivered as planned can help ensure that the IEP is being carried out appropriately.

- The regular progress reports that the law requires will help parents and schools monitor the child's progress toward his or her annual goals. It is important to know if the child is not making the progress expected—or if he or she has progressed much faster than expected. Together, parents and school personnel can then address the child's needs as those needs become evident.

## *Reviewing and Revising the IEP*

The IEP team must review the child's IEP at least once a year. One purpose of this review is to see whether the child is achieving his or her annual goals. The team must revise the child's individualized education program, if necessary, to address the following:

- The child's progress or lack of expected progress toward the annual goals and in the general curriculum

- Information gathered through any reevaluation of the child

- Information about the child that the parents share

- Information about the child that the school shares (for example, insights from the teacher based on his or her observation of the child or the child's class work)

- The child's anticipated needs

- Other matters

Although the IDEA requires this IEP review at least once a year, in fact the team may review and revise the IEP more often. Either the parents or the school can ask to hold an IEP meeting to revise the child's IEP. For example, the child may not be making progress toward his or her IEP goals, and his or her teacher or parents may become concerned. On the other hand, the child may have met most or all of the goals in the IEP, and new ones may need to be written. In either case, the IEP team would meet to revise the IEP.

### Look at Those Factors Again!

When the IEP team is meeting to conduct a review of the child's IEP and, as necessary, to revise it, members must again consider all of the factors discussed previously. This includes the following:

- The child's strengths
- The parents' ideas for enhancing their child's education
- The results of recent evaluations or reevaluations
- How the child has done on state- and district-wide tests

The IEP team must also consider the "special factors," as listed earlier.

### What If Parents Don't Agree with the IEP?

There are times when parents may not agree with the school's recommendations about their child's education. Under the law, parents have the right to challenge decisions about their child's eligibility, evaluation, placement, and the services that the school provides to the child. If parents disagree with the school's actions—or refusal to take action—in these matters, they have the right to pursue a number of options. Some of the options are as follows.

**Try to reach an agreement:** Parents can talk with school officials about their concerns and try to reach an agreement. Sometimes the agreement can be temporary. For example, the parents and school can agree to try a plan of instruction or a placement for a certain period of time and see how the student does.

**Ask for mediation:** During mediation, the parents and school sit down with someone who is not involved in the disagreement and try to reach an agreement. The school may offer mediation, if it is available as an option for resolving disputes prior to due process.

**Ask for due process:** During a due process hearing, the parents and school personnel appear before an impartial hearing officer and present their sides of the story. The hearing officer decides how to solve the problem. (Note: Mediation must be available at least at the time a due process hearing is requested.)

**File a complaint with the state education agency:** To file a complaint, generally parents write directly to the state education agency (SEA) and say what part of IDEA they believe the school has violated. The agency must resolve the complaint within sixty calendar days. An extension of that time limit is permitted only if exceptional circumstances exist with respect to the complaint.

## Office of Special Education Programs Monitoring

The U.S. Department of Education's Office of Special Education Programs (OSEP) regularly monitors states to see that they are complying with IDEA. Every two years OSEP requires that states report progress toward meeting established performance goals that, at a minimum, address the performance of children on assessments, dropout rates, and graduation rates. As part of its monitoring, the department reviews IEPs and interviews parents, students, and school staff to find out the following information:

- Whether, and how, the IEP team made the decisions reflected in the IEP

- Whether those decisions and the IEP content are based on the child's unique needs, as determined through evaluation and the IEP process

- Whether any state or local policies or practices have interfered with decisions of the IEP team about the child's educational needs and the services that the school would provide to meet those needs

- Whether the school has provided the services listed in the IEP

# Updates in the Individualized Education Program with IDEA 2004

When Congress reauthorized IDEA 2004, they made significant changes to Individualized Education Programs (IEPs) in several areas, including:

- Content of IEP;

- IEP meeting attendance;
- IEPs by agreement;
- Review and revision of IEPs;
- Transition;
- Alternate means of participating in meetings.

This part of the chapter will provide you with an overview of changes in the law about IEPs and IEP meetings under IDEA 2004.

### Content of IEPs

Some requirements for the contents of IEPs changed with IDEA 2004 while other requirements remained the same. Here is a summary of changes between IDEA 97 and IDEA 2004.

**Present levels of performance:** In IDEA 97, IEPs were required to include "a statement of the child's present levels of educational performance."

Under IDEA 2004, the child's IEP must include "a statement of the child's present levels of academic achievement and functional performance."

Present levels of academic achievement and functional performance are objective data from assessments.

**Annual goals:** Under IDEA 97, IEPs were required to include a "statement of measurable annual goals, including benchmarks or short-term objectives." IDEA 2004 eliminated the requirements for "benchmarks and short-term objectives" in IEPs—except that the IEPs of children who take alternate assessments must include "a description of benchmarks or short-term objectives."

IDEA 2004 added new language about "academic and functional goals." IEPs must now include "a statement of measurable annual goals, including academic and functional goals."

**Educational progress:** IDEA 97 required IEPs to include a statement about how the child's progress toward the annual goals would be measured, how the child's parents would be regularly informed about "their child's progress toward the annual goals," and whether the child's progress was sufficient.

Under IDEA 2004, the child's IEP must include "a description of how the child's progress toward meeting the annual goals . . . will be measured and when periodic reports on the progress the child is making toward meeting the annual goals (such as through the use of quarterly or other periodic reports, concurrent with the issuance of report cards) will be provided."

**Special education and related services:** IDEA 2004 includes important new language about research-based instruction.

The child's IEP must include "a statement of the special education and related services and supplementary aids and services, based on peer-reviewed research to the extent practicable, to be provided to the child . . . and a statement of the program modifications or supports for school personnel."

**Accommodations and alternate assessments:** IDEA 2004 contains new language about "individual appropriate accommodations" on state and district testing and new requirements for alternate assessments.

The child's IEP must include: "a statement of any individual appropriate accommodations that are necessary to measure the academic achievement and functional performance of the child on State and districtwide assessments" and " if the IEP Team determines that the child shall take an alternate assessment on a particular State or districtwide assessment of student achievement, a statement of why (AA) the child cannot participate in the regular assessment; and (BB) the particular alternate assessment selected is appropriate for the child."

**Transition:** Congress made extensive changes to the legal requirements for transition. IDEA 97 required "a statement of transition services needs" (beginning at age fourteen) and "a statement of needed transition services for the child" (beginning at age sixteen). The statement of transition services needs at age fourteen was eliminated.

Under IDEA 2004, the first IEP after the child is sixteen (and updated annually) must include: "appropriate measurable postsecondary goals based upon age appropriate transition assessments related to training, education, employment, and, where appropriate, independent living skills . . . and the transition services (including courses of study) needed to assist the child in reaching these goals. (Section 1414(d)(1)(A))

## *When IEP Team Members May Be Excused from IEP Meetings*

An IEP team member may be excused from attending an IEP meeting if the member's area of curriculum or service will not be discussed or modified and if the parent and school agree.

A member of the IEP team may also be excused if the member's area of curriculum or service will be discussed or modified, if the member submits a written report to the parent and the IEP team in advance, and if the parent provides written consent. (Section 1414(d)(1)(C))

## Developing the IEP

In developing the IEP, the IEP team shall consider:

- The child's strengths;
- The parent's concerns for enhancing the child's education;
- The results of the initial evaluation or most recent evaluation;
- The child's academic, developmental, and functional needs. (Section 1414(d)(3)(A))

The IEP team shall consider special factors for children:

- Whose behavior impedes learning;
- Who have limited English proficiency;
- Who are blind or visually impaired;
- Who are deaf or hard of hearing. (Section 1414(d)(3)(B))

## Educational Placements

The law about educational placements is in Section 1414(e). Parents are members of the team that decides the child's placement. The decision about placement cannot be made until after the IEP team, which includes the parent, reaches consensus about the child's needs, program, and goals.

Although the law is clear on this issue, the child's "label" often drives decisions about services and placement, leading school personnel to determine the child's placement before the IEP meeting.

These unilateral actions prevent parents from "meaningful participation" in educational decision making for their child. When Congress added this provision to the law in 1997, they sent a message to school officials that unilateral placement decisions are illegal.

## Reviewing and Revising the IEP

The IEP must be reviewed at least once a year to determine if the child is achieving the annual goals. The IEP team must revise the IEP to address:

470

- Any lack of expected progress;
- Results of any reevaluation;
- Information provided by the parents;
- Anticipated needs. (Section 1414(d)(4)(A))

### Revising IEP by Agreement, Without an IEP Meeting

IDEA 2004 changed the process by which IEPs can be amended or modified. If the parent and school agree to amend or modify the IEP, they may revise the IEP by agreement without convening an IEP meeting.

The team must create a written document that describes the changes or modifications in the IEP and note that, by agreement of the parties, an IEP meeting was not held. (Section 1414(d)(3)(D))

### Alternative Ways to Participate in Meetings

School meetings do not have to be face-to-face. IEP and placement meetings, mediation meetings, and due process (IEP) resolution sessions may be convened by conference calls or videoconferences. (Section 1414(f))

### Children Who Transfer: In-State and Out-of State

If a child transfers to a district in the same state, the receiving school must provide comparable services to those in the sending district's IEP until they develop and implement a new IEP. If a child transfers to another state, the receiving district must provide comparable services to those in the sending district's IEP until they complete an evaluation and create a new IEP. (Section 1414(d)(2)(C))

### Multi-Year IEPs

Fifteen states may request approval to implement optional "comprehensive, multi-year IEPs" for periods of no longer than three years. IEP review dates must be based on "natural transition points."

Parents have the right to opt out of this program. The parent of a child served under a multi-year IEP can request a review of the IEP without waiting for the "natural transition point." (Section 1414(d)(5))

Chapter 40

# *Treatment and Education of Autistic and Related Communication Handicapped Children (TEACCH) and Structured Teaching*

## *Chapter Contents*

Section 40.1—Autism Teaching Methods: TEACCH ............... 474

Section 40.2—Structured Teaching ........................................... 475

## Section 40.1

# *Autism Teaching Methods: TEACCH*

TEACCH (treatment and education of autistic and related communication handicapped children), developed at the University of North Carolina in the 1970s, is used by many public school systems. This method is often less intensive than applied behavior analysis (ABA) or verbal behavior programs in the preschool years. A TEACCH classroom is usually very structured, with separate, defined areas for each task, such as individual work, group activities, and play. It relies heavily on visual learning, a strength for many children with autism and pervasive developmental disorders. The children use schedules made up of pictures and/or words to order their day and to help them move smoothly between activities. Children with autism may find it difficult to make transitions between activities and places.

Children may sit at a workstation and be required to complete certain activities, such as matching pictures or letters. The finished assignments are then placed in a container. Children may use picture communication symbols—small laminated squares that contain a symbol and a word—to answer questions and request items from their teacher. The symbols help relieve frustration for nonverbal children while helping those who are starting to speak to recall and say the words they want.

TEACCH says that it respects the "the culture of autism," and embraces a philosophy that people with autism have "characteristics that are different, but not necessarily inferior, to the rest of us." It says, "the person is the priority, rather than any philosophical notion like inclusion, discrete trial training, facilitated communication, etc."

Drawbacks to this method: Social interaction and verbal communication may not be heavily stressed because TEACCH is more focused on accommodating a child's autistic traits than in trying to overcome them. Also, more research is needed into the effectiveness of TEACCH, especially in comparison to applied behavior analysis and other teaching methods. In contrast to the outcome studies of ABA published by Dr. O. Ivar Lovaas, TEACCH has not published comprehensive, long-term studies of its effectiveness in treating and educating children. Parents who want their child included with nondisabled peers may not be happy with a TEACCH program.

TEACCH, as originally developed in North Carolina, includes an array of services that may be missing from other public schools that have adopted this method for their autism classroom. You may wish to learn more about the North Carolina model to see how your school's program measures up.

## Section 40.2

# *Structured Teaching*

"Structured Teaching: Strategies for Supporting Students with Autism" by Susan Stokes, written under a contract with CESA 7 and funded by a discretionary grant from the Wisconsin Department of Public Instruction, 2000. The text of this document may be found online at http://www.specialed.us/autism/structure/str10.htm; accessed October 16, 2006.

Structured teaching is an intervention philosophy developed by the University of North Carolina, Division TEACCH (treatment and education of autistic and related communication handicapped children). Structured teaching is an approach in instructing children with autism. It allows for implementation of a variety of instructional methods (e.g., visual support strategies, picture exchange communication system [PECS], sensory integration strategies, discrete trial, music/rhythm intervention strategies, Greenspan's Floortime, etc.). The following information outlines some important considerations for structured teaching to occur. It is one of many approaches to consider in working with children with autism.

Eric Schopler, founder of Division TEACCH in the early 1970s, established the foundation for structured teaching in his doctoral dissertation[2] by demonstrating that people with autism process visual information more easily than verbal information.

## What Is Structured Teaching?

Structured teaching[1] is based upon an understanding of the unique features and characteristics associated with the nature of autism.

Structured teaching describes the conditions under which a person should be taught rather than "where" or "what" (i.e., "learning how to learn").

Structured teaching is a system for organizing their environments, developing appropriate activities, and helping people with autism understand what is expected of them.

Structured teaching utilizes visual cues that help children with autism focus on the relevant information, which can, at times, be difficult for the person with autism to distinguish from the nonrelevant information.

Structured teaching addresses challenging behaviors in a proactive manner by creating appropriate and meaningful environments that reduce the stress, anxiety, and frustration that may be experienced by children with autism. Challenging behaviors may occur due to the following characteristics of autism:

- Language comprehension difficulties
- Expressive language difficulties
- Social relations difficulties
- Sensory processing difficulties
- Resistance to change
- Preference for familiar routines and consistency
- Organizational difficulties
- Difficulty attending to relevant stimuli
- Distractibility

Structured teaching greatly increases a child's independent functioning (i.e., without adult prompting or cueing), which will assist him throughout life.

This section will address the features of a structured teaching approach. It is important to remember that to effectively use the features of this approach, the individual's strengths and needs must be taken into consideration.

# Primary Components of Structured Teaching

## Physical Structure

Physical structure refers to the way in which we set up and organize the person's physical environment: It emphasizes where and how we place the furniture and materials[1] in the various environments including classrooms, playground, workshop/work area, bedroom, hallways, locker/cubby areas, and so on.

Close attention to physical structure is essential for a number of reasons:

- Physical structure provides environmental organization for people with autism.

- Clear physical and visual boundaries help the person to understand where each area begins and ends.

- The physical structure minimizes visual and auditory distractions.

The amount of physical structure needed is dependent on the level of self-control demonstrated by the child, not his cognitive functioning level. As students learn to function more independently, the physical structure can be gradually lessened.[5]

Example: A high-functioning child with autism may display limited self-control. He will need a more highly structured environment than a lower-functioning child displaying better self-control.

Physical structure consists of a number of components, including location, design and layout, and organization.

**Location:** Physical structure should be considered in any environment in which the person with autism interacts, including classrooms, playground, workshop/work area, bedroom, hallways, locker/cubby areas, etc.

**Design and layout:** A number of points are important in design and layout:

- *Clear visual and physical boundaries:* Each area of the classroom (or environment) should be clearly, visually defined through the arrangement of furniture (e.g., bookcases, room dividers, office panels, shelving units, file cabinets, tables, rugs, etc.) and use of boundary markers, such as carpet squares or colored floor tape. Children with autism typically do not automatically segment

477

their environments like typically developing children. Large, wide-open areas can make it extremely difficult for children with autism to understand what is to occur in each area, where each area begins and ends, and how to get to a specific area by the most direct route. By strategically placing furniture to clearly visually define specific areas, it will decrease the child's tendency to randomly wander or run from area to area. Visual physical boundaries can also be further defined within a specific area. Example: During group story time, a carpet square or taped-off square can provide the child with autism clear visual cues as to the physical boundaries of that activity. Floor tape can also be used in gym class to indicate to the child with autism the area in which he should stay to perform certain motor skills, like warm-up exercises. Example: Color-coded placemats (according to each child's assigned color) can be used for snack or mealtimes. The placemats will visually and physically define each child's "space" (and food items) on the table. These visual cues will help children with autism better understand their environment, as well as increase their ability to become more independent in their environment and less reliant on an adult for direction.

- *Minimize visual and auditory distractions:* Visual distractions can be minimized:

  - By painting the entire environment (walls, ceilings, bulletin boards, etc.) a muted color (e.g., off-white);

  - By limiting the amount of visual "clutter" which is typically present in most classrooms in the form of art projects, seasonal decorations, and classroom materials;

  - By placing sheets or curtains to cover shelves of classroom materials, as well as other visually distracting equipment (e.g., computer, copy machine, TV/VCR, etc.);

  - By storing unnecessary equipment and materials in another area. Example: In the play area, limit the number of appropriate toys that the children can use and then, on a weekly basis, rotate in "new" toys, while putting away the "old" ones.

  - Through the use of natural lighting from windows to reduce visually distracting fluorescent lighting;

  - By controlling the amount of light through the use of blinds, curtains, or shades, thus creating a warm and calm environment;

478

- By placing study carrels and individual student work areas, bordered by a wall or corner of the classroom, away from group work tables, to reduce environmental visual distractions;

- By carefully considering where the child with autism will sit in the regular education classroom. Example: Tony, a student with autism, was seated in the front of the class, facing away from the door or windows and away from shelves with instructional materials in order to minimize visual distractions.

- Through the use of carpeting, lowered ceilings, and acoustical tiles, by turning off the P.A. system (or covering it with foam to mute the sound) and by using headphones for appropriate equipment, such as the computer or tape players, to reduce auditory distractions.

- *Appropriate instructional, independent, recreation and leisure areas in each physically structured environment:* In a classroom setting, these areas may include a small group work area; an independent work area; a 1:1 work area; a play/recreation/leisure area; a sensory motor area; and a crash/quiet area. At home, these areas may include an independent work area; a play area; and a crash/quiet area. Again, these specific areas should have clear visual boundaries to define each area for the child with autism. It is also important to keep in mind the various distractions that may be present in each area, and make accommodations accordingly.

**Organization:** A physically structured environment must be extremely organized to effectively implement a structured teaching approach. Adequate storage of various materials (not in view of the students), which can also be easily accessed by the adults in the environment, is critical.

Example: A sectioned-off storage area (with high dividing units to keep materials out of sight of the students) within the classroom can be very helpful to keep the environment "clutter and distraction-free" yet provide easy access to needed materials.

Students with autism can also be taught to keep the physical environment structured and organized through the use of pictures, color-coding, numbers, symbols, and so on.

Example: In the play area, pictures of the toys can be placed on the shelves to provide structure when putting things away.

479

## *Visual Schedules*

A daily visual schedule is a critical component in a structured environment. A visual schedule will tell the student with autism what activities will occur and in what sequence.

Visual schedules are important for children with autism because they do the following:

- Help address the child's difficulty with sequential memory and organization of time.

- Assist children with language comprehension problems to understand what is expected of them.[5]

- Lessen the anxiety level of children with autism, and thus reduce the possible occurrence of challenging behaviors, by providing the structure for the student to organize and predict daily and weekly events. Schedules clarify that activities happen within a specific time period (e.g., understanding that "break time" is coming, but after "work time") and also alert the student to any changes that might occur.

- Assist students in transitioning independently between activities and environments by telling them where they are to go next.[5] Visual schedules can be used in all environments (e.g., classroom, gym, occupational therapy, speech/language therapy, home, Sunday school, etc.).

- Are based on a "first-then" strategy (that is, "first you do ___, then you do ___"), rather than an "if-then" approach (i.e., "if you do ___, then you can do___"). This first-then strategy allows the "first" expectation (whether a task, activity, or assignment) to be modified, as needed. The modification is in terms of task completion and amount of prompting, in order to accommodate the student's daily fluctuations in his or her ability to process incoming information. Then he or she can move on to his or her next visually scheduled task/activity. Example: A student is having particular difficulty completing a math worksheet, due to anxiety, sensory processing difficulties, communication, difficulty generalizing, internal/external distracters, change, and so on. The assignment can be modified so that the child only has to complete three math problems first, and then he has a sensory break, as indicated on his visual schedule.

- Can incorporate various social interactions into the student's daily schedule (e.g. showing completed work to a teacher/parent for social reinforcement, requiring appropriate social greetings).

- Can increase a student's motivation to complete less desired activities by strategically alternating more-preferred with less-preferred activities on the student's individual visual schedule. Example: By placing computer time after math, the student may be more motivated to complete math knowing that computer time will be next.

A visual schedule for a student with autism must be directly taught and consistently used. Visual schedules should not be considered as "crutches" for students with autism, from which they should gradually be "weaned." Instead, these individual visual schedules should be considered as "prosthetic" or "assistive technology" devices. For the student with autism, the consistent use of a visual schedule is an extremely important skill. It has the potential to increase independent functioning throughout his life—at school, at home and in the community.

**Developing visual schedules:** In general, schedules should be arranged from a "top-to-bottom" or "left-to-right" format, including a method for the student to manipulate the schedule to indicate that an activity is finished or "all done" (cross or mark off with a dry erase marker, place the item in an "all done" envelope or box, check off the item, draw a line through the scheduled activity, etc.).

A minimum of two scheduled items should be presented at a time so that the student begins to understand that events and activities happen in a sequential manner, not in isolation.

Schedules can be designed using a variety of formats, depending upon the needs of the individual student (object schedule, three-ring binder schedule, clipboard schedule, manila file folder schedules, dry erase board schedules, Velcro strip across the top of the desk, etc.).

Various visual representation systems can be used for an individual visual schedule including real objects, photographs (e.g., "Picture This" software program or own photos), realistic drawings, a commercial picture system (e.g., "Boardmaker" software program), or written words or lists.

**Individual schedule:** It is necessary to develop an individual schedule for the child with autism in addition to the general classroom schedule.

An individual schedule will give the child with autism important information in a visual form that he or she can readily understand.

Another consideration when individualizing a schedule for a student with autism is the length of the schedule (number of activities).

The length of the schedule may need to be modified due to the student becoming increasingly obsessed and/or anxious regarding an upcoming scheduled activity, or due to difficulty in processing "too much" information presented at once.

Example: A particular student "obsesses" over recess. If at the beginning of his day he sees "recess" scheduled later in the morning, he will continue to be obsessed with "going out for recess," resulting in increased anxiety and distractibility for the rest of the morning activities until recess. The student's schedule could be created with a few activity items at a time, up until recess. Again, individualization is the key to success.

**Check schedule:** Some students may need a "check schedule" visual physical prompt to teach them to independently check their schedule, as well as learn the importance of their schedule.

Example: "Check schedule" visual prompts can be made by writing the student's name on laminated colored paper strips or using popsicle sticks or poker chips with a large check printed on the chip.

The "check schedule" prompts are visual and physical cues (as opposed to adult prompts) given to the student for any transition in his daily activities, to cue him to check his schedules.

A child who relies too heavily on adult prompts rather than using "check schedule" prompts with his or her schedule, may have more difficulty understanding the importance of his or her schedule and have limited success in using it.

**Transitions:** Some students may need to transition to the next scheduled activity by taking their scheduled item (card or object) off their individual schedule and carrying this with them to the next activity/location. This may be due to the child's increased distractibility in maneuvering through the environment. The distractibility, or inability to sustain attention throughout the transition, is independent of the child's cognitive functioning level or verbal skills.

Example: Some nonverbal students with autism, who function at a younger cognitive level, do not require transition schedule cards to get to the next scheduled activity. On the other hand, certain higher-functioning students with autism require a transition card to get to the next scheduled activity, due to their increased distractibility.

### Teaching Components

Teaching components include work systems and visual structure.

**Work systems:** This refers to the systematic and organized presentation of tasks and materials in order for students to learn to work independently, without adult directions or prompts. It is important to note that "work systems" can reflect any type of task(s) or activities (e.g., academic, daily living skills, recreation and leisure, etc.). Each "work system," regardless of the nature of the specific task or activity, should address the following four questions:

- What is the work to be done? What is the nature of the task? (e.g., sorting by colors; adding/subtracting two-digit numbers, making a sandwich, brushing teeth, etc.).

- How much work? Visually represent to the student exactly how much work is to be done. If the student is to cut out only ten soup can labels, don't give him or her a whole stack and expect the child to independently count and/or understand that he or she is to cut out only ten soup can labels for the task to be considered complete. Seeing the whole stack of labels—even if told that he or she is going to cut only ten—can cause a child with autism a great deal of frustration and anxiety in not being able to understand exactly how much work to complete. Remember, students with autism rely upon their visual channel to process information; therefore, seeing a whole stack of work to complete can prove overwhelming. Provide only the materials the student will need for the specific task or activity in order to decrease his or her possible confusion in understanding exactly how much and what work is to be done.

- When am I finished? The student needs to independently recognize when he or she is finished with a task or activity. The task itself may define this, or the use of timers or visual cues, such as a red dot, to indicate where to stop on a particular worksheet, has proven effective.

- What comes next? Items such as physical reinforcers, highly desired activities, break times or free choices are highly motivating toward task completion. In some cases, being "all done" with the task motivates the child enough to complete it.

Experience with structured teaching and the use of "work systems" has shown that a student's overall productivity increases when the student has a way of knowing how much work there is to do, as well as when it is to be finished.[1] Use of a "work system" helps to organize the child with autism through use of a structured and systematic approach to completing various tasks independently.

Examples of various types of work systems, from easiest to most difficult, include:

- *Left to right sequence—finished box/basket/folder to the far right:* This is the most concrete level of "work systems" and involves placing items to be completed to the left of the person's workspace (e.g., a shelf, folder, basket/tub, etc.). The student is taught to take the items from the left, complete them at his or her work space in front of him or her, and then place the completed work to the right in an "all done" box, folder, or basket.

- *Matching—color, shape, alphabet, number:* This would be a higher level skill, in that the person must complete his or her "work jobs" in a sequential order by matching color, shape, alphabet letter, or number coding system. Example: The student has a sequence strip of individual numbers 1–10 Velcroed on his or her desk or work space. The student also has multiple "work jobs" located on his or her left. To complete tasks in this work system (matching), the student takes the number "1" off his or her number strip and matches it to the number "1" located on one of the work jobs. This is the job/task/activity he or she must complete first. The student continues matching numbers to tasks in order to complete those tasks (work jobs) in a specified sequential order.

- *Written system:* This is the highest level of the work system. It would involve a written list of "work jobs" to be completed in sequential order.

**Visual structure:** This is the process of incorporating concrete visual cues into the task or activity itself. By doing so, the student will not have to rely on the teacher's verbal or physical prompts in order to understand what to do.[2] The student can use his or her strong visual skills to get meaning from the task/activity without adult assistance. Thus, these visual cues increase the student's ability to work successfully and independently.

Students with autism tend to have difficulty processing the most obvious information in their environments, and at times they may become overly focused or attentive to insignificant or irrelevant details. In order to help students with autism identify and focus on the significant and relevant details of a task or activity, their daily activities and tasks need to be modified to incorporate the following:

- *Visual instructions:* A student should be able to sequentially complete a task or activity by looking at the visual instructions given. Visual instructions will help the student to combine and organize a series of steps to obtain a desired outcome.[2] Visual instructions may include the following forms:

- The materials of the task define the task (e.g., putting rings on a stick with the rings located in a container on the left, and the stick standing upright on the right—again following the left-to-right sequence)

- A cut-out or outline jig (e.g., an outline of a plate and silverware to direct the person where to place the silverware on a placemat)

- A picture jig (e.g., a picture of various toys or clothing items in specific locations for the child to match the real object, in order to learn to put away his or her belongings)

- Written instruction (e.g., written steps to complete a task or sequenced activity such as the morning routine or spelling work.)

- Product sample or model (e.g., a completed art project)

- *Visual organization:* Visual organization refers to the task of presenting the materials and space in an organized manner so that the sensory input or extra stimulation are reduced. Visual organization can be achieved through the following adaptations:

  - Use containers to organize materials (e.g., placing the various materials of an activity into separate containers or arranging alphabet letters to be matched by standing them upright in a foam tray, rather than having them bunched together in a single container).

  - Limit the area (e.g., use masking tape to enclose specific areas for a student to vacuum).

- *Visual clarity:* The purpose of visual clarity is to highlight the important information, concepts, and specific parts of the instruction and key materials.[1] The nature of the task is designed to prompt the student to focus on the important details of the "work job" (task/activity/assignment). These details are highlighted through colors, pictures, numbers, or words. Providing visual clarity promotes student independence rather than relying upon adult guidance.[2] The most concrete level of visual clarity is achieved by limiting the materials needed to complete the task successfully (e.g., removing unnecessary, irrelevant, or extra materials).[2] Examples of visual clarity include the following:

- Color coding (e.g., assign each student a specific color and consistently use this color to teach the child to identify his or her environmental belongings more readily, including work areas, cubby space/locker, small group chair, snack/lunch seat, communication books, and so on)

- Labeling (e.g., for sorting tasks, highlighting openings on containers to make them more visually obvious)

Through the use of a visually structured teaching method, a student with autism can learn to complete various tasks and activities independently, without an adult's physical or verbal prompt. Therefore many students with autism can engage in "independent work sessions" for various periods of time throughout their day, in any environment (home, school, work), and on any skill area, such as academic/curricular, daily living skills, recreation and leisure, and so on).

## *Conclusion*

The structured teaching approach allows the student with autism to learn a process of focusing upon and following visual cues in various situations and environments, in order to increase his or her overall independent functioning. It is important to note that various instructional interventions, such as sensory integration, picture exchange communication system (PECS), Greenspan's Floortime, discrete trial, and the like, can easily be incorporated into the structured teaching approach.

1. Division TEACCH. *Division TEACCH Training Manual*. Revised January 1998. Chapel Hill, NC.

2. Division TEACCH. *Visually Structured Tasks: Independent Activities for Students with Autism and Other Visual Learners*. March 1996. Chapel Hill, NC.

3. Harris, Sandra L. and Jan S. Handleman. *Preschool Programs for Children with Autism*. Autism, Pro-Ed, 1994.

4. Johnson, Kathleen. "Autism 101" Training. CESA 6, Oshkosh, WI. March 16–17, 2000.

5. "Structured Teaching," 15 August 1998. Division TEACCH, Chapel Hill, NC http://www.unc.edu/depts/teacch.

6. Trehin, Paul. "Some Basic Information about TEACCH," Autisme France. 23 March 2000. http://www.unc.edu/depts/teacch.

Chapter 41

# School Transitions and the Autistic Child: Planning for Successful Transitions across Grade Levels

Transition is a natural part of all educational programs. Students with and without disabilities are expected to adjust to changes in teachers, classmates, schedules, buildings, and routines. The transition from one grade to the next can be especially challenging for the student with an autism spectrum disorder. However, these students can more easily make this shift if careful planning and preparation occurs. Following are suggestions for facilitating a smooth transition.

Preparation for transition should begin early in the spring. Whether a student is moving to a new classroom or to a new building, it is helpful to identify the homeroom teacher or general or special educator who will have primary responsibility for the student.

Once the receiving teacher is identified, involve this person in the annual case conference process so that he or she may gain information about the student's current level of functioning and can provide input into projected goals.

Written transition plans may facilitate the student's successful movement. A meeting should be conducted to allow key participants to exchange relevant information. Responsibilities and timelines for individuals involved in the transition should be clearly stated.

"Planning for Successful Transitions across Grade Levels," by Cathy Pratt, © 2000 Indiana Resource Center for Autism. Reprinted with permission. The text of this document may be found online at http://www.iidc.indiana.edu/irca/education/transpln.html; accessed September 29, 2006.

Either during the annual case conference or at the transition planning meeting, information should be exchanged about effective instructional strategies, needed modifications and adaptations, positive behavior support strategies, and methods of communication. The receiving teacher should learn about the strategies that have worked in the past so that precious time is not lost at the beginning of the new school year.

The receiving teacher may find it helpful to observe the student in his or her current classroom or school setting. This will provide important insight into the student's learning style and needed supports.

Instructional assistants who will be involved in the student's daily education should be identified, educated, and informed about their role in the student's education.

Many teachers may not have previous experience with students with autism spectrum disorders. Therefore, they will need basic information about autism spectrum disorders and about how autism impacts the student with whom they will be working. Student-specific information about learning styles, communication systems, medical issues, and behavior supports is also critical. Remember to include cafeteria workers, custodians, bus drivers, the school secretary, and the school nurse in the training. Classmates of the new student also may need information. This should be provided in a respectful manner and without stigmatizing the student with autism spectrum disorders.

Before entering a new school, work to alleviate any anxieties the student with autism spectrum disorders may have about the new setting. Preparation for this move can be facilitated by providing the student with a map of the school, a copy of his or her schedule for the fall, a copy of the student handbook and rules, and a list of clubs and extracurricular activities.

Develop a videotape about the new school and provide written information about specific situations so that the student can learn and rehearse for the change at his or her own pace.

Visitations should be conducted to allow the student and his or her family to meet relevant school staff, to locate the student's locker, and to become familiar with the school culture.

Identify key people or a mentor the student can contact if she or he is having a difficult time adjusting or understanding a certain situation. It may also be helpful to find a location where the student can go to relax and to regroup. Provide the student with a visual menu of coping strategies.

Parents should receive information about bus schedules, parent-teacher organizations, and available resources (e.g., counselors, social workers, nurses).

Prior to the new school year, it will be helpful to establish methods and a schedule for communicating between home and school. Suggestions for maintaining ongoing communication include journals, daily progress notes, mid-term grades, scheduled appointments or phone calls, informal meetings, report cards, or parent-teacher conferences.

Once in the new school, ask for peers who are willing to help the student with the transition and acclimation to the new school. By gaining the support of a friend without a disability, the student with an autism spectrum disorder may have greater access to social opportunities during and after school.

The ultimate goal is to promote a successful experience for both the student and the rest of the school community. By systematically addressing the transition process, students with autism spectrum disorders can be prepared to participate in their new school experience.

Chapter 42

# Transition Planning for Life after High School: A Team Effort

## Introduction

The completion of high school is the beginning of adult life. Entitlement to public education ends, and young people and their families are faced with many options and decisions about the future. The most common choices for the future are pursuing vocational training or further academic education, getting a job, and living independently.

For students with disabilities, these choices may be more complex and may require a great deal of planning. Planning the transition from school to adult life begins, at the latest, during high school. In fact, transition planning is required, by law, to start once a student reaches fourteen years of age, or younger, if appropriate. This transition planning becomes formalized as part of the student's Individualized Education Program (IEP).

Transition services are intended to prepare students to make the transition from the world of school to the world of adulthood. In planning what type of transition services a student needs to prepare for adulthood, the IEP team considers areas such as postsecondary education or vocational training, employment, independent living, and community participation. The transition services themselves are a coordinated set of activities that are based on the student's needs and

Reprinted from "Transition Planning: A Team Effort," National Dissemination Center for Children with Disabilities (NICHCY), updated 2002. "Changes in the Law with IDEA 2004" is reprinted from "Topic: Secondary Transition," U.S. Department of Education, Office of Special Education Programs, February 1, 2007.

that take into account his or her preferences and interests. Transition services can include instruction, community experiences, the development of employment and other post-school adult living objectives, and (if appropriate) the acquisition of daily living skills and functional vocational assessment.

The student and his or her family are expected to take an active role in preparing the student to take responsibility for his or her own life once school is finished. Where once school provided a centralized source of education, guidance, transportation, and even recreation, after students leave school, they will need to organize their own lives and needs and navigate among an array of adult service providers and federal, state, and local programs. This can be a daunting task, one for which the student and his or her family need to be prepared.

This transition summary provides ideas and information on how students, families, school personnel, service providers, and others can work together to help students make a smooth transition. In particular, this chapter focuses on creative transition planning and services that use all the resources that exist in communities, not just the agencies that have traditionally been involved. This chapter also provides the following items:

- Definitions of some terms used in transition planning

- Lists of individuals and agencies that can help the IEP team create a successful transition plan

- Guides to finding the groups and agencies that provide transition services

- Examples of creative transition plans

- Ways to improve the transition system by working at the community level.

## Brief Legal Overview[1]

If students are to mature into independent, productive adults and become increasingly responsible for their actions and accomplishments, they need to acquire the skills that are of value in the world of adulthood. The Individuals with Disabilities Education Act (IDEA) acknowledges this and contains provisions meant to encourage student involvement and shared decision making.

Since 1990, transition services have been a requirement of law for students who are sixteen years or older, or younger if deemed appropriate by the IEP team. The services are planned at the IEP meeting, to which students must be invited. Thus, the 1990 IDEA legislation provided students with an enormous new opportunity to be involved in planning their own education, to look into the future, to voice their preferences and concerns and desires, to be heard, and to share in making decisions that so directly affect them.

Under the reauthorization of the IDEA in 1997 (IDEA 97), this involvement was expanded. In addition to transition services beginning at age sixteen, a statement of transition service needs is required at age fourteen. At this time, and updated annually thereafter, the IEP team looks at the child's courses of study (such as advanced placement courses or vocational education programs) and determines whether or not those courses of study are leading the student to where the student needs to be upon graduation. What other courses might be indicated, given the student's goals for life after secondary school? Beginning to plan at age fourteen, with an eye to necessary coursework, is expected to help students plan and prepare educationally. Then, at age sixteen, or younger if appropriate, transition services are delivered in a wide range of areas.

IDEA 97 also outlined procedures for the transfer of parental rights to the student when he or she reaches the age of majority under state law. Both the parents and the student must be notified of any transfer of rights that will take place at that time. Students are to receive the notification at least one year before they reach the age of majority. A statement must be included in the IEP that the student has been informed of the rights, if any, that will transfer to the student on reaching the age of majority. After the student attains the age of majority, if rights transfer, the school must provide any notice required by the law (e.g., procedural safeguards notice, notice regarding an upcoming IEP meeting) to both the student and the parents. In states where rights transfer, all other rights accorded to the parents transfer to the student. (If the student is determined incompetent under state law, then the rights remain with the parents.)

Many students, however, may not have the ability to provide informed consent with respect to their educational program, although they have not been determined under state law to be incompetent. To protect the interests of these children, IDEA 97 provides that each state that transfers rights needs to establish procedures for appointing the parents (or another appropriate individual, if the parents are not available) to represent the student's educational interests.

This transfer of rights is obviously an enormous step forward toward empowering students as adults and encouraging them to inform themselves about and become deeply involved in their education and particularly in planning for their future. Educators will need to provide additional training and opportunities for students to understand the impact of this responsibility.

## Changes in the Law with IDEA 2004

The reauthorized Individuals with Disabilities Education Act (IDEA) was signed into law on December 3, 2004, by President George W. Bush. The provisions of the act became effective on July 1, 2005, with the exception of some of the elements pertaining to the definition of a "highly qualified teacher" that took effect upon the signing of the act. The final regulations were published on August 14, 2006. This section addresses significant changes from preexisting regulations to the final regulatory requirements regarding secondary transition.

The IDEA 2004 regulations stipulate the following changes:

1.  Add "further education" of children with disabilities to the IDEA's purposes. The purposes of IDEA include ensuring that all children with disabilities have available to them a free appropriate public education (FAPE) that emphasizes special education and related services designed to meet their unique needs and prepare them for further education, employment, and independent living.

2.  Refer to a "child" instead of a "student." The definition of "transition services" is changed to refer to a "child," rather than a "student," with a disability.

3.  Change the definition of "transition services." The term "transition services" means a coordinated set of activities for a child with a disability that:

    *   Is designed to be within a results-oriented process that is focused on improving the academic and functional achievement of the child with a disability to facilitate the child's movement from school to post-school activities, including postsecondary education, vocational education, integrated employment (including supported employment), continuing and adult education, adult services, independent living, or community participation;

    *   Is based on the individual child's needs, taking into account the child's strengths, preferences, and interests; and

- Includes instruction, related services, community experiences, the development of employment and other post-school adult living objectives, and, if appropriate, acquisition of daily living skills and functional vocational evaluation.

4. Require changes to performance goals and indicators. The state has established goals for the performance of children with disabilities in the state that address graduation rates and dropout rates, as well as such other factors as the state may determine.

5. Establish an exception to requirements for evaluation before a change in eligibility. The evaluation described in Section 300.305(e)(1) [see 20 U.S.C. 1414(c)(5)(B)(i)] is not required before the termination of a child's eligibility under Part B due to graduation from secondary school with a regular diploma, or due to exceeding the age eligibility for FAPE under state law. For a child whose eligibility under Part B terminates under circumstances described above, the local educational agency (LEA) shall provide the child with a summary of the child's academic achievement and functional performance, which shall include recommendations on how to assist the child in meeting the child's postsecondary goals.

6. Change the secondary transition requirements in the IEP. Beginning not later than the first IEP to be in effect when the child turns sixteen, or younger if determined appropriate by the IEP Team, and updated annually thereafter, the IEP must include:

- Appropriate measurable postsecondary goals based upon age-appropriate transition assessments related to training, education, employment, and, where appropriate, independent living skills;

- The transition services (including courses of study) needed to assist the child in reaching those goals; and

- Beginning not later than one year before the child reaches the age of majority under state law, a statement that the child has been informed of the child's rights under Part B, if any, that will transfer to the child on reaching the age of majority under Section 300.520 [see 20 U.S.C. 1415(m)].

7. Add requirement to invite child to IEP team meeting when purpose includes "consideration of postsecondary goals." The LEA

must invite a child with a disability to attend the child's IEP team meeting if a purpose of the meeting will be the consideration of the postsecondary goals for the child and the transition services needed to assist the child in reaching those goals under Section 300.320(b).

8. Add development and implementation of transition programs to list of permissible uses of state-level funds under Part B. States may use funds reserved under Section 300.704(b)(1) for the development and implementation of transition programs, including coordination of services with agencies involved in supporting the transition of students with disabilities to postsecondary activities.

9. Delete requirement that an LEA take other steps if an invited agency does not attend an IEP meeting during which transition services will be discussed. If a purpose of a child's IEP team meeting will be the consideration of postsecondary goals for the child and the transition services needed to assist the child in reaching those goals, the LEA, to the extent appropriate, and with consent, must invite a representative of any participating agency that is likely to be responsible for providing or paying for transition services to attend the child's IEP team meeting. However, if the participating agency does not attend the meeting, the LEA is no longer required to take other steps to obtain participation of an agency in the planning of any transition services.

10. Add requirement for consent prior to inviting a representative of any participating agency likely to be responsible for providing or paying for transition services to attend a child's IEP team meeting. To the extent appropriate, with the consent of the parents or a child who has reached the age of majority, in implementing the requirements of Section 300.321(b)(1), the public agency must invite a representative of any participating agency that is likely to be responsible for providing or paying for transition services.

## Transition Teams

This section looks at ways to create effective transition teams. Collaboration between team members and participating agencies is an essential part of the process.

## What Is Collaboration?

There are basically four ways in which people can interact to establish or improve services and plan for young adults preparing for transition from school to post-school activities. Let us look at these methods briefly.

**Networking:** Through networking, people gain an awareness of available resources and discover how to access or refer individuals to those services. An example of networking might be a transition coordinator talking with local business owners to identify possible job training sites for students. While networking is an essential step in collaboration, it will not be enough for students who have complex transition service needs.

**Service coordination:** Service coordination assists in the selection and scheduling of services. In coordinating, people arrange for a student with disabilities to receive specific services from different agencies (for example, one agency making a phone call to another agency to determine their respective roles and to schedule activities).

**Cooperation:** With cooperation, people look for ways to support and complement one another's transition services. For example, an adult services agency may accept a student's recent test results from his or her school to determine the student's eligibility for services. This would prevent the student from being tested twice and would save the adult services agency time and expense.

**Collaboration:** Collaboration begins with networking, coordination, and cooperation and then requires team members to share decisions, responsibility, and trust. It requires that team members invest time and energy to come up with options and design strategies for carrying out these plans. Because collaboration requires lots of time and energy, it is impossible to make all decisions collaboratively. In some instances, the desired result can be achieved through networking, coordination, or cooperation. Working together, or collaboratively, invites participation of multiple service providers and the use of multiple resources. See the student stories in the following text for examples of collaboration in action.

## Individual Transition Team Members

Many different individuals come together to help the student plan for transition. Typically, transition planning is handled by members of the IEP team, with other individuals becoming involved as needed. It's important to involve a variety of people, for they will bring their unique perspectives to the planning table. The team draws upon the expertise of the different members and pools their information to make decisions or recommendations for the student.

Who are some of the individuals who may be part of the transition team? Naturally, the student and his or her family are core members of the team. They keep the whole team grounded and focused on the goals and on finding services and developing a plan that will benefit the youth with disabilities. When the purpose of the IEP meeting is to discuss transition, the student must be invited to attend. If there is no way he or she can come to the meeting, then the school must take other steps to make sure that the student's preferences and interests are considered in the plan that is developed.

Other members of the team include those normally on the IEP team (special education and general education teachers, related service providers, administrators, and others as appropriate), plus transition specialists, who may be well informed about resources and adult services in the community.

In addition, representatives that have traditionally provided post-high-school services should be involved. This may include the following:

- **The vocational rehabilitation (VR) agency:** The VR agency has traditionally been a primary player in determining the way transition services are delivered. VR has its own eligibility requirements. Therefore, not all students receiving special education services can receive VR services.

- **Service agencies for students with mental retardation or mental health concerns such as the Mental Health Agency:** Depending on the student's individual needs, it may be important for the transition team to include representatives from service agencies addressing mental retardation or mental health. The services provided by these agencies, however, vary greatly from community to community due to differences in local funding and priorities.

- **Independent living centers (ILCs):** ILCs are nonresidential, community- based agencies that are run by people with various disabilities. ILC services vary from place to place.

- **Social Security Administration:** Social Security Administration programs provide financial assistance or work incentives to eligible people with disabilities, based upon federal guidelines.

## Common Community Agencies and the Services They May Offer

Vocational rehabilitation agencies assist persons with cognitive, sensory, physical, or emotional disabilities to attain employment and increased independence. Funded by federal and state money, VR agencies typically operate regional and local offices. VR services typically last for a limited period of time and are based on an individual's rehabilitation plan. If needed, an individual with disabilities can request services at a later time, and a new rehabilitation plan will be developed.

Examples of employment services provided by VR agencies are as follows:

- Vocational guidance and counseling
- Medical, psychological, vocational, and other types of assessments to determine vocational potential
- Job development, placement, and follow-up services
- Rehabilitation, technological services and adaptive devices, tools, equipment, and supplies

Examples of postsecondary services provided by VR agencies are as follows:

- Apprenticeship programs, usually in conjunction with the Department of Labor
- Vocational training
- College training toward a vocational goal as part of an eligible student's financial aid package

Examples of adult and independent living services provided by VR agencies are as follows:

- Housing or transportation supports needed to maintain employment
- Interpreter services
- Orientation and mobility services

Mental health and mental retardation agencies provide a comprehensive system of services responsive to the needs of individuals with mental illness or mental retardation. Federal, state, and local funding are used to operate regional offices; local funding is often the primary source. Services are provided on a sliding payment scale.

Examples of employment services provided by these agencies are as follows:

- Supported and sheltered employment

- Competitive employment support for those who need minimal assistance

Examples of adult and independent living services provided by mental health and mental retardation agencies are as follows:

- Case management services to access and obtain local services

- Therapeutic recreation, including day activities, clubs, and programs

- Respite care

- Residential services (group homes and supervised apartments)

Independent living centers (ILCs) help people with disabilities to achieve and maintain self-sufficient lives within the community. Operated locally, ILCs serve a particular region. ILCs may charge for classes, but advocacy services are typically available at no cost.

Examples of employment services provided by ILCs are as follows:

- Information and referral services

- Connecting students with mentors with disabilities

Examples of postsecondary services provided by ILCs are as follows:

- Information and referral services

- Connecting students with mentors with disabilities

Examples of adult and independent living services provided by ILCs are as follows:

- Advocacy training

- Auxiliary social services (e.g., maintaining a list of personal care attendants)

- Peer counseling services

- Housing assistance

- Training in skills of independent living (attendant management, housing, transportation, career development)

- Information and referral services

- Connecting with mentors

The Social Security Administration operates the federally funded program that provides benefits for people of any age who are unable to do substantial work and have a severe mental or physical disability. Several programs are offered for people with disabilities, including Social Security Disability Insurance (SSDI), Supplemental Security Income (SSI), Plans to Achieve Self-Support (PASS), Medicaid, and Medicare.

Examples of employment services provided by the Social Security Administration include work incentive programs such as the following:

- Cash benefits while working (e.g., student-earned income)

- Medicare or Medicaid while working

- Help with any extra work expenses the individual has as a result of the disability

- Assistance to start a new line of work

Examples of postsecondary services provided by the Social Security Administration include the following:

- Financial incentives for further education and training

Examples of adult and independent living services provided by the Social Security Administration include the following:

- Medical benefits

- Can use income as basis for purchase or rental of housing

Other individuals or agencies may serve as one-time or ongoing consultants to the team, sharing a particular expertise or insight, while others may be valuable sources of specific information that helps the team plan and make decisions. Consider the useful information to be gained from any of the following:

- Postsecondary education and training providers such as representatives from colleges or trade schools, who can help the student explore types of training available as well as remind the group that lifelong learning for all individuals is important

- Department of Labor job services agencies, which offer transition services and employment programs, although not usually with a disability focus

- School to Work Opportunities Act (STWOA) program representatives, who can tell the team about job training available under STWOA to help students prepare for their first job or further education and training

- Community leaders such as religious leaders, directors of recreation programs, and county extension agents, who may help the team address a particular need that a student has

- Community recreation centers such as Boys Clubs, YMCA, or 4-H clubs, which may provide job counseling and youth development activities

- Employers, who can provide training and job opportunities and who can explain the expectations that the business community has for future workers

### *Potential Consultants to the Transition Team*

Additional potential consultants to the transition team include the following:

- **Adult education representative:** Provides information about lifelong education options

- **Advocacy organization(s) representative:** May offer self-advocacy training or support groups for young adults

- **Assistive technology representative:** Provides expertise on devices that can open doors to opportunities

- **At-risk/prevention specialist:** Offers counseling and support on teen pregnancy, alcohol, and drugs

- **Business-education partnership representative:** Provides links between schools and local businesses and industry

- **Community action agency representative:** May link team to resources for traditionally underrepresented groups

- **Correctional education staff:** Provides incarcerated youth with continued learning opportunities

- **Dropout prevention representative:** Provides youth with alternative to dropping out of school

- **Employer:** Offers insight into expectations; promotes hiring of people with disabilities

- **Employment specialist:** Provides job development, placement, coaching

- **Extension service agent:** Offers programs in parenting, homemaking, independent living

- **Guidance counselor:** Provides information on curriculum, assessment, graduation requirements, and college

- **Health department/school nurse:** Provides guidance on community health services and health care advice

- **Higher education representative:** Provides information on postsecondary services to students with disabilities

- **Housing agency representative:** Assists in developing housing options

- **Leisure program representative:** Knows available program options within the community

- **Literacy council representative:** Coordinates volunteers to teach basic reading and writing skills

- **Local government representative:** Funds many local services; can provide information on local services

- **Local disability representative:** Provides information and training (often serves all disabilities, not just one)

- **Parent training and information center representative:** Provides training on transition planning and advocacy services to families

- **Religious community member:** Can provide social support to young adults and their families

- **Residential service provider:** Can help access specialized housing

- **Social worker:** Provides guidance and arranges for case management, support, and respite care

- **Special Olympics representative:** Provides sports training, competition, and recreational opportunities for youth

- **Therapists:** Provide behavioral, physical, occupational, and speech services in the community

- **Transportation representative:** Offers expertise about transportation options and training

- **United Way representative:** Funds many community programs that may offer options for young adults

- **Very Special Arts representative:** Provides information on art programs and opportunities for youth

- **Vocational educator:** Provides job training; teachers work-related skills

- **YMCA/YWCA:** Offers recreation and leisure programs

Team members do not necessarily have to come from social service agencies. Students and their families may also invite a relative, friend, or advocate who can provide emotional support, access to their personal networks, or other unique expertise. If possible, it is also helpful to have team members from similar language and cultural backgrounds as the student. These members can help the team understand how cultural or language issues impact the transition process. Some typical transition outcomes, such as going away to college, getting a paying job, moving out of the family home, and making decisions independently of the family are valued differently by different cultures.

It is very important to invite service representatives and other individuals identified as transition consultants to IEP meetings that will be focused on only transition. They do not need to be at every IEP meeting of the student. If they cannot attend the meetings focusing on transition, talk to them about the IEP and bring their ideas or comments to the meeting.

### Creating the Transition Plan

After the IEP team identifies the student's preferences and interests and identifies the agencies and resources that may be helpful in planning the student's transition, it's time to sit down and figure out a way to make all the pieces fit together. This takes time, creativity, and patience, but the rewards are worth the effort. Remember that other people have done this before. Consult school professionals, disability groups, parent organizations, and other families for their suggestions.

Planning an effective transition can involve many different individuals and agencies. The student stories below illustrate the types of collaboration involved in creative planning. They show plans for three different components that every transition plan should include: plans for employment, plans for education and/or training after high school, and plans for living independently. Following these student stories are sections that show the steps that a transition team may need to take in order to meet the student's goals.

### Marcia's Employment Path

Marcia, a twenty-year-old student with mild cognitive disabilities and a mild hearing impairment, has a transition goal of full-time employment upon graduation this year. Marcia has a one-year-old child. Marcia's transition planning team includes her and her family, the vocational educator, special educator, vocational rehabilitation counselor, mental retardation caseworker, hearing specialist, social worker, and occupational therapist.

Starting at age seventeen, Marcia began exploring job opportunities through job shadowing and internship experiences. Both Marcia and her parents reported that she liked working with people, that she liked working inside, and that she would prefer an office setting. Marcia's vocational education teacher observed her in a simulated work experience and reported that Marcia followed instructions when given visual cues from a co-worker. The vocational educator and vocational rehabilitation counselor identified a small business that needed office assistance. Marcia, working with the vocational rehabilitation counselor and her special education teacher, set up a job interview at the small business and was successful at obtaining a part-time job as an administrative aide.

The counselor/special educator team observed the work setting and identified the work and social demands of the job. The IEP transition team identified that Marcia would need the following supports to work: visual cues outlining the steps of the job; a co-worker to assure safety (for example, in an emergency); monitoring for errors; a flashing light on the telephone; transportation training; and child care for her son. The special educator and rehabilitation counselor provided training to the employer and other employees, who, in turn, agreed to provide the natural supports Marcia needed and develop the visual clues for the steps of the job.

The occupational therapist and the family developed a plan for Marcia to learn how to travel using the city buses. The social worker identified a good low-cost child care setting, and the Department of Social Services agreed to cost-share these services with Marcia (who receives SSI) until one year after graduation. The social worker also agreed to coordinate Marcia's participation in a parenting class offered by the Health Department. The IEP team recommended a consultation with a representative from the Social Security Administration (SSA) to provide guidance on benefits and the use of any work incentives.

The local school agreed to provide a job coach initially, and the Department of Mental Retardation Services agreed to pick up this cost six months prior to graduation. The rehabilitation counselor, who specializes in working with students with hearing impairments, agreed to act as job monitor for this placement and to follow up with adult education or the Literacy Council for Marcia's continued education options. The rehabilitation counselor continued to work with Marcia, and by the time she exited school Marcia had secured a full-time position at the business.

**Planning for employment (Marcia's Plan):** Things that this student needs include the following:

- **Assessment** that identifies current strengths, needs, interests, and preferences for post-school employment, independent living, and postsecondary training and/or education.

- **Development** of job and job placement options and awareness of skills needed.

- **Matching** of student and job.

- School- and work-based **training and preparation**.

- **Placement** and **follow-along**.

Actions the high school transition team may recommend to meet these needs include the following:

- Assessment

  - Interview youth regarding vocational interests and preferences (use other methods to assess interests and preferences of nonverbal students)

  - Conduct situational assessment (observation in a work setting) to assess endurance, strength, aptitude, social skills, interests, interactions

- Conduct formal vocational evaluation by a trained evaluator
- Self-assessment
- Develop student's awareness of different jobs
- Discuss health care issues that may impact employment

- Development
  - Analyze local labor market (contact employment services for state and request information for the region; contact local vocational advisory council; contact local chamber of commerce; review local want ads; contact employment agencies) to identify job openings and local labor needs
  - Get a range of work experiences: explorations, job shadowing, mentoring, and internships
  - Identify community programs offering job placement or training
  - Build network of employer and community program contacts
  - Provide training to employers on issues related to employees with disabilities

- Matching
  - Analyze the demands and expectations of the job site (e.g., duties, skill requirements, hours, location, transportation, wages, benefits, social skills)
  - List the supports the student needs to be successful on the job
  - Match the student's assessment and the list of needed supports to the job demands, including transportation to the job
  - Identify current gaps and needs for success
  - Identify needed natural supports, job accommodations, adaptive equipment, and support services

- Training and preparation
  - Provide instruction to youth on job-seeking skills
  - Provide community-based work experiences related to career development
  - Identify potential service providers

507

- Provide natural supports and accommodations
- Provide instruction and training (pre-employment or on-the-job)
- Placement and follow-along
  - Work with employer to determine employee's response to the job demands and identify strategies to capitalize on strengths and minimize limitations
  - Provide natural supports and accommodations
  - Monitor progress and readiness for job advancement
  - Monitor changing need for natural supports
  - Make adjustments, as needed

### *Carlos's Plan for College*

Carlos, a sixteen-year-old junior in high school with a significant learning disability, plans to attend college upon graduation. Carlos loves working with computers and demonstrates skill and interest in using computers for graphic design. (Carlos's team includes him and his family, guidance counselor, independent living center representative, postsecondary education support services provider, and a student with a learning disability who had graduated two years ago and is currently attending college.)

Since Carlos is interested in pursuing a career involving computers, but is still undecided about what he would like to major in, the guidance counselor provided a list of colleges that offer a variety of computer-related degrees, including graphic design, programming, and management information systems. Carlos agreed to attend the local College Fair, and his family agreed to take him to visit campuses and observe and inquire regarding the support Carlos may need.

The team agreed that, in order to be successful in college, Carlos would need a college that offered small class size, student mentoring services, and note-taking services. The team agreed that Carlos had depended on others to advocate for him. They recommended that Carlos improve his self-advocacy skills. The representative from the Center for Independent Living invited Carlos to participate in their next self-advocacy program as a means of meeting this transition service need, and the school division agreed to pay for the costs of this service.

The postsecondary service provider told Carlos, his family, and the other professionals that a local college was offering an orientation for new students that would give Carlos an idea of the demands of the college setting. Funding for this was possibly available from the local advocacy group representing individuals with learning disabilities. The special educator reported that the advocacy group was looking for individuals to apply to their program. The guidance counselor set up an appointment with the family, to discuss options for college financial assistance.

**Planning for education after high school (Carlos's plan):** Things that this student needs include the following:

- **Assessment** that identifies strengths, needs, interests, and preferences for postsecondary education

- **Development** of postsecondary education options

- **Matching** of student and postsecondary education setting

- **Preparation** for postsecondary education

- **Placement** and **follow-along**

Actions the high school transition team may recommend to meet these needs include the following:

- Assessment
  - Assess student's self-advocacy skills, academic preparation, and college bound test scores
  - Assess student's technical skills, social skills, independent living skills
  - Interview youth regarding educational setting interests and preferences—size, setting, programs (use other methods to assess interests and preferences if student is nonverbal)
  - Identify youth's long-term career goals
  - Develop a list of supports student needs to achieve postsecondary education goals
  - Discuss health care issues that may impact student in postsecondary setting
  - Identify needed natural supports, academic or physical accommodations, and support services

- Development
  - Visit campuses
  - Participate in college night
  - Have college students with disabilities talk to youth
  - Research colleges and universities that offer special services to students with disabilities
  - Discuss financial issues
  - Discuss preferred location of college
- Matching
  - Analyze the demands and expectations of the postsecondary education setting—accessibility, support services availability, academic rigor, social culture, independent living setting
  - Match the student's assessment and list of needed supports to the demands of the postsecondary education setting
- Preparation
  - Provide developmental academic support and coursework needed to prepare for postsecondary education goals
  - Assist youth with applications, interviews, and test preparation
  - Identify potential service providers
  - Develop natural supports
  - Provide self-advocacy training
- Placement and follow-along
  - Monitor progress in the postsecondary setting
  - Monitor changing need for natural supports
  - Monitor changing need for services
  - Advocate for changes and adjustments, as needed

### Mark's Independence

Mark, a twenty-year-old youth with mental retardation, will be finishing high school next year. Mark has long expressed a strong desire to live independently after leaving high school. His older brother has his own apartment, and Mark associates living on his own with being an adult. Living independently is part of Mark's transition plan, which also includes employment and attending a community recreation program for adults with disabilities.

Two years ago Mark's family, working on the advice of the other IEP team members, put him on a waiting list to be matched with other individuals who are looking for housing. Over the past three years, the IEP team has worked on improving Mark's advocacy and independent living skills. Mark's family contacted the local Arc and was able to connect with a mentor to help Mark strengthen his self-advocacy skills. The occupational therapist at school focused on improving the critical living skills Mark needed to live on his own.

At the beginning of this school year, Mark's family contacted the county agency that serves adults with disabilities. The agency assigned a service coordinator (sometimes called a case manager) to work with Mark and his IEP team. The service coordinator, along with the IEP team, determined the level and types of support Mark needed, and arranged for the necessary supports he needed to keep a job and live with others. The IEP team, including Mark's family and the service coordinator, determined that Mark could live with individuals with other disabilities in a house or apartment on a cost-share basis as long as he received daily assistance. A residential support person would visit Mark every day to monitor that his needs were being met, to help with finances and nutrition, and to set up recreational activities.

Mark also would need training on how to use the city transit system, so he could travel independently from home to job and the community recreation center. His IEP team established an IEP goal for Mark to learn how to use public transportation. The Department of Rehabilitative Services counselor reported that rehabilitation services could assist Mark in purchasing the assistive devices he will need on the job. The service coordinator agreed to monitor Mark's integration into the community over the year following graduation.

**Planning for living independently (Mark's plan):** Things that this student needs include the following:

- **Assessment** that identifies strengths, needs, interests, and preferences for adult and independent living, including recreation and leisure

- **Development** of adult living placement options, including recreation and leisure (not needed immediately, but for planning purposes)

511

- **Matching** of youth to adult living placement options, including recreation and leisure

- **Training** and **preparation** for adult living

- **Placement** and **follow-along**

Actions the high school transition team may recommend to meet these needs include the following:

- Assessment

  - Interview youth and family regarding adult and independent living interests and preferences (use other methods to assess interests and preferences if student is nonverbal)

  - Observe youth in independent living or recreational setting

  - Interview youth and family regarding medical needs

  - Interview youth and family regarding financial plans

  - Identify transportation skills and needs

  - Develop a list of supports student needs to be successful

  - Identify needed natural supports, accommodations, and support services

- Development

  - Analyze adult living options in the local area (for example, group homes, supported living homes, roommates)

  - Analyze locality for leisure/recreation options in the local area

  - Coordinate with other families and youth looking for adult living options

  - Provide training and education for families and youth regarding living and financial options for transition-aged youth

  - Analyze community for transportation options

- Matching

  - Analyze the demands and expectations of the adult living and community participation options

  - Match the student's assessment and list of supports to the demands and expectations of these options

- Training and preparation
  - Provide instruction to prepare youth to enter identified adult living and community options
  - Identify potential service providers for needed supports and accommodations
  - Develop natural supports
  - Provide opportunities to participate in the community in the identified settings
- Placement and follow-along
  - Monitor progress
  - Monitor changing need for natural supports
  - Monitor changing need for services
  - Make adjustments, as needed

## How to Find Resources in Your Community

Creating a dynamic transition plan like the three described here is not easy. Keep in mind that in many places needed services have long waiting lists or are simply unavailable. Unlike school services, adult services are not mandated by federal law. Transition team members must keep digging, networking broadly, and thinking creatively in order to help each young adult live as productively, independently, and happily as possible. Knowing a wide range of possible contributors will be the key to creating a collaborative transition plan with supports tailored to an individual's needs.

Your school district should have much information on transition services that are typically used, such as transportation services and housing. Team members should talk with special education teachers and administrators, as well as parents who have already gone through the transition process with their son or daughter. Team members can then focus their efforts on personalizing and supplementing with other nontraditional services and resources to meet the student's transition goals. It is important that transition teams look beyond familiar agencies and services when exploring supports for individuals with disabilities. Yet the team must also be selective and choose supports that reflect the individual student's needs.

Sometimes, finding transition services or options resembles detective work. Transition team members, especially the parents, students, and special educators, may need to make phone calls to agencies and organizations and take notes. The white, blue, and yellow pages of the local phone book are a good tool for discovering transition resources. The following section provides some helpful hints on how to find possible service providers or programs.

Modern technology can enhance planning. For example, local libraries have information on local government, and many now have computers with internet access. Increasingly, agencies and organizations use websites and e-mail to find and share information. Some of the terms listed below may also be useful in key word searches on the internet.

## *Let Your Fingers Do the Walking in Transition Planning*

**White pages:** The table of contents may include references such as "Community Service Numbers" or "Disabilities, Services for Individuals with."

Some of the headings you will find that might relate to the varying service needs of youth with disabilities include the following:

- Adult Protection
- Disabilities Services
- Education
- Employment
- Financial Aid
- Handicapped/Disabled
- Housing
- Human Rights
- Human Services
- Mental Health and Mental Retardation
- Recreational/Social Development
- Rehabilitation
- Social Security Administration
- Social Services
- Transportation
- Volunteer Opportunities

**Blue pages:** Local, state, and federal government listings can always be found in the blue pages of the phone book. Local listings might have some of the following headings:

- Employment Opportunities and Information
- Housing
- Human Resource Management
- Mayor's Office on Disability
- Social Services

State listings might have some of the following headings:

- Children
- Clinics
- Education
- Health Services
- Housing
- Labor
- Libraries
- Museums and Theaters
- Social Services

Local, state, and federal government listings will include numbers for all state and government agencies. Examples of these would be as follows:

- Employment Commission
- Medicaid
- Mental Health
- Mental Retardation
- Rehabilitation Services
- Social Services
- Transitional Living Center
- Transportation Department
- Vocational Evaluation Center

**Yellow pages.** Check out the index of commonly used terms. Using key words, here are a few examples of what you might find:

- *Disability:* Access Unlimited; Adult Care Services; Assisted Living; Charter's Mobility Center; Paradapt Services

- *Associations:* Arc; Boy Scouts; Families for Children with Mental Health Concerns; Information and Referral—United Way; Learning Disabilities Council; Neighborhood Housing Services

- *Mental Health:* Alliance for the Mentally Ill

Part of transition planning involves collecting information from the community to use for both immediate needs and anticipated needs. However, sometimes making a "cold" phone call to get information can be intimidating. The following phone interview guide will give you some ideas on how to gather information.

Some state disability rights agencies provide information and referral services. National information services, such as the National Dissemination Center for Children with Disabilities (NICHCY) and the National Center on Secondary Education and Transition, offer websites to provide users with easy access to information. Every state has a parent training and information center, known as the PTI, where people can call to get information on agencies and services within their state. PTIs also offer training in transition planning, as do other major disability groups such as the Arc, United Cerebral Palsy (UCP), Centers for Independent Living, and others.

## Transition Services Phone Interview Guide

When you are starting your cold calling and search for service providers, start with agencies that can refer you to other organizations, such as vocational rehabilitation or an independent living center.

Name of Organization

Name of Person You Spoke with

Position

Address

Phone Number

Fax Number

Date Contacted

Sample phone script:

"Hello, this is (your name). I am a (teacher, parent, family member, administrator, coordinator) of a youth (young adult) who is" [OR if you are the student, then "I am"] (exploring career options, exploring where to live after graduation, interested in a recreational program, or whatever fits your ultimate goals). I am looking for information to help in planning for my (own, son's, daughter's, family member's, student's) future. I found your organization through (another agency, the yellow pages, a publication) and I am interested in learning more about what services you provide (or what your organization does). Could you tell me who in your organization I should talk to about this? Thank you.

Please tell me about your agency/organization. Who do you serve? What services do you offer?

How does one get involved with your agency/organization? Are there special eligibility or admission requirements? How does one apply?

Are there costs involved in participating in your agency's or organization's programs? If so, how much are they? Do you offer special rates?

Do you have any ideas about how your agency or organization might help meet a need such as: [Describe a specific problem or need that you might have, for example: youth has a visual disability and needs assistance changing buses; youth has physical disability and is interested in playing a sport; teen parent with a learning disability needs child care so that she can go to work after school; and so forth.]

Could you refer me to some other people, agencies, or organizations that might offer some services to meet this need?

Do you have any written materials describing your agency (or organization)? If so, could you please send them to me [your name] at [your address]? Thank you for speaking with me today. This information is very helpful in planning my (own, student's, son's, daughter's) future as a member of our community. Best wishes for fulfilling your agency's (or organization's) mission.

## Community-Level Transition Teams

While many people are involved in helping improve transition services for students at an individual level, there is a movement to improve the transition system at the community level. Many states have created community groups that help with planning at the local level. They may be called by different names, such as "community transition team," "interagency community council," or "local transition advisory group." No matter what they're called, these teams usually include representatives from disability-related agencies and the community who come together with the mission of improving the transition of young adults with disabilities from school to adult life. The idea behind developing these community transition teams has been that they are operated locally and therefore are able to:

- Share resources and funding,
- Hold information fairs,
- Try out new ways of serving youths and young adults, and
- Help change or influence policies and procedures.

Transition teams can be a strong force within the community. Their primary purpose is to assess how a community's transition services system works and to develop policies and procedures to make this system work better. They can identify the best ways to meet the needs of youth with disabilities leaving the local schools within their community. They can promote actions through school boards and other governmental entities in areas such as policy and funding.

To find out if your community has a transition team and how you can get involved, contact one of the following:

- Your local school or school district's department of special education: Ask to talk to the person in charge of the transition of students with disabilities in the district.
- Your state's Parent Training and Information Center (PTI)
- Your State Transition Systems-Change Project

If a community-level transition team does not already exist in your area, you can take steps to create one. When participating agencies and the community at large support community transition teams, they have the potential to create a well-connected, culturally diverse, and very responsive transition services system. Here are some steps you can take to get a community transition team started:

- **Find out what your community is already doing.** Assess the range of transition services going on in your school and community by talking with school professionals, parents, and community and parent groups.

- **Identify areas that need improvement.** Decide what

transition services are lacking and which of these service gaps you want to address.

- **Make a plan.** Talk with school professionals, parents, community and parent groups, and others about ways to address these service gaps (e.g., starting a career development center at school, holding information meetings, doing research on other communities' transition systems).

- **Measure your success.** Agree on what you will use to determine if your efforts are successful (e.g., every student will be involved in at least three job shadowing experiences, the school district will hold two transition information fairs each year).

## Conclusion: Taking the First Steps

To improve transition results for young people with disabilities, individual transition team members and community transition team members must work creatively. Many services exist in every community. If transition team members cultivate relationships with these resources and combine successful teamwork methods with the services available in their community, they will be able to create dynamic individual plans. Here are some starting steps.

### Students

- Write down your long-term goals and what you think you need to do to reach these.

- Read your IEP and transition plan and decide if the plan is being implemented.

- Tell your teachers you want to lead your own IEP meeting and ask them to help you learn what to do.

- Learn about your civil rights under the law, such as the Americans with Disabilities Act.

- Learn about your disability, how to explain to people your strengths, and how to ask for reasonable accommodations.

- Practice job interviews and/or asking for accommodations.

- Talk with your doctor and parents about your health care needs so you will be ready to take responsibility for them.

- Ask your teacher how to get involved with your community's transition team.

## Family Members

- Observe your son or daughter's independent living skills, work behaviors, social involvement, dreams, and hopes.

- Call your child's teachers and ask that transition services, including financial planning, be addressed at your next meeting.

- Help your child learn about his or her disability and how to ask for the supports he or she needs.

- Give your child responsibility for chores at home.

- Role-play different situations with your child (e.g., interviews).

- Discuss your child's medical needs with him or her and facilitate discussions with your doctor.

- Introduce your child to adult role models with disabilities.

- Look in your phone book and Yellow Pages and identify three new possible resources to help your son or daughter's transition to adult activities.

## School or Agency Administrators

- Evaluate transition services in your system.

- Look into establishing or strengthening your community transition team.

- Make a phone call to develop a new community agency contact.

- Find some funding to share across agencies or for service development.

- Set up a meeting with staff members to learn each person's expertise in transition.

- Develop a cooperative agreement with another agency specifying how to coordinate transition.

- Encourage your staff to be creative in problem solving.

## Special Educators

- Talk to students and families about transition services.

- Ask to attend a conference, workshop, or other learning opportunity related to transition.

- Teach students about their civil rights under the law, such as the Americans with Disabilities Act.

- Pledge to conduct collaborative, needs-based IEP meetings that empower youth and families.

- Provide youth with step-by-step activities that familiarize them with the IEP process and prepare them to take active roles.

- Call the local rehabilitation counselor or mental retardation case manager and coordinate a meeting.

- Use the phone interview guide presented earlier in this publication and call one community agency or resource.

### *Vocational Educators/Educators*

- Contact a special educator and find out when IEPs are scheduled for your current or future students.

- Offer to provide a tour of your program and share your knowledge and expertise in job competencies, job development, and job placement.

- Identify one student receiving special education services and work with him or her to provide vocational counseling to help define realistic career goals.

- Develop a plan to coordinate your work-study program with all the special education community-based work programs.

### *Guidance Counselors*

- Create a workshop for students on self-advocacy skills that would promote success in postsecondary education or employment settings.

- Ask to attend a workshop, in-service, or other training to learn about community agencies and resources.

- Ask a college representative about services for students with disabilities.

### *Community Agency Service Providers*

- Attend a workshop, in-service, or other training to learn about community agencies and resources.

- Develop a folder that contains some of the wealth of information you have about community resources and how to access them, and share with IEP team members, transition councils, families, students, and administrators.

- Identify three things that could help you actively participate in the IEP process when appropriate, and share these with the high school administrator or special educator/transition specialist.

### *Vocational Rehabilitation Counselors*

- Schedule regular office hours at schools with which you work.

- Support activities and use of assistive technology for students in high school that result in employment.

- Serve on a local transition committee.

- Share your knowledge of the job market and job assessments.

### *Any of the Above*

- Identify two ways you can add to the collaborative transition planning process; share this with administrators, special educators/transition specialists, or other service providers.

- Offer to take the lead to develop a community transition resource directory for your community.

- Most of all, take any one proactive step in your community toward collaborative transition planning and observe the results.

You can work to improve the system of transition services both at the individual level and in your community. It's worth it!

## Notes

1. This legal overview was taken directly from the approved OSEP IDEA 97 Training Package, Module 9, pp. 9-11 through 9-13. This document is available from NICHCY.

Chapter 43

# Postsecondary Education for People with Autism

## Chapter Contents

Section 43.1—Preparing for Postsecondary Education
If You Have Disabilities: Know Your Rights
and Responsibilities ........................................... 524

Section 43.2—Lessons Learned: A Parent's Report
Regarding Her Son's First Year at College ....... 530

Section 43.1

# Preparing for Postsecondary Education If You Have Disabilities: Know Your Rights and Responsibilities

Reprinted from "Students with Disabilities Preparing for Postsecondary Education: Know Your Rights and Responsibilities," U.S. Department of Education, June 2006.

More and more high school students with disabilities are planning to continue their education in postsecondary schools, including vocational and career schools, two- and four- year colleges, and universities. As a student with a disability, you need to be well informed about your rights and responsibilities as well as the responsibilities postsecondary schools have toward you. Being well informed will help ensure you have a full opportunity to enjoy the benefits of the postsecondary education experience without confusion or delay.

This section explains the rights and responsibilities of students with disabilities who are preparing to attend postsecondary schools. It also explains the obligations of a postsecondary school to provide academic adjustments, including auxiliary aids and services, to ensure the school does not discriminate on the basis of disability.

The Office for Civil Rights (OCR) in the U.S. Department of Education enforces Section 504 of the Rehabilitation Act of 1973 (Section 504) and Title II of the Americans with Disabilities Act of 1990 (Title II), which prohibit discrimination on the basis of disability. Practically every school district and postsecondary school in the United States is subject to one or both of these laws, which have similar requirements.[1]

Although both school districts and postsecondary schools must comply with these same laws, the responsibilities of postsecondary schools are significantly different from those of school districts.

Moreover, you will have responsibilities as a postsecondary student that you do not have as a high school student. OCR strongly encourages you to know your responsibilities and those of postsecondary schools under Section 504 and Title II. Doing so will improve your opportunity to succeed as you enter postsecondary education.

The following questions and answers provide more specific information to help you succeed.

### As a student with a disability leaving high school and entering postsecondary education, will I see differences in my rights and how they are addressed?

Yes. Section 504 and Title II protect elementary, secondary, and postsecondary students from discrimination. Nevertheless, several of the requirements that apply through high school are different from the requirements that apply beyond high school. For instance, Section 504 requires a school district to provide a free appropriate public education (FAPE) to each child with a disability in the district's jurisdiction. Whatever the disability, a school district must identify an individual's education needs and provide any regular or special education and related aids and services necessary to meet those needs as well as it is meeting the needs of students without disabilities.

Unlike your high school, your postsecondary school is not required to provide FAPE. Rather, your postsecondary school is required to provide appropriate academic adjustments as necessary to ensure that it does not discriminate on the basis of disability. In addition, if your postsecondary school provides housing to nondisabled students, it must provide comparable, convenient, and accessible housing to students with disabilities at the same cost.

Other important differences you need to know, even before you arrive at your postsecondary school, are addressed in the remaining questions.

### May a postsecondary school deny my admission because I have a disability?

No. If you meet the essential requirements for admission, a postsecondary school may not deny your admission simply because you have a disability.

### Do I have to inform a postsecondary school that I have a disability?

No. However, if you want the school to provide an academic adjustment, you must identify yourself as having a disability. Likewise, you should let the school know about your disability if you want to ensure that you are assigned to accessible facilities. In any event, your disclosure of a disability is always voluntary.

## What academic adjustments must a postsecondary school provide?

The appropriate academic adjustment must be determined based on your disability and individual needs. Academic adjustments may include auxiliary aids and modifications to academic requirements as are necessary to ensure equal educational opportunity. Examples of such adjustments are arranging for priority registration; reducing a course load; substituting one course for another; providing note takers, recording devices, sign language interpreters, extended time for testing, and, if telephones are provided in dorm rooms, a TTY in your dorm room; and equipping school computers with screen-reading, voice recognition, or other adaptive software or hardware.

In providing an academic adjustment, your postsecondary school is not required to lower or effect substantial modifications to essential requirements. For example, although your school may be required to provide extended testing time, it is not required to change the substantive content of the test. In addition, your postsecondary school does not have to make modifications that would fundamentally alter the nature of a service, program or activity or would result in undue financial or administrative burdens. Finally, your postsecondary school does not have to provide personal attendants, individually prescribed devices, readers for personal use or study, or other devices or services of a personal nature, such as tutoring and typing.

## If I want an academic adjustment, what must I do?

You must inform the school that you have a disability and need an academic adjustment. Unlike your school district, your postsecondary school is not required to identify you as having a disability or assess your needs.

Your postsecondary school may require you to follow reasonable procedures to request an academic adjustment. You are responsible for knowing and following these procedures. Postsecondary schools usually include, in their publications providing general information, information on the procedures and contacts for requesting an academic adjustment. Such publications include recruitment materials, catalogs, and student handbooks, and are often available on school websites. Many schools also have staff whose purpose is to assist students with disabilities. If you are unable to locate the procedures, ask a school official, such as an admissions officer or counselor.

### *When should I request an academic adjustment?*

Although you may request an academic adjustment from your postsecondary school at any time, you should request it as early as possible. Some academic adjustments may take more time to provide than others. You should follow your school's procedures to ensure that your school has enough time to review your request and provide an appropriate academic adjustment.

### *Do I have to prove that I have a disability to obtain an academic adjustment?*

Generally, yes. Your school will probably require you to provide documentation that shows you have a current disability and need an academic adjustment.

### *What documentation should I provide?*

Schools may set reasonable standards for documentation. Some schools require more documentation than others. They may require you to provide documentation prepared by an appropriate professional, such as a medical doctor, psychologist, or other qualified diagnostician. The required documentation may include one or more of the following: a diagnosis of your current disability; the date of the diagnosis; how the diagnosis was reached; the credentials of the professional; how your disability affects a major life activity; and how the disability affects your academic performance. The documentation should provide enough information for you and your school to decide what is an appropriate academic adjustment.

Although an Individualized Education Program (IEP) or Section 504 plan, if you have one, may help identify services that have been effective for you, it generally is not sufficient documentation. This is because postsecondary education presents different demands than high school education, and what you need to meet these new demands may be different. Also, in some cases the nature of a disability may change.

If the documentation that you have does not meet the postsecondary school's requirements, a school official must tell you in a timely manner what additional documentation you need to provide. You may need a new evaluation in order to provide the required documentation.

### *Who has to pay for a new evaluation?*

Neither your high school nor your postsecondary school is required to conduct or pay for a new evaluation to document your disability and need for an academic adjustment. This may mean that you have to pay or find funding to pay an appropriate professional for an evaluation. If you are eligible for services through your state vocational rehabilitation agency, you may qualify for an evaluation at no cost to you.

### *Once the school has received the necessary documentation from me, what should I expect?*

The school will review your request in light of the essential requirements for the relevant program to help determine an appropriate academic adjustment. It is important to remember that the school is not required to lower or waive essential requirements. If you have requested a specific academic adjustment, the school may offer that academic adjustment or an alternative one if the alternative would also be effective. The school may also conduct its own evaluation of your disability and needs at its own expense.

You should expect your school to work with you in an interactive process to identify an appropriate academic adjustment. Unlike the experience you may have had in high school, however, do not expect your postsecondary school to invite your parents to participate in the process or to develop an IEP for you.

### *What if the academic adjustment we identified is not working?*

Let the school know as soon as you become aware that the results are not what you expected. It may be too late to correct the problem if you wait until the course or activity is completed. You and your school should work together to resolve the problem.

### *May a postsecondary school charge me for providing an academic adjustment?*

No. Furthermore, it may not charge students with disabilities more for participating in its programs or activities than it charges students who do not have disabilities.

### *What can I do if I believe the school is discriminating against me?*

Practically every postsecondary school must have a person—frequently called the Section 504 coordinator, ADA coordinator, or disability services coordinator—who coordinates the school's compliance with Section 504 or Title II or both laws. You may contact this person for information about how to address your concerns.

The school must also have grievance procedures. These procedures are not the same as the due process procedures with which you may be familiar from high school. However, the postsecondary school's grievance procedures must include steps to ensure that you may raise your concerns fully and fairly and must provide for the prompt and equitable resolution of complaints.

School publications, such as student handbooks and catalogs, usually describe the steps you must take to start the grievance process. Often, schools have both formal and informal processes. If you decide to use a grievance process, you should be prepared to present all the reasons that support your request.

If you are dissatisfied with the outcome from using the school's grievance procedures or you wish to pursue an alternative to using the grievance procedures, you may file a complaint against the school with OCR or in a court.

Students with disabilities who know their rights and responsibilities are much better equipped to succeed in postsecondary school. We encourage you to work with the staff at your school because they, too, want you to succeed. Seek the support of family, friends, and fellow students, including those with disabilities. Know your talents and capitalize on them, and believe in yourself as you embrace new challenges in your education.

## Notes

1.  You may be familiar with another federal law that applies to the education of students with disabilities—the Individuals with Disabilities Education Act (IDEA). That law is administered by the Office of Special Education Programs in the Office of Special Education and Rehabilitative Services in the U.S. Department of Education. The IDEA and its Individualized Education Program (IEP) provisions do not apply to postsecondary schools. This section does not discuss the IDEA or state and local laws that may apply.

Section 43.2

# Lessons Learned: A Parent's Report Regarding Her Son's First Year at College

Reprinted from "First Year of College: Lessons Learned," © 2003 Coulter Video. Reprinted with permission. Julie Coulter is the writer of "The College Prep Portfolio," which helps students prepare throughout high school to apply for college. You can find more articles on her website at www .coultervideo.com.

My husband and I began a new phase in life when our son left home to attend college. After struggling with attention deficit disorder (ADD) and Asperger syndrome through special education programs in a mainstream environment for thirteen years, he had graduated from high school successfully. We're proud of his hard work and the steps he took to get to college. We're very grateful to all the high school teachers who helped our son prepare for college. We're also very thankful for college programs for students with special needs.

Students and parents have many decisions to make as they evaluate college programs. We visited several colleges and our son applied to four schools. He chose to attend a small liberal arts college with special services programs and without traditional fraternity and sorority life. He also chose to live on campus.

Many special needs students have had a hard time socially in high school and are ready for a change and to make a fresh start. Parents can help a student approach these changes with a positive attitude and outlook. Parents can also help a student start off the new experience on the "right foot" by helping their son or daughter plan and organize for a new life on campus. Our son was looking forward to this change and to exercising his independence from us. We have to keep reminding ourselves that our children need to learn to function independently. Many parents struggle with giving up control of their student's day-to-day activities and encouraging independence. After our son's first week at college and hearing him tell me "Go get a job! Go make a quilt!" I realized quickly that I had been "fired" from one role and had a new role to play.

## First Semester Preparation—Living on Campus

When students decide to live on campus, they have to decide whether to have a roommate or request a single room. Our son decided to have a roommate in spite of the recommendation from the high school child study team for a single room. He completed the survey sent by the college to determine his likes and dislikes, sleep habits, whether he is messy or neat, and musical taste. He also had to indicate the type of dorm he preferred: single sex or co-ed, smoking or nonsmoking, alcohol free or alcohol allowed (for those over age twenty-one). The college staff assigned our son a roommate who also has Asperger syndrome. After he had been in school for a few weeks, I asked, "How's your roommate doing?" He replied, "I don't know! We're two guys with Asperger, Mom—we don't talk!" Students may need some guidance in interpersonal relationships to help them get along in the dorm. Our son had an experience with another student, who also has Asperger syndrome, who began to hang out in a particular student's room to play a computer game he liked. The student with Asperger syndrome did not understand when he had become a nuisance to the other student, who did not want to have constant visitors in his room. Our son learned to put on his headphones when his neighbors blasted music he did not want to hear.

## Dorm Room Organization

If your student will live on campus and struggles with organization, you may need to help arrange his or her dorm room before leaving the campus. Students need to limit the amount of "stuff" that they take to the dorm! Many students can use the campus computer labs rather than having a computer in their room. We visited several colleges that provided computers to students as a part of their tuition fee.

Our son's dorm room was small, the desk did not easily accommodate a computer and printer, and we quickly filled the available closet and storage areas. We made many trips to stores and a lumberyard to buy organizing bins, stacking shelves, and wood. We added sections of wood to raise the bed up (the bed risers we had purchased didn't fit the bed) and placed bins under the bed for books. We added wood to the desk to build surfaces with different heights to accommodate the computer and printer and still leave a space for writing. We had not thought to take tools with us so we recommend carrying your toolbox along! We admired the handiwork of two students who had built loft frames and hoisted their beds up on the frames and put their desks under the beds. We bought laundry hampers, detergent, a small ironing board, and an iron. Later, our son found out that irons were not allowed in the dorm. If students will have to use a hall bathroom, they will need a caddy to carry personal grooming items back and forth between their rooms and the bathroom. We also bought closet organizers to make the best use of the small closet space.

## Personal Records

We organized a binder for our son to keep important information such as medical information, insurance forms, important addresses and phone numbers, preprinted mail labels for family members and postage stamps, bank account records, a "to do" list and calendar listing of family birthdays.

## Students, Counselors, and Self-Advocacy

A thoughtful college counselor recently reminded me that unlike high school, colleges have to "provide access, not success." I think this difference between high school and college is important for students to understand. Transition programs in high school vary tremendously and many students with special needs have not learned to advocate for themselves. Many students have depended upon parents for all interaction between school staff and are not experienced in discussing the accommodations they need in the classroom. The students must learn to advocate for themselves, by practicing explaining their special needs and their classroom accommodations, as they will have to communicate with new professors every semester.

The college counselors and advisors may recognize the level of the student's self-advocacy skills as they interview the student. Both college counselors and academic advisors can assist students by providing written documentation of "things to do" to reinforce the responsibility of the student in assuring his or her needs for accommodations are met in the classroom. Talking with counselors and professors will also assist the student in getting ready for the workplace and learning when and how to discuss Asperger syndrome with future employers.

Many students with Asperger syndrome go to college carrying their "baggage" of primary and secondary school experiences, which has shaped their attitude and their view of the world. They may have struggled academically and socially. If they experienced teasing, they may be wary of other students and reluctant to seek help if they encounter problems. The special services staff can help students with

Asperger syndrome by establishing anti-hazing guidelines on campus and giving students a list of people to contact and a place to go for help if hazing occurs. Our son received several crank phone calls, which he reported to the dorm's resident director. The resident director held a dorm meeting and advised everyone that students who participated in this type of behavior could be expelled from school. College counselors and parents can encourage students to seek out counseling if needed.

## Medication Management

Parents and students need to discuss how to manage students' medication while they are in college. Students need to know how to maintain their medication supply and may have to find a new physician if they are away from home. Changes in medication may not be a good idea for first semester—as we discovered the hard way! Parents should make sure that the student knows how to access student health services on campus.

## Preparing College Staff

Students and parents need to find out if the teaching staff of the college has knowledge of Asperger syndrome, either during the application process or upon acceptance and determination to attend a specific school. At our son's school, Dorothy Wells, the director of disability services, provides a binder of teaching tips to professors for all disabilities represented by the student population and she wrote a new section to cover Asperger syndrome. If needed, the student can provide documentation or resources to the college staff on Asperger syndrome and autism spectrum disorders. Ms. Wells also conducted an in-service for staff, including residential dorm personnel, to review the needs of students with Asperger syndrome, and suggested ways of handling potential problems in the classrooms and dorms. If the college has part-time or adjunct professors, the special services staff may have a harder time getting the information to all personnel.

## Special Education Services and Academic Advisors

Usually, colleges have a separate process for students to apply for special education services. Colleges may request a copy of the high school Individualized Education Program (IEP) but depend more upon educational and psychological testing results to determine a student's eligibility for services. Colleges need to see recent test data, preferably completed during the student's senior year.

During high school, the family depended upon the case manager to communicate classroom accommodations for students with the teaching staff. In college, the student has to take over the communication part of that role. The college special services personnel need to explain the "Letter of Accommodation" process to students. These letters go to professors to detail the classroom accommodations for which the student has demonstrated a need. Such needs are determined by the special services staff based on the educational and psychological testing data. The student must take his or her classroom schedule to special services staff, who will then prepare the "Letter of Accommodation" for professors. The student is responsible for providing the letter to each of his or her professors. Students need to learn that they must provide the information to the professor about their disability and their need for accommodations in the classroom. Some students prefer to provide information about their strengths and weaknesses to their professors in writing. The students are responsible for repeating this process during every semester's registration process.

The students also need a clear understanding of the type of special education services provided by the college. Some programs require mandatory attendance by the student and cost an additional amount based on the services provided. Some colleges provide the services to all students who have demonstrated the need for accommodation at no extra charge. If the student has demonstrated a need for special assistance such as a note-taker, then he or she must provide a copy of his or her schedule to the special services staff so that the college can arrange to provide that service. At our son's school, if a student who has a note-taker decides to cut class, the note-taker leaves the class after waiting fifteen minutes. Having a note-taker doesn't give a student a free ride! Students will need to locate academic resource centers and obtain a written explanation of the type of services available for students. Our son resisted seeking help from the resource center in spite of our weekly pleas for him to get help. He did not understand the meaning of "academic resource center" and thought that it meant psychological counseling, so he refused to go for help. He also was tired of "special ed" and just wanted to be a regular student.

As many students with Asperger syndrome have problems with change and transitions, college staff can assist these students when they arrive on campus by providing clear written information prior to their arrival so that they have the opportunity to read and study the information with their family before arriving on campus. This packet should include: schedules of orientation programs, maps of campus, directions for checking into dorms, explanation of the class registration process, outlining the academic advisor role, and course selection. The college should invite students to meet the special services personnel during the orientation to campus. The students need a clear understanding of the registration process and alternatives to take if they cannot get into the classes they originally chose. During orientation for parents, the college staff will need to explain to parents and students the Family Educational Rights and Privacy Act (FERPA) law and the waiver that students can sign which will allow college staff to talk to parents about their student, if needed. The college can also provide contact information for school staff to the parents.

During our son's freshman orientation, the staff used the vehicle of a scavenger hunt game to help the students locate the buildings on campus, which only encouraged the students to run around quickly to finish the scavenger hunt rather than actually learning what happened in each building. We suggest a tour of the academic resource center and a written guide to explain the services available to students, including special software, computer programs, and tutoring. The students with Asperger syndrome may not ask questions or seek help.

Students need help in understanding the academic course selection and advising process. We spent a lot of energy and time dealing with so many nonacademic issues that we did not spend enough time preparing our son for the choice of academic courses. We helped him create a basic plan, which had to change when he registered. Advisors will assist the students in choosing academic courses and how to develop a two- or four-year plan for their academic program. The student needs to ask his or her advisor what to do in case a course needs changing and about the calendar deadline for those changes. Taking a lighter class load may help the student adjust to college life. As we visited colleges, we found that many regular education students take longer than four years to complete their degree programs. The special needs student who takes a lighter class load may need to attend college for ten semesters. Students also need to learn how to calculate grade point average and need to know the expected grade point average needed for graduation.

Students may need to meet with the special services staff after the first month of school to check on their status and adjustment to college life and their ability to communicate with school staff. The special services staff and the academic advisor cannot require a student to visit them, they can only ask the student to come!

## Communication with Students

Students will need to communicate with the college staff and their families on a regular basis and will need to understand how to use the telephone system, internet connection, and mail services on campus. Students need to learn how their college staff will provide information to them. As many colleges today use e-mail and internet for most of their communication, students need to learn to check their campus e-mail on a regular basis. Many professors use e-mail to notify students of changes in coursework or test schedules. Some students, like our son, who was not used to using e-mail regularly, may need a reminder to answer their mother's e-mail!

## Campus Social Life

Students with Asperger syndrome may need extra help in locating extracurricular activities on campus. Both parents and special services staff may need to get involved to make sure that the student has connected to a group of friends and provide suggestions if needed. We know of several colleges that provide a peer advisor or "Big Sister" program to assist all freshmen students adjust to college life by designating a student from an upper class to guide them.

## Career Assistance

The unemployment level among adults with Asperger syndrome is high. My husband and I feel that students need encouragement to seek assistance from the college career center. These students need help in exploring the work world either through a job on campus or through an internship off campus. The special services staff can recommend that students meet the career counselor on campus. The career center can help students find summer employment in their field of interest as well as jobs after graduation.

## Declaring Independence

Our son was ready to declare his independence more than I realized. He has thoroughly enjoyed being on his own. The first year is almost over and our son told me yesterday he had made plans for next year to room with his new friend and already purchased his dorm contract. He wants a co-ed dorm next year because he's "tired of immature guy stuff"! I think he's doing fine!

Chapter 44

# Adults with Autism Spectrum Disorders: Living and Working Arrangements

## Chapter Contents

Section 44.1—Living Arrangements for Adults with
        Autism Spectrum Disorders .............................. 538
Section 44.2—Accommodating Employees with Asperger
        Syndrome ............................................................ 540

Section 44.1

# Living Arrangements for Adults with Autism Spectrum Disorders

Excerpted from "Autism Spectrum Disorders (Pervasive Developmental Disorders)," National Institute of Mental Health, National Institutes of Health, July 11, 2006.

Some adults with autism spectrum disorders (ASD), especially those with high-functioning autism or with Asperger syndrome, are able to work successfully in mainstream jobs. Nevertheless, communication and social problems often cause difficulties in many areas of life. They will continue to need encouragement and moral support in their struggle for an independent life.

Many others with ASD are capable of employment in sheltered workshops under the supervision of managers trained in working with persons with disabilities. A nurturing environment at home, at school, and later in job training and at work, helps persons with ASD continue to learn and to develop throughout their lives.

The public schools' responsibility for providing services ends when the person with ASD reaches the age of twenty-two. The family is then faced with the challenge of finding living arrangements and employment to match the particular needs of their adult child, as well as the programs and facilities that can provide support services to achieve these goals. Long before your child finishes school, you will want to search for the best programs and facilities for your young adult. If you know other parents of ASD adults, ask them about the services available in your community. If your community has little to offer, serve as an advocate for your child and work toward the goal of improved employment services. Learn as much as possible about the help your child is eligible to receive as an adult.

## Living Arrangements for the Adult with an Autism Spectrum Disorder

**Independent living:** Some adults with ASD are able to live entirely on their own. Others can live semi-independently in their own home or apartment if they have assistance with solving major problems, such as personal finances or dealing with the government agencies that provide services to persons with disabilities. This assistance can be provided by family, a professional agency, or another type of provider.

**Living at home:** Government funds are available for families that choose to have their adult child with ASD live at home. These programs include Supplemental Security Income (SSI), Social Security Disability Insurance (SSDI), Medicaid waivers, and others. Information about these programs is available from the Social Security Administration (SSA). An appointment with a local SSA office is a good first step to take in understanding the programs for which the young adult is eligible.

**Foster homes and skill-development homes:** Some families open their homes to provide long-term care to unrelated adults with disabilities. If the home teaches self-care and housekeeping skills and arranges leisure activities, it is called a "skill-development" home.

**Supervised group living:** Persons with disabilities frequently live in group homes or apartments staffed by professionals who help the individuals with basic needs. These often include meal preparation, housekeeping, and personal care needs. Higher-functioning persons may be able to live in a home or apartment where staff visit only a few times a week. These persons generally prepare their own meals, go to work, and conduct other daily activities on their own.

**Institutions:** Although the trend in recent decades has been to avoid placing persons with disabilities into long-term-care institutions, this alternative is still available for persons with ASD who need intensive, constant supervision. Unlike many of the institutions years ago, today's facilities view residents as individuals with human needs and offer opportunities for recreation and simple but meaningful work.

Section 44.2

# Accommodating Employees with Asperger Syndrome

Excerpted from "Employees with Asperger Syndrome,"
Job Accommodation Network, January 2007.

## Asperger Syndrome and the Americans with Disabilities Act

### Is Asperger Syndrome a Disability under the ADA?

The Americans with Disabilities Act (ADA) does not contain a list of medical conditions that constitute disabilities. Instead, the ADA has a general definition of disability that each person must meet (EEOC, 1992). Therefore, some people with Asperger syndrome will have a disability under the ADA and some will not.

A person has a disability if he or she has a physical or mental impairment that substantially limits one or more major life activities, has a record of such an impairment, or is regarded as having such an impairment (EEOC, 1992). To be a disability covered by the ADA, the impairment must substantially limit one or more major life activities. These are activities that an average person can perform with little or no difficulty. Examples are: walking, seeing, speaking, hearing, breathing, learning, performing manual tasks, caring for oneself, and working. These are examples only. Other activities such as sitting, standing, lifting, or reading are also major life activities (EEOC, 1992).

Most courts have agreed with the activities listed by the EEOC. For example, in Brown v. Cox Medical Centers, 286 F.3d 1040 (8th Cir. 2002), the court noted that the "ability to perform cognitive functions" is a major life activity. In Gagliardo v. Connaught Laboratories, Inc., 311 F.3d 565 (3d Cir. 2002), the court held that "concentrating and remembering (more generally, cognitive function)" are major life activities (Fram, 2004).

## Accommodating Employees with Asperger Syndrome

Note: People with Asperger syndrome may experience some of the limitations discussed in the following, but seldom develop all of them. Also, the degree of limitation will vary among individuals. Be aware that not all people with Asperger syndrome will need accommodations to perform their jobs and many others may need only a few accommodations. The following is only a sample of the possibilities available. Numerous other accommodation solutions may exist.

### Questions to Consider

1. What limitations is the employee with the Asperger syndrome experiencing?

2. How do these limitations affect the employee and the employee's job performance?

3. What specific job tasks are problematic as a result of these limitations?

4. What accommodations are available to reduce or eliminate these problems? Are all possible resources being used to determine possible accommodations?

5. Has the employee with Asperger syndrome been consulted regarding possible accommodations?

6. Once accommodations are in place, would it be useful to meet with the employee with Asperger syndrome to evaluate the effectiveness of the accommodations and to determine whether additional accommodations are needed?

7. Do supervisory personnel and employees need training regarding Asperger syndrome?

### Accommodation Ideas

**Reading, speaking, and communicating:** Individuals with Asperger syndrome may have difficulty communicating with co-workers or supervisors. For people with Asperger syndrome, poor communication may be the result of underdeveloped social skills, lack of experience or exposure in the workforce, shyness, intimidation, behavior disorders, or low self-esteem. Some suggestions to alleviate problems with reading, speaking, and communicating are as follows:

- Provide advance notice of topics to be discussed in meetings to help facilitate communication

- Provide advance notice of date of meeting when employee is required to speak to reduce or eliminate anxiety

- Allow employee to provide written response in lieu of verbal response

- Allow employee to have a friend or co-worker attend meeting to reduce or eliminate the feeling of intimidation

**Time management:** Individuals with Asperger syndrome may experience difficulty managing time, particularly if involved in an enjoyable or exciting task. This limitation can affect their ability to complete the task within a specified timeframe. It may also be difficult to prepare for, or to begin, less-desirable work activities. Following are some suggestions for alleviating problems with time management:

- Divide large assignments into several small tasks

- Set a timer to make an alarm after assigning ample time to complete a task

- Provide a checklist of assignments

- Supply an electronic or handheld organizer, and train on how to use effectively

- Use a wall calendar to emphasize due dates

**Impulsivity:** Individuals with Asperger syndrome may exhibit overactivity or impulsive behavior. This could be disruptive to the work environment or could inhibit efficient and effective work performance. Some suggestions for avoiding difficulties with impulsivity are as follows:

- Provide structured breaks to create an outlet for physical activity

- Use a job coach to teach or reinforce techniques to control impulsivity

- Allow the employee to work from home

- Review conduct policy with employee

- Adjust method of supervision to better prepare employee for feedback, disciplinary action, and other communication about job performance

- Use services of the Employee Assistance Program (EAP) if available

- Provide private workspace where employee will not disturb others by tapping, humming, or fidgeting

**Stress management:** Individuals with Asperger syndrome may have difficulty managing stress in the workplace. Situations that create stress can vary from person to person, but could likely involve heavy workloads, unrealistic timeframes, shortened deadlines, or conflict among co-workers. Following are some suggestions to aid in stress management:

- Provide praise and positive reinforcement
- Refer to EAP
- Allow employee to make telephone calls to doctors (and others) for support
- Provide sensitivity training for workforce
- Allow the presence and use of a support animal
- Modify work schedule

**Maintaining concentration:** Individuals with Asperger syndrome may experience decreased concentration, which can be attributed to auditory distractions (that can be heard) or visual distractions (that can be seen). People with Asperger syndrome report intolerance to distractions such as office traffic, employee chatter, and common office noises such as fax tones and photocopying. Some suggestions for maintaining concentration are as follows:

- To reduce auditory distractions:
  - Purchase a noise-canceling headset
  - Hang sound absorption panels
  - Provide a white noise machine
  - Relocate employee's office space away from audible distractions
  - Redesign employee's office space to minimize audible distractions

To reduce visual distractions:

  - Install space enclosures (cubicle walls)

- Reduce clutter in the employee's work environment
- Redesign employee's office space to minimize visual distractions
- Relocate employee's office space away from visual distractions

**Organization and prioritization:** Individuals with Asperger syndrome may have difficulty getting or staying organized, or have difficulty prioritizing tasks at work. This is likely the result of limited executive functions, which are cognitive skills required to prepare and execute complex behavior like planning, goal setting, and task completion. Following are suggestions for alleviating problems with organization and prioritization:

- Develop color-code system for files, projects, or activities
- Use weekly chart to identify daily work activities
- Use the services of a professional organizer
- Use a job coach to teach or reinforce organization skills
- Assign a mentor to help employee
- Allow supervisor to prioritize tasks
- Assign new project only when previous project is complete
- Provide a "cheat sheet" of high-priority activities, projects, people, and so on

**Social skills:** People with Asperger syndrome may have difficulty exhibiting appropriate social skills on the job. This might manifest itself as interrupting others when working or talking, demonstrating poor listening skills, not making eye contact when communicating, or inability to correctly read body language or understand innuendo. This can affect the person's ability to adhere to conduct standards, work effectively with supervisors, or interact with co-workers or customers. Following are some suggestions for alleviating problems with social skills:

- Behavior on the job:
  - Review conduct policy with employee to reduce incidents of inappropriate behavior
  - Provide concrete examples to explain inappropriate behavior
  - Provide concrete examples to explain consequences

- Recognize and reward appropriate behavior to reinforce appropriate behavior

- Provide a job coach to help understand different social cues

- Use training videos to demonstrate appropriate behavior in workplace

- Encourage all employees to model appropriate social skills

- Use role-play scenarios to demonstrate appropriate behavior in workplace

- Working effectively with supervisors:

  - Provide detailed day-to-day guidance and feedback

  - Offer positive reinforcement

  - Identify areas of improvement for employee in a fair and consistent manner

  - Provide clear expectations and the consequences of not meeting expectations

  - Give assignments verbally, in writing, or both, depending on what would be most beneficial to the employee

  - Establish long-term and short-term goals for employee

  - Adjust supervisory method by modifying the manner in which conversations take place, meetings are conducted, or discipline is addressed

- Interacting with co-workers:

  - Provide sensitivity training to promote disability awareness

  - Allow employee to work from home when feasible

  - Help employee "learn the ropes" by providing a mentor

  - Make employee attendance at social functions optional

  - Allow employee to transfer to another workgroup, shift, or department

  - Encourage employees to minimize personal conversation, or move personal conversation away from work areas

**Memory:** Individuals with Asperger syndrome may experience memory deficits that can affect their ability to complete tasks, remember job duties, or recall daily actions or activities. This could be caused by a side effect from medications. It could also be due to disinterest in the activity or misunderstanding the activity's level of importance. Some suggestions to alleviate troubles with memory are as follows:

- Provide written instructions
- Allow additional training time for new tasks
- Offer training refreshers
- Prompt employee with verbal cues
- Use a flowchart to describe the steps involved in a complicated task (such as powering up a system, closing down the facility, logging into a computer, etc.)
- Provide pictorial cues
- Use sticky notes as reminders of important dates or tasks
- Safely and securely maintain paper lists of crucial information such as passwords
- Allow employee to use voice-activated recorder to record verbal instructions
- Provide employee directory with pictures or use name tags and door/cubicle name markers to help employee remember co-workers' names
- Encourage employee to ask (or e-mail) with work-related questions

**Multitasking:** Individuals with Asperger syndrome may experience difficulty performing many tasks at one time. This difficulty could occur regardless of the similarity of tasks, the ease or complexity of the tasks, or the frequency of performing the tasks. Some suggestions to aid with multitasking are as follows:

- Separate tasks so that each can completed one at a time
- Create a flowchart of tasks that must be performed at the same time, carefully labeling or color-coding each task in sequential or preferential order
- Provide individualized/specialized training to help employee learn techniques for multitasking (e.g., typing on computer while talking on phone)
- Identify tasks that must be performed simultaneously and tasks that can be performed individually

- Provide specific feedback to help employee target areas of improvement

- Remove or reduce distractions from work area

- Supply proper working equipment to complete multiple tasks at one time, such as workstation and chair, lighting, and office supplies

- Explain performance standards such as completion time or accuracy rates

## References

American Psychiatric Association. (1994). *Diagnostic and statistical manual of mental disorders* (4th ed.). Washington, D.C.

Center for Disease Control and Prevention (2006). *How common are Autism spectrum disorders?* Retrieved January 8, 2007, from http://www.cdc.gov/ncbddd/autism/asd_common.htm

Equal Employment Opportunity Commission. (1992). *A technical assistance manual on the employment provisions (title I) of the Americans with Disabilities Act.* Retrieved October 28, 2005, from http://www.jan.wvu.edu/links/ADAtam1.html

Fram, David. (2004). *Resolving ADA workplace questions: How courts and agencies are dealing with employment issues.* National Employment Law Institute Publication, 17th edition.

Klin, A., Volkmar, F.R, & Sparrow, S.S. (2000). *Asperger syndrome.* New York, Guilford Press.

National Institute of Mental Health. (2006). *Autism spectrum disorders (pervasive developmental disorders).* Retrieved January 8, 2007, from http://www.nimh.nih.gov/publicat/autism.cfm#intro

# Chapter 45

# *Estate Planning for Parents of Autistic Children*

Estate planning is an important aspect of a family plan for any parent and it takes on even greater significance for the parent of a special needs child. This article explores the tax and non-tax reasons why estate planning is important.

There are many components to an estate plan. It may be as basic as a will, power of attorney, and health care proxy carefully coordinated with an individual's assets. It could also be as complex as a special needs trust, insurance trust, family limited partnership, or grantor retained annuity trust. This chapter focuses on the basics of any estate plan.

## *A Will*

Wills are important for multiple reasons. A will allows an individual to select beneficiaries, establish the times at which beneficiaries receive the assets, and the fiduciaries who administer the estate and any trusts created under the will. For the parent of a young child, a will is critical. In the absence of a designated guardian under a will, the court must determine who will be guardian of the person and property of a minor child (i.e., who will raise the child). This is a decision that any parent, but especially the parent of a special needs child, must carefully consider. Further, a will is important to ensure that

---

In this chapter: "The Importance of Estate Planning," by Lori I. Wolf, Esq., and Steven D. Leipzig, Esq. *Exceptional Parent Magazine*, November 2004, pp. 26–28. © 2004 EP Global Communications. All rights reserved.

assets are not placed in a child's hands before the child is responsible enough to invest and use the assets prudently.

For the parent of a special needs child, a will is especially important. Leaving assets (through intestate succession—by state law where a person dies without a will—or through a will) outright to a special needs child can result in the disqualification of the child from receiving Medicaid and other government assistance. With a properly structured will, assets allocated to a special needs child can be held in a trust that does not affect the child's eligibility for these governmental benefits. Under New Jersey law, the trustee for the special needs child's trust could be allowed to use trust income and principal to benefit the child for any reason the trustee deems appropriate. Alternatively, the trust can be structured as a supplemental needs or luxury trust, where the assets can be used for luxury items such as travel, books, and other items that are not provided for by Medicaid. In the state of New York, only the latter, supplemental needs trust, allowing assets to be used for expenses not otherwise covered by Medicaid, will protect the beneficiary's Medicaid eligibility. Each state's laws and regulations differ, but clearly it is important to have a very careful plan that evaluates how best to protect both the child and the availability of government assistance where appropriate.

A special needs trust can be a trust created during a parent's lifetime or a testamentary trust (i.e., a trust created under the parent's will). The advantage of establishing a stand-alone lifetime trust is that the trust can be used as the recipient of gifts from the parent and from grandparents, aunts and uncles, and others. This gifting can accomplish tax planning for a family. That trust can establish a parent's hopes and goals for a child and his or her care.

One issue that a parent developing a plan must face is how to allocate assets among children, based on the different children's needs. Factors to consider include the potential ability of each child to earn a living, the likely financial needs of each child, and the assets available. A special needs child may be less likely than other children to be self-supporting as an adult, but may also have less of a need for large sums of money, since his or her lifestyle may be modest and at least partially funded by government aid. One possible solution is to leave a specific dollar amount to a special needs trust (taking care that the appropriate amount will be available to the special needs child before assets are allocated to other children), with the remaining assets divided among the other children. This maximizes the likelihood that the appropriate amount will be available to the special needs child, while making sure that the special needs child does not receive significantly more than he or she needs (thereby tying up assets until the child's death).

Thought must also be given as to who is best qualified to make financial decisions on behalf of a child. The trustee (and successors) should meet two key characteristics: he or she should be someone who the parent trusts implicitly and someone who has some financial savvy. A third factor important in deciding upon the trustee of a special needs trust is designating someone who is sensitive to the unique needs of the beneficiary.

In developing an estate plan, consideration must be given to the tax consequences of the plan. This is important so that the assets available to pass to a special needs child and other family members can be maximized.

The federal estate tax is imposed on the value of assets less liabilities at the date of a person's death. Currently, the federal estate tax ranges from 45 percent and incrementally increases to a maximum rate of 48 percent. Under recent tax legislation, the maximum tax rate will be gradually reduced to 45 percent in 2009. In 2010, there will be a repeal of the federal estate tax, and the estate tax will return in 2011 with a maximum rate of 55 percent.

There are two important concepts that are critical to understanding how the federal estate tax works. First, there is the unlimited marital deduction, which means that all of the assets one leaves to his or her surviving spouse are exempt from federal estate taxes.

The second important concept involves the applicable exclusion. The applicable exclusion permits an individual to leave up to $1.5 million of assets through a combination of lifetime gifts and testamentary bequests, without paying federal estate taxes on this amount. Congress recently passed legislation that will increase the estate tax applicable exclusion to $2 million in 2006 and to $3.5 million in 2009. There will be a full repeal of the federal estate tax in 2010, and a complete return to 2002 law, with a $1 million applicable exclusion, in 2011. The gift tax applicable exclusion will remain permanently at $1 million.

In many states there is also a state estate tax that must be considered in connection with planning. Under recent legislation passed in the state of New Jersey, there is a new state estate tax imposed on assets in excess of $675,000 passing to someone other than a spouse. In New York, the exempt amount is $1 million.

In connection with an estate plan, it is important for a married individual to take into consideration the tax laws and the potential to minimize taxes by taking advantage of the unlimited marital deduction while maximizing the use of each spouse's applicable exclusion. This will help maximize the moneys available to children at the surviving spouse's death. The net effect of this planning is that, with a $1.5 million applicable exclusion, a married couple with proper planning can leave up to $3 million transfer tax- free to children.

## Power of Attorney

A power of attorney allows an individual to appoint people to manage his or her assets and make investment decisions on his or her behalf. Having this document avoids the necessity of having to go to court to get someone appointed as a guardian if an individual cannot manage his or her own affairs. This document is important for all individuals. For a special needs child who is capable of making decisions, it is important for this individual to have a power of attorney giving someone the power to make financial decisions on his or her behalf where appropriate.

A power of attorney can be effective immediately (in which case it is not impacted by a subsequent disability or incapacity). Alternatively, a power of attorney can be prepared so it is only effective on disability or incapacity.

## Health Care Proxies

Health care proxies serve two purposes. First, this document asserts an individual's desire to be free from the use of life-sustaining or prolonging procedures and medications if the individual becomes irreversibly or terminally ill. Second, the health care proxy can direct a health care agent appointed to make a wide range of medical and health care decisions if the individual is unable to articulate his or her own preferences.

Again, this is an important document for all individuals, including a special needs child who is capable of appointing an individual to act on his or her behalf where appropriate.

## Insurance

Insurance is an important asset used in connection with an estate plan. Insurance can be used to ensure that sufficient assets are available to provide adequate income to the surviving spouse, to provide for the lifetime care of the special needs child, and to provide sufficient assets to care for any other children until they finish schooling and are able to earn a living. This is critical for a young family with a special needs child who will need sufficient assets to maintain his or her care over an extended period of time. The beneficiary of an insurance policy should be coordinated with the estate plan. If estate taxes are a concern due to the size of an estate, the parents can have his or her insurance owned by and payable to a trust for his or her designated beneficiaries to remove the insurance from the parent's taxable estate.

Estate planning is essential for any parent, but takes on additional significance for the parent of a child with special needs. In addressing the plan, a parent should make sure he or she is being counseled by an attorney with experience handling the sensitive issues accompanying a special needs child.

Reprinted with the expressed consent and approval of *Exceptional Parent*, a monthly magazine for parents and families of children with disabilities and special health care needs. Subscriptions cost is $39.95 per year for twelve issues. To subscribe call 877-372-7368. EP Global Communications, 416 Main Street, Johnstown, PA 15901.

# Part Eight

# Additional Help and Information

# Chapter 46

# *Glossary of Terms Related to Autism Spectrum Disorders*

**Angelman syndrome:** A genetic disorder caused by abnormal function of the gene UBE3A, located within a small region on chromosome 15. Characteristics include: developmental delay, lack of speech or minimal use of words; movement or balance disorder, usually ataxia of gait or tremulous movement of limbs, and any combination of frequent laughter or smiling; apparent happy demeanor; easily excitable personality, often with hand flapping movements; hypermotoric behavior; and short attention span.[2]

**applied behavior analysis:** An intervention that relies on the theory that rewarded behavior is more likely to be repeated than ignored behavior. This theory provides the foundation of several different methods of behavioral management often used with persons who have autism and other developmental disorders.[2]

**Asperger disorder:** A pervasive developmental disorder characterized by severe and enduring impairment in social skills and restrictive and repetitive behaviors and interests, leading to impaired social and occupational functioning but without significant delays in language development.[1]

The terms in this glossary were excerpted from *Stedman's Electronic Medical Dictionary* v.5.0, © 2000 Lippincott Williams and Wilkins [marked 1], and from the following publications from the National Institute of Child Health and Human Development: "Autism Overview: What We Know," NIH Publication No. 05-5592, May 2005; "Rett Syndrome," NIH Publication No. 06-5589, April 2006; and "Autism and Genes," NIH Publication No. 05-5590, May 2005 [marked 2].

**behavior management therapy:** A method of therapy that focuses on managing behavior—that is, changing unwanted behaviors through rewards and reinforcements and by confronting something that arouses anxiety, discomfort, or fear and overcoming the unwanted responses.[2]

**candidate gene:** A gene located in a chromosome region suspected of being involved in a disorder, whose protein product suggests that it could be the gene in question.[2]

**chromosomes:** One of the "packages" of genes and other DNA in the nucleus of a cell. Humans have twenty-three pairs of chromosomes, forty-six in all. Each parent contributes one chromosome to each pair, so children get half of their chromosomes from their mothers and half from their fathers.[2]

**congenital:** Existing from birth; not hereditary or inherited.[2]

**coprolalia:** Involuntary utterances of vulgar or obscene words; seen in Gilles de la Tourette syndrome.[1]

**cytogenetic:** Study of chromosomes using a specific method that involves staining a chromosome and examining it under a microscope.[2]

**developmental screening:** A check-up similar to the physical check-up a child gets from a health care provider, but that focuses on a child's social, emotional, and intellectual development. This screening monitors and charts development to make sure that the child is developing as expected for his or her age.[2]

**echolalia:** Involuntary parrotlike repetition of a word or sentence just spoken by another person.[1]

**electrocardiogram (ECG):** A test that records and measures the electrical activity of the heart. Measures the rate and regularity of the heartbeats, the presence of any damage to the heart, and the effects of drugs or devices used to regulate the heartbeat.[2]

**epidemiological studies:** Studies of the number of people with a disease(s), the locations of these people, the patterns of the disease(s), and what contributes to or causes the disease(s) or related events in certain groups.[2]

**epilepsy:** A brain disorder in which clusters of nerve cells, or neurons, in the brain sometimes signal abnormally. In epilepsy, the normal pattern of neuronal activity becomes disturbed, causing strange sensations, emotions, and behavior or sometimes convulsions, muscle spasms, and loss of consciousness.[2]

**fragile X syndrome:** The most common form of inherited mental retardation. A mutation in a single gene, the FMR1 gene on the X chromosome, causes the disorder, which can be passed from one generation to the next. Symptoms occur because the mutated gene cannot produce enough of a protein that is needed by the body's cells, especially cells in the brain, to develop and function normally.[2]

**fraternal twins:** Twins resulting from the fertilization of two separate eggs. Fraternal twins share about 50 percent of their genes, just like siblings who are born at different times.[2]

**gastroesophageal reflux:** Flow of the stomach contents back into the esophagus, which can result in heartburn and in esophageal damage.[2]

**gene:** Pieces of DNA. They contain the information for making a specific protein.[2]

**genome:** All the DNA contained in an organism or a cell; includes both the DNA and chromosomes within the nucleus and the DNA outside the nucleus.[2]

**hereditary:** A gene or trait passed down from parent to offspring.[2]

**homeobox genes:** Genes found in almost all animals that control how and where parts of the body develop. Active very early in life, acting like a movie director by telling other genes when to act and when to stop in building the body.[2]

**hot spots:** Areas on chromosomes where mutations, activity, or recombination occurs with unusually high frequency.[2]

**hyperlexia:** In mentally retarded children, the presence of relatively advanced reading ability.[1]

**identical twins:** Twins formed from the splitting of the same fertilized egg, so they share 100 percent of their genetic material.[2]

**Individualized Education Plan:** A written set of instruction goals, or specific skills, for every child in a special education program that is required by law. The document is an agreement between the school and the family about a child's educational goals. The Individualized Education Plan (IEP) is reviewed every year and, if needed, changed to meet a child's new or changing needs.[2]

**Landau-Kleffner syndrome:** Childhood disorder characterized by generalized and psychomotor seizures associated with acquired aphasia; multifocal spikes and spike and wave discharges in the electroencephalogram.[1]

**linkage disequilibrium:** An association of genes or markers near each other on a chromosome that is more than would be expected by chance. Linked genes and markers tend to be inherited together.[2]

**mental retardation:** A term used when a person has certain limitations in mental functioning and in skills such as communicating, taking care of him- or herself, and social skills.[2]

**mutation:** A permanent structural change in DNA. In most cases, DNA changes either have no effect or cause harm, but some mutations improve an organism's survival.[2]

**neurotransmitter:** A substance that transmits nerve impulses between nerve cells.[2]

**obsessive-compulsive disorder (OCD):** A disorder characterized by recurrent, unwanted thoughts (obsessions) and repetitive behaviors or an urgent need to perform "rituals" (compulsions).[2]

**occupational therapy:** Therapeutic use of self-care, work, and recreational activities to increase independent function, enhance development, and prevent disability; may include adaptation of tasks or environment to achieve maximum independence and optimum quality of life.[1]

**pervasive developmental disorders:** A group of mental disorders of infancy, childhood, or adolescence characterized by distortions in the acquisition of the multiple basic psychologic functions necessary for the elaboration of social skills, language skills, and imagination; also characterized by restricted or stereotypical activities and interests.[1]

**Prader-Willi syndrome:** An uncommon inherited disorder characterized by mental retardation, decreased muscle tone, short stature, emotional liability, and an insatiable appetite that can lead to life-threatening obesity. Caused by a missing part on the paternally derived chromosome 15.[2]

**prevalence:** The number of people in a given population who have a certain condition or disease.[2]

**proteins:** Large molecules made up of one or more chains of amino acids. Proteins perform a wide variety of activities in the cell and in the body.[2]

**replicate:** Describes a situation in which many studies that use the same methods and steps have gotten the same outcome, suggesting that a finding is likely to be true.[2]

**Rett syndrome:** Mostly caused by mutations in the MECP2 gene on the X chromosome, Rett syndrome is a disorder of brain development that occurs almost exclusively in girls. After a few months of apparently normal development, affected girls develop problems with language, learning, coordination, and other brain functions.[2]

**secretin:** A hormone, formed by the epithelial cells of the duodenum under the stimulus of acid contents from the stomach, that incites secretion of pancreatic juice; used as a diagnostic aid in the diagnosis of pancreatic exocrine disease.[1]

**seizures:** A sudden attack, often one of convulsions, as in epilepsy. Seizures don't necessarily involve movement or thrashing; they can also make someone seem as though he or she is frozen, or unmoving.[2]

**selective serotonin reuptake inhibitor:** A class of chemical compounds that selectively, to varying degrees, inhibit the reuptake of serotonin by presynaptic neurons and are posited to exert their antidepressant effect by this mechanism.[1]

**serotonin:** A neurotransmitter that is found especially in the brain, blood serum, and stomach lining of mammals.[2]

**stereotyped behaviors:** Actions that are repeated without change.[2]

**susceptibility:** The state of being predisposed to, of being sensitive to, or of lacking the ability to resist manifestations of something (such as a pathogen, familial disease, or a drug); a person who is susceptible is more likely to show symptoms of a disorder.[2]

**Tourette syndrome:** A tic disorder appearing in childhood, characterized by multiple motor tics and vocal tics present for more than one year.[1]

**tuberous sclerosis:** A rare, multi-system genetic disease that causes noncancerous tumors to grow in the brain and on other vital organs such as the kidneys, heart, eyes, lungs, and skin. It commonly affects the central nervous system and results in symptoms including seizures, developmental delay, behavioral problems, skin abnormalities, and kidney disease.[2]

**X-chromosome inactivation:** In females, the phenomenon by which one X chromosome is randomly inactivated in early embryonic cells; all descendant cells, then, also have that chromosome inactive.[2]

# Chapter 47

# How to Evaluate Health Information on the Internet

Millions of consumers are using the internet to get health information. And thousands of websites are offering health information. Some of those sites are reliable and up-to-date; some are not. How can you tell the good from the bad?

First, it's important to carefully consider the source of information and then to discuss the information you find with your health care professional. These questions and answers can help you determine whether the health information you find on the internet or receive by e-mail from a website is likely to be reliable.

## Questions and Answers: Evaluating Internet Health Information

### Who runs the website?

Any good health website should make it easy to learn who is responsible for the site and its information. On the U.S. Food and Drug Administration's (FDA) website, for example, the FDA is clearly noted on every major page, along with a link to the site's home (main) page, www.fda.gov.

Information about who runs the site can often be found in an "About Us" or "About This Website" section, and there's usually a link to that section on the site's home page.

---

Reprinted from " How to Evaluate Health Information on the Internet," U.S. Food and Drug Administration, December 2005.

## What is the purpose of the website?

Is the purpose of the site to inform? Is it to sell a product? Is it to raise money? If you can tell who runs and pays for the site, this will help you evaluate its purpose. Be cautious about sites trying to sell a product or service.

Quackery abounds on the internet. Look for these warning signs and remember the adage "If it sounds too good to be true, it probably is":

- Does the site promise quick, dramatic, miraculous results? Is this the only site making these claims?

- Beware of claims that one remedy will cure a variety of illnesses, that it is a "breakthrough," or that it relies on a "secret ingredient."

- Use caution if the site uses a sensational writing style (lots of exclamation points, for example).

- A health website for consumers should use simple language, not technical jargon.

- Get a second opinion. Check more than one site.

## What is the original source of the information on the website?

Always pay close attention to where the information on the site comes from. Many health and medical websites post information collected from other websites or sources. If the person or organization in charge of the site did not write the material, the original source should be clearly identified. Be careful of sites that don't say where the information comes from.

Good sources of health information include the following:

- Sites that end in ".gov," sponsored by the federal government, like the U.S. Department of Health and Human Services (www.hhs.gov), the FDA (www.fda.gov), the National Institutes of Health (www.nih.gov), the Centers for Disease Control and Prevention (www.cdc.gov), and the National Library of Medicine (www.nlm.nih.gov)

- ".edu" sites, which are run by universities or medical schools, such as Johns Hopkins University School of Medicine and the University of California at Berkeley Hospital, health system, and other health care facility sites, like the Mayo Clinic and Cleveland Clinic

- ".org" sites maintained by not-for-profit groups whose focus is research and teaching the public about specific diseases or conditions, such as the American Diabetes Association, the American Cancer Society, and the American Heart Association

- Medical and scientific journals, such as the *New England Journal of Medicine* and the *Journal of the American Medical Association*, although these aren't written for consumers and could be hard to understand

- Sites whose addresses end in ".com" are usually commercial sites and are often selling products.

### *How is the information on the website documented?*

In addition to identifying the original source of the material, the site should identify the evidence on which the material is based. Medical facts and figures should have references (such as citations of articles in medical journals). Also, opinions or advice should be clearly set apart from information that is "evidence-based" (that is, based on research results).

### *How is information reviewed before it is posted on the website?*

Health-related websites should give information about the medical credentials of the people who prepare or review the material on the website.

### *How current is the information on the website?*

Websites should be reviewed and updated on a regular basis. It is particularly important that medical information be current, and that the most recent update or review date be clearly posted. These dates are usually found at the bottom of the page. Even if the information has not changed, it is helpful to know that the site owners have reviewed it recently to ensure that the information is still valid. Click on a few links on the site. If there are a lot of broken links, the site may not be kept up-to-date.

### *How does the website choose links to other sites?*

Reliable websites usually have a policy about how they establish links to other sites. Some medical websites take a conservative approach and do not link to any other sites; some link to any site that asks or pays for a link; others link only to sites that have met certain criteria. Look for the website's linking policy, often found in a section titled "About This Website."

## What information about its visitors does the website collect, and why?

Websites routinely track the path visitors take through their sites to determine what pages are being used. However, many health-related websites ask the visitor to "subscribe" or "become a member." In some cases, this may be done so they can collect a fee or select relevant information for the visitor. In all cases, the subscription or membership will allow the website owners to collect personal information about their visitors.

Many commercial sites sell "aggregate" data about their visitors to other companies—what percentage are women with breast cancer, for example. In some cases, they may collect and reuse information that is personally identifiable, such as a visitor's zip code, gender, and birth date.

Any website asking users for personal information should explain exactly what the site will and will not do with the information. The FDA website, for example, spells this out in its Privacy Statement. Be sure to read and understand any privacy policy or similar language on the site, and don't sign up for anything you don't fully understand.

## How does the website manage interactions with visitors?

There should always be a way for visitors to contact the website owners with problems, feedback, and questions. The FDA's website provides contact information on its Contact Us page.

If the site hosts a chat room or other online discussion areas, it should tell its visitors about the terms of using the service. Is the service moderated? If so, by whom, and why? It is always a good idea to spend time reading the discussion without joining in, to feel comfortable with the environment, before becoming a participant.

## Can the accuracy of information received in an e-mail be verified?

Carefully evaluate e-mail messages. Consider the origin of the message and its purpose. Some companies or organizations use e-mail to advertise products or attract people to their websites. The accuracy of health information may be influenced by the desire to promote a product or service.

### Is the information that's discussed in chat rooms accurate?

Assessing the reliability of health information that you come across in discussion groups or chat rooms on the internet is at least as important as it is for websites. Although these groups can sometimes provide good information about specific diseases or disorders, they can also perpetuate misinformation. Most internet service providers don't verify what is discussed in these groups, and you have no way of knowing the qualifications or credentials of the other people online. Sometimes people use these groups to promote products without letting on that they have a financial stake in the business. It's best to discuss anything you learn from these groups with your health care professional.

## A Quick Checklist

You can use the following checklist to help make sure that the health information you are reading online can be trusted:

- Can you easily see who sponsors the website?
- Is the sponsor a government agency, a medical school, or a reliable health-related organization, or is it related to one of these?
- Is there contact information?
- Can you tell when the information was written?
- Is your privacy protected?
- Does the website make claims that seem too good to be true? Are quick, miraculous cures promised?

Chapter 48

# Resources for Information about Autism Spectrum Disorders

## General

### American Speech-Language-Hearing Association (ASHA)
10801 Rockville Pike
Rockville, MD 20852-3279
Toll-Free: 800-638-8255
Phone: 301-897-5700
Fax: 301-571-0457
TTY: 301-897-0157
Website: http://www.asha.org
E-mail: actioncenter@asha.org

### Association for Science in Autism Treatment
389 Main Street
Suite 202
Malden, MA 02148
Phone: 781-397-8943
Fax: 781-397-8887
Website: http://www.asatonline.org
E-mail: info@asatonline.org

### Autism Information Center
Centers for Disease Control and Prevention
Toll-Free: 800-311-3435
Phone: 404-639-3534
Website: www.cdc.gov/ncbddd/autism

The information in this chapter was compiled from various sources deemed accurate. All contact information was verified and updated in March 2007. Inclusion does not imply endorsement. This list is intended to serve as a starting point for information gathering; it is not comprehensive.

**Autism National Committee (AUTCOM)**
P.O. Box 429
Forest Knolls, CA 94933
Website: http://www.autcom.org

**Autism Network for Hearing and Visually Impaired Persons**
7510 Ocean Front Avenue
Virginia Beach, VA 23451
Phone: 757-428-0019
Fax: 757-428-0019

**Autism Network International (ANI)**
P.O. Box 35448
Syracuse, NY 13235-5448
Website: http://ani.autistics.org

**Autism Patient Center**
Website: http://www.patientcenters.com/autism

**Autism-PDD Resources Network**
Website: http://www.autism-pdd.net

**Autism Research Foundation**
c/o Moss-Rosene Lab
Suite W701
715 Albany Street
Boston, MA 02118
Phone: 617-414-7012
Website: http://www.ladders.org
E-mail: tarf@ladders.org

**Autism Research Institute (ARI)**
4182 Adams Avenue
San Diego, CA 92116
Phone: 619-281-7165
Fax: 619-563-6840
Website: http://www.autismresearchinstitute.com

**Autism Society of America**
7910 Woodmont Avenue
Suite 300
Bethesda, MD 20814-3067
Toll-Free: 800-3AUTISM (328-8476)
Phone: 301-657-0881
Fax: 301-657-0869
Website: http://www.autism-society.org

**Autism Society of Northwest Ohio**
4848 Dorr Street
Toledo, OH 43615
Phone: 419-578-ASNO (2766)
Fax: 419-536-5038
Website: http://www.asno.org

**Autism Speaks**
2 Park Avenue, 11th Floor
New York, NY 10016
Phone: 212-252-8584
Fax: 212-252-8676
Website: http://www.autismspeaks.org
E-mail: contactus@autismspeaks.org

**Center for Autism and Related Disorders (CARD)**
19019 Ventura Boulevard
Suite 300
Tarzana, CA 91356
Phone: 818-345-2345
Fax: 818-758-8015
Website: http://
www.centerforautism.com
E-mail: CARDHeadquarters
@centerforautism.com

**Center for the Study of Autism**
c/o Autism Research Institute
4182 Adams Avenue
San Diego, CA 92116
Website: http://www.autism.org

**Cure Autism Now (CAN) Foundation**
5455 Wilshire Boulevard
Suite 2250
Los Angeles, CA 90036-4234
Toll-Free: 888-8AUTISM
(828-8476)
Phone: 323-549-0500
Fax: 323-549-0547
Website: http://
www.cureautismnow.org
E-mail: info@cureautismnow.org

**Indiana Resource Center for Autism**
Indiana Institute on Disability
and Community
2853 E. Tenth Street
Bloomington, IN 47408-2696
Phone: 812-855-6508
TTY: 812-855-9396
Fax: 812-855-9630
Website: www.iidc.indiana.edu/
irca

**MAAP Services for Autism, Asperger's, and PDD**
P.O. Box 524
Crown Point, IN 46308
Phone: 219-662-1311
Fax: 219-662-0638
Website: http://
www.maapservices.org
E-mail: info@maapservices.org

**National Dissemination Center for Children with Disabilities**
U.S. Department of Education,
Office of Special Education Pro-
grams
P.O. Box 1492
Washington, DC 20013-1492
Toll-Free: 800-695-0285
Fax: 202-884-8441
Website: http://www.nichcy.org
E-mail: nichcy@aed.org

**National Institute of Child Health and Human Development (NICHD)**
NICHD Clearinghouse
P.O. Box 3006
Rockville, MD 20847
Phone: 800-370-2943
Fax: 301-984-1473
Website: www.nichd.nih.gov/
autism
E-mail:
NICHDinformationresourcecenter
@mail.nih.gov

**National Institute of Mental Health (NIMH)**
National Institutes of Health, DHHS
6001 Executive Boulevard, Room 8184, MSC 9663
Bethesda, MD 20892-9663
Toll Free: 866-615-NIMH (6464)
Phone: 301-443-4513
TTY: 866-415-8051
Fax: 301-443-4279
Website: http://
www.nimh.nih.gov
E-mail: nimhinfo@nih.gov

**National Institute on Deafness and Other Communication Disorders Information Clearinghouse**
1 Communication Avenue
Bethesda, MD 20892-3456
Toll-Free: 800-241-1044
TTY/TDD: 800-241-1055
Website: http://
www.nidcd.nih.gov
E-mail: nidcdinfo@nidcd.nih.gov

**National Institutes of Health Autism Research Network**
Website: www
.autismresearchnetwork.org/AN

**National Organization for Rare Disorders (NORD)**
P.O. Box 1968
Danbury, CT 06813-1968
Toll-Free: 800-999-NORD (6673)
Phone: 203-744-0100
TDD: 203-797-9590
Fax: 203-798-2291
Website: http://
www.rarediseases.org
E-mail: orphan@rarediseases.org

**New York Families for Autistic Children**
95-16 Pitkin Avenue
Ozone Park, NY 11417
Phone: 718-641-3441
Fax: 718-641-4452
Website: http://www.nyfac.org

**Organization for Autism Research**
2000 North 14th Street
Suite 480
Arlington, VA 22201
Phone: 703-243-9710
Website: http://
www.researchautism.org

**Professional Development in Autism Center**
Phone: 206-221-3139
Website: http://
depts.washington.edu/pdacent/

### Southwest Autism Research and Resource Center

Campus for Exceptional Children
300 N. 18th Street
Phoenix, AZ 85006-4103
Phone: 602-340-8717
Fax: 602-340-8720
Website: http://www.autismcenter.org
E-mail: sarrc@autismcenter.org

### Talk About Curing Autism (TACA)

P.O. Box 12409
Newport Beach, CA 92658-2409
Phone: 949-640-4401
Fax: 949-640-4424
Website: http://www.tacanow.com

### Yale Child Study Center

Yale Social Learning Disabilities Project
230 South Frontage Road
New Haven, CT 06520
Phone: 203-764-8326
Website: http://www.autism.fm

## Angelman Syndrome

### Angelman Syndrome Foundation

4255 Westbrook Drive
Suite 216
Aurora, IL 60504
Toll-Free: 800-432-6435
Phone: 630-978-4245
Fax: 630-978-7408
Website: http://www.angelman.org
E-mail: info@angelman.org

## Applied Behavior Analysis

### Cambridge Center for Behavioral Studies, Autism Section

336 Baker Avenue
Concord, MA 01742-2107
Phone: 978-369-CCBS (2227)
Fax: 978-369-8584
Website: http://www.behavior.org/autism/index.cfm

### Center for Autism and Related Disorders (CARD)

19019 Ventura Boulevard
Suite 300
Tarzana, CA 91356
Phone: 818-345-2345
Fax: 818-758-8015
Website: http://www.centerforautism.com
E-mail: CARDHeadquarters@centerforautism.com

## Asperger Syndrome

### Asperger Syndrome and High Functioning Autism Association

P.O. Box 916
Bethpage, NY 11714-0916
Phone: 516-470-0360
Website: http://www.ahany.org

### Asperger Syndrome Education Network (ASPEN)

9 Aspen Circle
Edison, NJ 08820
Phone: 732-321-0880
Website: http://www.aspennj.org
E-mail: info@aspennj.org

## Online Asperger Syndrome Information and Support (O.A.S.I.S.)

Website: http://www.aspergersyndrome.org

## Auditory Processing Disorder

### American Academy of Audiology (AAA)

11730 Plaza America Drive
Suite 300
Reston, VA 20190
Toll-Free: 800-222-2336
Phone: 703-790-8466
Fax: 703-790-8631
Website: http://www.audiology.org
E-mail: info@audiology.org

### American Speech-Language-Hearing Association (ASHA)

10801 Rockville Pike
Rockville, MD 20852
Toll-Free: 800-638-8255
Phone: 301-897-5700
Fax: 301-571-0457
TTY: 301-897-0157
Website: http://www.asha.org
E-mail: actioncenter@asha.org

## Feingold Diet

### Feingold Association of the United States

554 East Main Street, Suite 301
Riverhead, NY 11901
Toll-Free: 800-321-3287
Phone: 631-369-9340
Fax: 631-369-2988
Website: http://www.feingold.org

## Floor Time

### Floortime Foundation

4938 Hampden Lane, Suite 229
Bethseda, MD 20814
Website: http://www.floortime.org
E-mail: info@floortime.org

## Fragile X Syndrome

### Conquer Fragile X Foundation

P.O. Box 128
Palm Beach, FL 33480
Phone: 561-833-3457
Fax: 877-833-8791
Website: http://www.cfxf.org
E-mail: mail@cfxf.org

### Fragile X Research Foundation

45 Pleasant Street
Newburyport, MA 01950
Phone: 978-462-1866.
Fax: 978-463-9985
Website: http://www.fraxa.org
E-mail: info@fraxa.org

### National Fragile X Foundation

P.O. Box 190488
San Francisco, CA 94119
Toll-Free: 800-688-8765
Phone: 925-938-9300
Fax: 925-938-9315
Website: http://www.fragilex.org
E-mail: NATLFX@FragileX.org

## Hippotherapy

**American Hippotherapy Association**
136 Bush Road
Demascus, PA. 18415
Toll-Free: 888-851-4592
Fax: 570-224-4462
Website: http://www.
americanhippotherapyassociation
.org
E-mail: info
@americanhippotherapyassociation
.org

**North American Riding for the Handicapped Association, Inc. (NARHA)**
P.O. Box 33150
Denver, CO 80233
Toll-Free: 800-369-7433
Phone: 303-452-1212
Fax: 303-252-4610
Website: http://www.narha.org

## Irlen Method

**Irlen Institute**
5380 Village Road
Long Beach, CA 90808
Toll Free: 800-554-7536
Phone: 562-496-2550
Website: http://www.irlen.com
E-mail: irlen@irlen.com

## Landau-Kleffner Syndrome

**American Speech-Language-Hearing Association (ASHA)**
10801 Rockville Pike
Rockville, MD 20852-3279
Toll-Free: 800-638-8255
Phone: 301-897-5700
Fax: 301-571-0457
TTY: 301-897-0157
Website: http://www.asha.org
E-mail: actioncenter@asha.org

**Epilepsy Foundation**
8301 Professional Place
Landover, MD 20785-7223
Toll-Free: 800-EFA-1000
(332-1000)
Phone: 301-459-3700
Fax: 301-577-2684
Website: http://
www.epilepsyfoundation.org
E-mail: postmaster@efa.org

**National Aphasia Association**
350 Seventh Avenue
Suite 902
New York, NY 10001
Toll-Free: 800-922-4NAA (4622)
Phone: 212-267-2814
Fax: 212-267-2812
Website: http://www.aphasia.org
E-mail: naa@aphasia.org

## National Organization for Rare Disorders (NORD)
P.O. Box 1968
Danbury, CT 06813-1968
Toll-Free: 800-999-NORD (6673)
Phone: 203-744-0100
TDD: 203-797-9590
Fax: 203-798-2291
Website: http://
www.rarediseases.org
E-mail:
orphan@rarediseases.org

## Music Therapy

### American Music Therapy Association
8455 Colesville Road
Suite 1000
Silver Spring, MD 20910
Phone: 301-589-3300
Fax: 301-589-5175
Website: http://
www.musictherapy.org
E-mail: info@musictherapy.org

## Nonverbal Learning Disorder

### NLD on the Web!
Website: http://
www.nldontheweb.org

### NLD Ontario
Website: http://
www.nldontario.org
E-mail: info@nldontario.org

## Occupational Therapy

### American Occupational Therapy Association
4720 Montgomery Lane
P.O. Box 31220
Bethesda, MD 20824-1220
Phone: 301-652-AOTA (2682)
Fax: 301-652-7711
TDD: 800-377-8555
Website: www.aota.org

## Prader-Willi Syndrome

### Prader-Willi Syndrome Association
5700 Midnight Pass Road
Suite 6
Sarasota, FL 34242
Toll-Free: 800-926-4797
Phone: 941-312-0400
Website: http://
www.pwsausa.org
E-mail: national@pwsausa.org

## Rett Syndrome

### International Rett Syndrome Association (IRSA)
9121 Piscataway Road
Suite 2B
Clinton, MD 20735
Toll-Free: 800-818-RETT (7388)
Phone: 301-856-3334
Fax: 301-856-3336
Website: http://
www.rettsyndrome.org
E-mail:
admin@rettsyndrome.org

## Rett Syndrome Research Foundation (RSRF)
4600 Devitt Drive
Cincinnati, OH 45246
Phone: 513-874-3020
Fax: 513-874-2520
Website: http://www.rsrf.org
E-mail: monica@rsrf.org

## Savant Syndrome

### Wisconsin Medical Society
330 E. Lakeside Street
Madison, WI 53715
Toll-Free: 866-442-3800
Fax: 608-442-3802
Website: http://www
.wisconsinmedicalsociety.org/
savant/

## Sibling Issues

### Autism Siblings
18337 Grevillea Avenue
Redondo Beach, CA 90278
Toll-Free: 877-456-3210
Fax: 310-793-6067
Website: http://
www.autismsiblings.org
E-mail:
autismsiblings@earthlink.net

### Sibling Support Project
6512 23rd Avenue NW, #213
Seattle, WA 98117
Phone: 206-297-6368
Fax: 509-752-6789
Website: http://
www.siblingsupport.org
E-mail:
donmeyer@siblingsupport.org

## Social Stories

### Gray Center for Social Learning and Understanding
4123 Embassy Drive SE
Kentwood, MI 49546
Phone: 616-954-9747
Fax: 616-954-9749
Website: http://
www.thegraycenter.org
E-mail: info@thegraycenter.org

## Son-Rise Program

### Autism Treatment Center of America
The Option Institute
2080 S. Undermountain Road
Sheffield, MA 01257
Toll-Free: 877-766-7473
Phone: 413-229-2100
Fax: 413-229-8931
Website: http://www
.autismtreatmentcenter.org

## TEACCH

### Division TEACCH
Phone: 919-966-2174
Fax: 919-966-4127
Website: http://www.teacch.com
E-mail: TEACCH@unc.edu

## Tuberous Sclerosis

### Epilepsy Foundation
8301 Professional Place
Landover, MD 20785-7223
Toll-Free: 800-EFA-1000
(332-1000)
Phone: 301-459-3700
Fax: 301-577-2684
Website: http://
www.epilepsyfoundation.org
E-mail: postmaster@efa.org

### Tuberous Sclerosis Alliance
801 Roeder Road, Suite 750
Silver Spring, MD 20910
Toll-Free: 800-225-6872
Phone: 301-562-9890
Fax: 301-562-9870
Website: http://
www.tsalliance.org
E-mail: info@tsalliance.org

## Williams Syndrome

### Williams Syndrome Foundation
University of California
Irvine, CA 92697-2300
Phone: 949-824-7259
Website: http://
www.williamssyndrome.org
E-mail: hlenhoff@uci.edu

# Index

# *Index*

Page numbers followed by 'n' indicate a footnote. Page numbers in *italics* indicate a table or illustration.

## A

AAA *see* American Academy of Audiology
ABA *see* applied behavior analysis
ABC *see* Aberrant Behavior Checklist; Autism Behavior Checklist
Aberrant Behavior Checklist (ABC) 245
Abrams, Phillip 416n
absence seizures
  described 173
  heredity 174
acetylcholine 123–25
Achenbach Child Behavior Checklist (CBCL) 245
ACNP *see* American College of Neuropsychopharmacology
ACTH *see* adrenocorticotropic hormone
Adderall 289
ADHD *see* attention deficit hyperactivity disorder
ADI-R *see* Autism Diagnostic Interview - Revised
ADOS *see* Autism Diagnostic Observation Schedule
adrenocorticotropic hormone (ACTH) 176
"After the Diagnosis: Moving Forward with Confidence" (First Signs, Inc.; Waltz) 257n
"After the Diagnosis: Ten Things Parents Need to Do When Facing Autism Spectrum Disorders" (First Signs, Inc.; Waltz) 254n
age factor
  Angelman syndrome 153
  autism behavioral symptoms 7
  childhood explanations 260–63
  educational services 12
  fathers, autistic children 128–30
  Landau-Kleffner syndrome 155
  nonverbal learning disabilities 38–39
  Tourette syndrome 163
  tuberous sclerosis 134
Ages and Stages Questionnaire 226
Ahearn, William H. 348n
AIT *see* Berard Auditory Integration Training
Alexander, Duane 113, 117

581

Amaral, David 107–8, 119, 121–23
American Academy of Audiology
    (AAA), contact information 574
American College of
    Neuropsychopharmacology (ACNP),
    oxytocin publication 360n
American Hippotherapy Association,
    contact information 575
American Music Therapy Association
    autism therapy publication 383n
    contact information 576
American Occupational Therapy
    Association
    autism treatment publication 379n
    contact information 576
American Speech-Language-Hearing
    Association (ASHA), contact
    information 569, 574, 575
Americans with Disabilities Act (ADA)
    Asperger syndrome 540
amygdala
    autism studies 119–23
    depicted *111*
Anafranil (clomipramine) 289, 357
Anderson, George M. 130
Angelman, Harry 153, 154
Angelman syndrome
    chromosome 15 82
    defined 557
    information resource 573
    overview 153–55
"Angelman Syndrome" (Edelson) 153n
Angelman Syndrome Foundation,
    contact information 573
"Angelman Syndrome Information
    Page" (NINDS) 153n
angiomyolipomas, tuberous
    sclerosis 136
ANI *see* Autism Network
    International
animal therapy 286–87
anti-anxiety medications,
    described 14
antibodies, autism 103–4
anticonvulsant medications
    described 50
    infantile spasms 176
    Landau-Kleffner syndrome 155
    seizures 357

antidepressant medications
    attention deficit hyperactivity
        disorder 358
    autism 356–57
    described 14, 49–50
    *see also* selective serotonin
        reuptake inhibitors
antipsychotic medications
    behavioral problems 357
    described 14, 50
anxiety disorders
    medications 356–57
    Tourette syndrome 165
APEQ *see* Autism Phenotype
    Events Questionnaire
applied behavior analysis (ABA)
    defined 557
    described 11, 281–82, 297–99
    information resources 573
    tuberous sclerosis 144
Archart-Treidhel, Joan 123n
"Are Autism Cases on the Rise in
    U.S.?" (ScoutNews, LLC) 20n
ARI *see* Autism Research Institute
art therapy 286
ASD *see* autism spectrum
    disorders
ASHA *see* American Speech-
    Language-Hearing Association
Ashwood, Paul 104, 105–6
ASIEP-2 *see* Autism Screening
    Instrument for Educational
    Planning
ASPEN *see* Asperger Syndrome
    Education Network
Asperger, Hans 23, 52
Asperger syndrome
    college life 530–36
    defined 34, 557
    described 4
    diagnostic criteria 35–36
    employee accommodations
        540–47
    gender factor 23–24
    information resources 573–74
    overview 51–57
Asperger Syndrome and High
    Functioning Autism Association,
    contact information 573

Asperger Syndrome Education Network (ASPEN), contact information 573
"Asperger Syndrome Fact Sheet" (NINDS) 51n
assistive technology therapists, autism treatment 269
Association for Science in Autism Treatment, contact information 569
ATEC *see* Autism Treatment Evaluation Checklist
Ativan (lorazepam) 289, 358
atonic seizures, described 173–74
attention deficit hyperactivity disorder (ADHD)
  described 35
  diagnostic criteria 41–42
  medications 357–58
  overview 193–99
  Tourette syndrome 165, 168
  tuberous sclerosis 137
"Attention Deficit Hyperactivity Disorder and Autism" (National Autistic Society) 193n
Attwood, Tony 260n
atypical autism *see* pervasive developmental disorder not otherwise specified
"Auditory Integration Training (AIT)" (National Autistic Society) 326n
auditory processing disorder (APD)
  information resources 574
  overview 187–91
"Auditory Processing Disorder in Children" (NIDCD) 187n
Auditory Sequential Memory Test 244
augmentative and alternative communication support 311–12
auras, focal seizures 173
AUTCOM *see* Autism National Committee
autism
  causes 48, 75–87, 99–126
  coping strategies 254–56
  defined 34
  diagnosis guidelines 226–32
  diagnostic criteria 35, 47–48
  estate planning 549–53

autism, continued
  overview 3–18, 46–51
  signs 7–10, 46–47
  treatment 11–15, 49–50, 271–73
    health care teams 267–70
    overview 275–92
"Autism and Airport Travel Safety Tips" (Debbaudt) 438n
"Autism and Environmental Exposures" (Center for Children's Health and the Environment) 99n
"Autism and Genes" (NICHD) 77n, 557n
Autism Behavior Checklist (ABC) 234
Autism Diagnostic Interview - Revised (ADI-R) 150, 229, 233, 237
Autism Diagnostic Observation Scale - Generic 229
Autism Diagnostic Observation Schedule (ADOS) 143, 150, 233–34, 237
"Autism Fact Sheet" (NINDS) 46n
Autism Information Center, contact information 569
Autism National Committee (AUTCOM)
  autism treatments publication 271n
  contact information 570
Autism Network for Hearing and Visually Impaired Persons, contact information 570
Autism Network International (ANI), contact information 570
Autism Outreach, Inc., applied behavior analysis publication 297n
"Autism Overview: What We Know" (NICHD) 3n, 557n
Autism Patient Center, website address 570
Autism-PDD Resources Network, website address 570
Autism Phenotype Events Questionnaire (APEQ) 244–45
Autism Research Foundation, contact information 570
Autism Research Institute (ARI)
  contact information 570
  Form E-2 Checklist 234–35

Autism Screening Instrument for Educational Planning (ASIEP-2) 233
Autism Screening Questionnaire 227
Autism Siblings, contact information 577
Autism Society Canada, publications
  safety concerns 405n
  sensory integration 324n
Autism Society of America
  contact information 570
  publications
    autism causes 75n
    autism treatments 275n
    family stresses 392n
Autism Society of Northwest Ohio, contact information 570
Autism Speaks, contact information 570
autism spectrum disorders (ASD)
  adult living arrangements 538–39
  described 4, 33
  overview 27–43
  signs 213–19
  treatment 11–15
  tuberous sclerosis 140–45
  see also individual disorders
"Autism Spectrum Disorders (Pervasive Developmental Disorders)" (NIMH) 213n, 271n, 356n, 538n
"Autism Spectrum Disorders: An Overview" (Kutscher) 27n
"Autism Spectrum Disorders: Pervasive Developmental Disorders" (NIMH) 110n
"Autism Teaching Methods: TEACCH (Treatment and Education of Autistic and Related Communication Handicapped Children)" (AutismWeb.com) 474n
Autism Treatment Center of America contact information 577
Autism Treatment Evaluation Checklist (ATEC) 235, 245
AutismWeb.com, teaching methods publication 474n
autistic disorder see autism
"The Autistic Savant" (Treffert) 205n
autistic savant, described 205–9
*The Autistic Spectrum Parents' Daily Helper* (Abrams; Henriques) 416n
autosomal dominant disorder, described 135

**B**

Baker, Michael 221n
Bartz, Jennifer 360
basal ganglia
  autism studies 124
  depicted *111*
bathing issues, autistic children 417–18
Bayley Scales of Infant Development, Second Edition (BSID-II) 238
Beery-Buktenica Developmental Test of Visual-Motor Integration - 4th Edition (VMI-4) 240
Behavioral Rating Inventory of Executive Functioning - Preschool (BRIEF-P) 243
behavioral symptoms
  autism 7, 280–81
  autism spectrum disorders 294–97
  medications 357
behavioral therapy
  Angelman syndrome 153, 155
  autism 11–12, 49
  fragile X syndrome 150
  Tourette syndrome 167
behavior management therapy, defined 558
Behavior Rating Inventory of Executive Functioning (BRIEF) 243
behavior therapists, autism treatment 269
benign epilepsy syndromes, described 175
benign infantile encephalopathy 175
benign neonatal convulsions 175
Bérard, Guy 326
Berard Auditory Integration Training (AIT) 324, 326–29
beta-hydroxybutyrate (BHB) 181
BHB see beta-hydroxybutyrate
biofeedback, epilepsy 182

"Biomedical and Dietary Approaches" (Autism Society of America) 275n
birth factors, autism 127–30
blood tests
  autism 107–8, 249
  epilepsy 177
  Tourette syndrome 166
Bourneville disease *see* tuberous sclerosis
brain areas, autism *111*, 113–16, 116–19
brain scans, epilepsy 176
brain stem, depicted *111*
brain tumors, tuberous sclerosis 136
BRIEF *see* Behavior Rating Inventory of Executive Functioning
BRIEF-P *see* Behavioral Rating Inventory of Executive Functioning - Preschool
Brigance Early Development Inventory 239
BRIGANCE Screens 226
BSID-II *see* Bayley Scales of Infant Development, Second Edition

**C**

café au lait spots, tuberous sclerosis 137
Cambridge Center for Behavioral Studies, Autism Section, contact information 573
CAN *see* Cure Autism Now Foundation
candidate gene, defined 558
CAPD *see* central auditory processing disorder
carbamazepine 357
CARD *see* Center for Autism and Related Disorders
cardiac rhabdomyomas, tuberous sclerosis 136, 138
CARS *see* Childhood Autism Rating Scale
casein-free diet 335–36, 348–53
case studies, transition plans 504–13
CAT scan *see* computed axial tomography scan

CBCL *see* Achenbach Child Behavior Checklist
CCTT *see* Children's Color Trails Test
CDC *see* Centers for Disease Control and Prevention
CDD *see* childhood disintegrative disorder
CELF-3 *see* Clinical Evaluation of Language Fundamentals - Third Edition
CELF-P *see* Clinical Evaluation of Language Fundamentals - Preschool
Center for Autism and Related Disorders (CARD)
  autism diagnosis publication 236n
  contact information 571, 573
Center for Children's Health and the Environment, environmental exposures, autism publication 99n
Center for the Study of Autism, contact information 571
Centers for Disease Control and Prevention (CDC), publications
  MMR vaccine, autism 89n
  parental factors, autism 127n
central auditory processing disorder (CAPD) 187
cerebellum, depicted *111*
cerebral cortex, depicted *111*
CGI *see* Clinical Global Impression
Charles, Jane 221–24
CHAT *see* Checklist for Autism in Toddlers; Childhood Autism Test
Checklist for Autism in Toddlers (CHAT) 227, 236
Child Development Inventories 226
Childhood Autism Rating Scale (CARS) 229, 234, 236
Childhood Autism Test (CHAT) 232–33
childhood disintegrative disorder
  defined 34
  diagnostic criteria 36
childhood disintegrative disorder (CDD), overview 68–70
"Childhood Disintegrative Disorder" (Yale Developmental Disabilities Clinic) 68n

childhood integrative disorder, autism 4

Children's Color Trails Test (CCTT) 243–44

"Children with Autism Have Distinctly Different Immune System Reactions" (University of California) 103n

chlorpromazine 357

cholinergic nicotine receptors 123–26

chromosome 7, Williams syndrome 163

chromosome 9, tuberous sclerosis 135

chromosome 15
Angelman syndrome 154, 557
autism 82
Prader-Willi syndrome 158, 560

chromosome 16, tuberous sclerosis 135

chromosomes
autism 24, 79, 81–83
defined 558
genes 77
hot spots, defined 559
Rett syndrome 65

classic autism *see* autism

Clinical Evaluation of Language Fundamentals - Preschool (CELF-P) 241

Clinical Evaluation of Language Fundamentals - Third Edition (CELF-3) 241

Clinical Global Impression (CGI) 245

clinical trials
autism 50–51
secretin 14–15
Tourette syndrome 170

clomipramine 167, 289, 356

clonic seizures, described 173

clonidine 167

clozapine 289

Clozaril (clozapine) 289

cognitive behavioral therapy, Asperger syndrome 56

colic, Williams syndrome 161

collaboration, described 497

Combating Autism Act (2006) 22

communication
autism 3, 78, 113–14
autism spectrum disorders 294
described 27–32
four stages 306–7
hyperlexia 202–4
overview 304–13
siblings 403
speech-language therapists 11–12
workplace 541–42

"Communication and Interaction" (National Autistic Society) 304n

communication disorders, overview 33–42

communication skills
autism spectrum disorders 215–16
nonverbal learning disabilities 38

complementary therapies, autism 286

complex motor tics, described 164

complex vocal tics, described 164

compulsions, described 560

computed axial tomography scan (CAT scan; CT scan)
autism 250
autism studies 110
epilepsy 176
savant syndrome 208
Tourette syndrome 166
tuberous sclerosis 138

computer-based auditory interventions, described 324–25

congenital, defined 558

Conquer Fragile X Foundation, contact information 574

conversation books, described 312–13

Conyers, Carole 436

Cooke, David A. 123n, 153n, 155n, 160n, 254n, 257n, 345n, 438n

coping strategies
autism 254–56
family issues 392–96
grocery store trips 434–36
grooming issues 416–27
medical appointments 436–37
siblings 397–404
travel concerns 438–40

coprolalia
defined 558
described 164

Corbett, Blythe 107
Cordero, José 127
corpus callosum
    autism studies 114–15
    depicted *111*
corticosteroids, Landau-Kleffner
    syndrome 155
Coulter, Julie 530n
counselors
    autism 49
    autism treatment 268–69
    transition plans 521–22
Courchesne, Eric 130
CT scan *see* computed axial
    tomography scan
cue cards, described 312
Cure Autism Now Foundation
    (CAN), contact information 571
cyclin-dependent
    kinase-like 5 gene 65
cytogenetic, defined 558
cytogenetic studies, autism 80–81, 82
cytokines, autism 105–506

**D**

Daily Life Therapy (Higashi) 376–78
"Daily Life Therapy: Higashi"
    (National Autistic Society) 376n
DAS *see* Differential Abilities Scale
Debbaudt, Dennis 438n
delayed matching to sample (DMTS)
    247–48
*dementia infantilis* 69
dental abnormalities, Williams
    syndrome 162
dental care, autistic children 424–27
Denver-II (DDST-II) 226
Depakote (valproic acid) 357
Department of Education *see* US
    Department of Education
"Dependent Measures" (CARD) 236n
depression
    medications 356–57
    Tourette syndrome 165, 168
Developmental, Individual-
    Difference, Relationship-Based
    method (DIR method) 283–84

developmental disabilities
    described 3, 78
    Williams syndrome 162
Developmental Neuropsychological
    Assessment (NEPSY) 244
Developmental Profile II 239
developmental screening, defined 558
Dexedrine 289
dextroamphetamine 167
"Diagnosing and Evaluating
    Autism: Part 1" (University
    of Florida) 248n
*Diagnostic and Statistical Manual
    of Mental Disorders, Fourth
    Edition (DSM-IV)*
    attention deficit hyperactivity
        disorder 193
    autistic disorders 33–34, 53
    fragile X syndrome 149
diazepam 358
diet and nutrition
    attention deficit hyperactivity
        disorder 195
    autism treatment 287, 291–92,
        332–44
    epilepsy 181
    Prader-Willi syndrome 158–60
Differential Abilities Scale
    (DAS) 239
dimethylglycine (DMG) 334–35
diphtheria-tetanus-pertussis vaccine,
    autism 104
DIR method *see* Developmental,
    Individual-Difference,
    Relationship-Based method
discrete trial teaching (DTT) 11, 298
Division TEACCH, contact
    information 577
DMG *see* dimethylglycine
DMTS *see* delayed matching to
    sample
DOE *see* US Department of
    Education
dolphin therapy 287
dopamine, behavioral problems 357
Down, J. Langdon 206–7
dressing issues, autistic children
    416–17
drop attacks, described 175

*DSM-IV see Diagnostic and Statistical Manual of Mental Disorders, Fourth Edition (DSM-IV)*
DTT *see* discrete trial teaching
dyskinesia, Tourette syndrome 167

# E

"Early Autism Diagnosis, Intervention Important" (Baker) 221n
early infantile autism, described 207
early intervention
  autism diagnosis 221–24
  fragile X syndrome 148
  legislation 11, 228
  Prader-Willi syndrome 159
  tuberous sclerosis 142
eating difficulties, autistic children 422–23
ECG *see* electrocardiogram
echolalia
  defined 558
  described 164, 222
Edelson, Stephen M. 153n, 155n, 160n
Eden, Guinevere 203
education
  autistic children 12–13
  legislation 11, 12, 450–54
  Tourette syndrome 138–69
  *see also* schools
Elavil 289
electrocardiogram (ECG), defined 558
electroencephalogram (EEG)
  autism 249
  epilepsy 176–77
  Tourette syndrome 166
"Employees with Asperger Syndrome" (Job Accommodation Network) 540n
environmental factors
  attention deficit hyperactivity disorder 195–96
  autism 5, 99–102, 106
epidemiological studies, defined 558
epidemiology, Tourette syndrome 170

epilepsy
  autism studies 122
  autistic spectrum disorders 15
  defined 558–59
  Landau-Kleffner syndrome 156
  overview 171–86
  seizures 561
  tuberous sclerosis 142
Epilepsy Foundation, contact information 575, 578
epiloia *see* tuberous sclerosis
estate planning, autism 549–53
expressive verbal language, described 28

# F

facial angiofibromas, tuberous sclerosis 137
facilitated communication
  described 286
  overview 317–22
"Facilitated Communication" (National Autistic Society) 317n
failure to understand, secondary problems 32
Family Educational Rights and Privacy ACT (FERPA) 535
family studies, autism 79
FAPE *see* free appropriate public education
"FAQs about MMR Vaccine and Autism" (CDC) 89n
fatty acids, autism treatment 338–39
FDA *see* US Food and Drug Administration
"FDA Approves the First Drug to Treat Irritability Association with Autism, Risperdal" (FDA) 359n
feeding tubes
  Prader-Willi syndrome 158
  Rett syndrome 62
Feingold Association of the United States, contact information 574
Feingold diet, information resource 574
FERPA *see* Family Educational Rights and Privacy ACT

financial considerations
autism treatment 12
occupational therapy 381
postsecondary education
527–28
Son-Rise program 369–70
stress management 383
first aid, seizures 185–86
First Signs, Inc., publications
autism diagnosis 254n, 257n
treatment teams 267n
"First Year of College: Lessons
Learned" (Coulter) 530n
Floor time
described 283–84
information resource 574
Floortime Foundation, contact
information 574
fluency teaching 298–99
fluoxetine 167, 289, 356
fluphenazine 357
fluvoxamine 167, 289, 356
fMRI *see* functional magnetic
resonance imaging
focal seizures
described 172–73
treatment 179
Food and Drug Administration
(FDA) *see* US Food and Drug
Administration
forehead plaques, tuberous
sclerosis 137
foster homes, adult living
arrangements 539
Fragile X Research Foundation,
contact information 574
fragile X syndrome
autism 7, 223
autism spectrum disorders 218
autistic spectrum disorders 15
defined 559
information resources 574
overview 146–52
"Fragile X Syndrome" (University
of Michigan) 146n
Frankel, Fred 429
fraternal twins
autism 223
defined 559

free appropriate public education
(FAPE) 494, 525
functional contextual assessment,
tuberous sclerosis 143
functional magnetic resonance
imaging (fMRI)
autism studies 114, 118
epilepsy 176

**G**

GABA pathway genes
*see* gamma-amino-butyric
acid pathway genes
GADS *see* Gilliam Asperger's
Disorder Scale
galantamine 125–26
Galson, Steven 359
gamma-amino-butyric acid pathway
genes (GABA pathway genes) 84–85
GARS *see* Gilliam Autism Rating
Scale
gastroesophageal reflux, defined 559
gaze direction, described 222
gender factor
autism 23–25, 89
autism statistics 6
autism studies 121–23
childhood disintegrative disorder 69
fragile X syndrome 146
Rett syndrome 58
savant syndrome 207
Tourette syndrome 163
generalized seizures, described 173–74
genes
Asperger syndrome 53–54
autism 5, 24, 77–87
autism spectrum disorders 20–21
CDKL5 65
defined 559
ENGRAILED2 54
FMR1 146, 149
GABA pathway 84–85
GABRB3 54
HOX 82
HOXA1 83–84
HOXD1 84
MECP2 59–60, 64–65, 561

genes, continued
  RELN 84
  Rett syndrome 59–60
  TSC1 134–35, 139–40
  TSC2 134–35, 139–40
  UBE3A 153, 557
genetic counseling, Tourette
  syndrome 168
genetic studies, Tourette
  syndrome 169
genetic testing
  autism 227, 250
  tuberous sclerosis 135
genome
  defined 559
  described 80
Geodon (ziprasidone) 357
Gilliam Asperger's Disorder Scale
  (GADS) 236–37
Gilliam Autism Rating Scale
  (GARS) 229, 234, 236
gluten-free diet 335–36, 348–53
Goldman-Fristoe-Woodcock Test of
  Auditory Discrimination 240–41
gonadal mosaicism, tuberous
  sclerosis 135
Grandin, Temple 285, 325
grandparents, stress sources
  394–95
Gray, Carol 284
Gray Center for Social Learning
  and Understanding
  contact information 577
Greenspan, Stanley 283
grooming issues, autistic children
  416–27
group homes, adult living
  arrangements 539
growth dysregulation hypothesis 112
guanfacine 167
*Guideline Summary: Practice
  Parameter - Screening and
  Diagnosis of Autism* (NGC) 226n
"A Guide to Improving Behaviors in
  Children with Autism Spectrum
  Disorders" (Stephens) 294n
"A Guide to the Individualized
  Education Program" (DOE) 449n
Gutstein, Steven 285

**H**

Hagerman, Randi 146n
Haldol (haloperidol) 357
haloperidol 166, 357
hamartin 135
Harchik, Alan 434n, 436n
health care proxies, estate
  planning 552
health care teams
  autism diagnosis 48
  autism treatment 267–70
  Rett syndrome 63–64
"Healthy Smiles for Children with
  Autism" (Rady Children's Hospital
  and Health Center) 424n
hearing tests, autism 249
heart problems, Williams
  syndrome 161
Heller, Theodore 69
Hellings, Jessica 410
"Helping Siblings Understand
  Autism and Encouraging
  Positive Relationships" (Mathew,
  et al.) 397n
Henriques, Leslie 416n
hereditary, defined 559
heredity
  Asperger syndrome 53–54
  autism 5, 48–49
  epilepsy 174
  fragile X syndrome 146
  Prader-Willi syndrome 157
  Rett syndrome 59–60
  Tourette syndrome 167–68
  tuberous sclerosis 135
hernias, Williams syndrome 162
HFA *see* high-functioning autism
high-functioning autism (HFA)
  described 34
  diagnosis 55
  diagnostic criteria 37
hippocampus
  depicted *111*
  epilepsy 175
hippotherapy, information
  resources 575
Hollander, Eric 360–62

homeobox genes
  autism 82, 83–84
  defined 559
hot spots, defined 559
"How Do the Behaviors Seen in
  Persons with Fragile X Relate to
  Those Seen in Autism?"
  (Hagerman) 146n
HPRT enzyme 412
hug machine, described 325
hyperacusis, Williams syndrome 162
hypercalcemia, Williams syndrome
  161
hyperlexia
  defined 559
  described 34
  diagnostic criteria 41
  overview 202–4
hypomelanic macules, tuberous
  sclerosis 137, 138

**I**

IBD *see* inflammatory bowel disease
*ICD-10 see International
  Classification of Diseases*
IDEA *see* Individuals with
  Disabilities Education Act
"IDEA 2004 Roadmap to the IEP: IEP
  Meetings, Content, Review and
  Revision, Placements, Transition,
  and Transfers" (Wright; Wright)
  449n
identical twins
  autism 223
  defined 559
idiot savant, described 206–7
IEP *see* individualized education
  plans; Individualized Education
  Program
IHC, puberty publication 441n
ILC *see* independent living centers
Illinois Autism/PDD Training and
  Technical Assistance Project,
  publications
  picture exchange communication
    system 314n
  social stories 300n

immune system, autism 103–8
"The Importance of Estate Planning"
  (Wolf; Leipzig) 549n
impulsivity, workplace 542–43
independent living centers (ILC) 498,
  500
Indiana Resource Center for Autism,
  contact information 571
individualized education plans
  (IEP)
  defined 559
  described 13, 278
  tuberous sclerosis 143
Individualized Education Program
  (IEP)
  Asperger syndrome 533
  high school 491
  overview 449–71
  postsecondary education 527
Individuals with Disabilities
  Education Act (IDEA; 1997) 11, 12,
  228, 278, 467–71, 492
Individuals with Disabilities
  Education Improvement Act
  (2004) 11, 12, 494–96
infantile spasms 175–76
inflammatory bowel disease (IBD)
  new variant 91
  vaccines 93–94
information processing,
  autism 310–11
inheritance *see* genes; heredity
Insel, Thomas R. 121
institutions, adult living
  arrangements 539
insurance coverage
  autism treatment 12
  estate planning 552–53
intentional communication,
  described 305
interactive communication
  boards, described 312
*International Classification of
  Diseases (ICD-10)* 52
International Rett Syndrome
  Association (IRSA), contact
  information 576
internet health information,
  overview 563–67

intractable epilepsy, described 172, 178
Irlen lenses 325
Irlen Institute, contact information 575
Irlen method, information resource 575
irritability, Williams syndrome 161
IRSA *see* International Rett Syndrome Association
"Is Eliminating Casein and Gluten from a Child's Diet a Viable Treatment for Autism?" (Ahearn) 348n

**J**

Job Accommodation Network, Asperger syndrome employees publication 540n
joint attention, described 31
Just, Marcel 113, 115–16
juvenile myoclonic epilepsy 175

**K**

Kanner, Leo 207
Kaufman, Raun 364
Kay, Shannon 435
ketogenic diet, epilepsy 181
ketosis, epilepsy 181
kidney disorders
  tuberous sclerosis 136
  Williams syndrome 162
Kitahara, Kiyo 376
Kutscher, Martin 27n

**L**

Lamictal (lamotrigine) 357
lamotrigine 357
Landau-Kleffner syndrome
  defined 560
  information resources 575–76
  overview 155–56
"Landau-Kleffner Syndrome" (Edelson) 155n

"Landau-Kleffner Syndrome Information Page" (NINDS) 155n
Language Processing Test - Revised (LPT-R) 242
language skills
  Asperger syndrome 51–52
  autism 7, 113
  communication 28–32
  early autism diagnosis 222
  hyperlexia 41
"Learning Approaches" (Autism Society of America) 275n
learning disorders, language-based 33
Leipzig, Steven D. 549n
Leiter International Performance Scale - Revised (LIPS-R) 238
Lennox-Gastaut syndrome 175
Leong, Sylvina 397n
limbic system, autism studies 112
linkage disequilibrium, defined 560
linkage ratios, autism 81
"The Link Between the Immune System and Autism" (University of California) 103n
Lippincott Williams and Wilkins, dictionary publication 557n
LIPS-R *see* Leiter International Performance Scale - Revised
literal verbal skills, described 28
lithium 358
"Living with Autism: Stress on Families" (Autism Society of America) 392n
lorazepam 358
Lovaas, O. Ivar 281, 475
low birth weight, Williams syndrome 161
LPT-R *see* Language Processing Test - Revised
Luvox (fluvoxamine) 289, 356

**M**

MAAP Services for Autism, Asperger's and PDD, contact information 571
magnesium supplements 332–33

magnetic resonance imaging (MRI)
  autism 250
  autism studies 110, 119–20
  epilepsy 176, 184
  fragile X syndrome 150
  savant syndrome 208
  Tourette syndrome 166
  tuberous sclerosis 138
magnetic resonance spectroscopy
  (MRS), epilepsy 177, 184–85
magnetoencephalogram (MEG),
  epilepsy 177, 184
Massachusetts General Hospital,
  autism screening tools publication
  232n
Mathew, Jenie 397n
measles mumps rubella vaccine
  (MMR vaccine)
  autism 21, 22, 76, 104
  overview 89–97
"Medical Appointments Can Be
  Made Less Challenging for
  Children with Autism"
  (Harchik) 436n
medical devices, epilepsy 180–81
medications
  Asperger syndrome 56
  autism spectrum disorders 13–14
  autism treatment 49–50, 287–90,
    356–62
  epilepsy 178–79
  Landau-Kleffner syndrome 155
  self-injurious behavior 410–11
  Tourette syndrome 166–67
MEG *see* magnetoencephalogram
melanin, tuberous sclerosis 137
melatonin, epilepsy 182
memory without reckoning 207
mental retardation
  autism 7
  autistic spectrum disorders 15,
    217
  defined 560
  savant syndrome 206
  tuberous sclerosis 137
mercury, autism 21
Merrill Palmer Scale of Mental
  Tests (MPSMT) 238–39
metabolic screening, autism 249

methyl-CpG-binding protein 2 gene
  59–60, 64–65
methylphenidate 167, 357
mineral supplements, autism
  treatment 290–91
Minshew, Nancy 117–19
MMR vaccine *see* measles mumps
  rubella vaccine
molluscum fibrosum, tuberous
  sclerosis 137
motor skills
  Asperger syndrome 51–52
  nonverbal learning disabilities 37
  Rett syndrome 62–63
motor therapies, sensory
  integration 324–25
motor tics, described 164–65
MPSMT *see* Merrill Palmer
  Scale of Mental Tests
MRI *see* magnetic resonance
  imaging
MRS *see* magnetic resonance
  spectroscopy
mTOR 135, 139, 140
musculoskeletal problems,
  Williams syndrome 162
music therapy
  described 286
  information resources 576
  overview 383–88
"Music Therapy and Individuals
  with Diagnoses on the Autism
  Spectrum" (American Music
  Therapy Association) 383n
mutation, defined 560
myoclonic encephalopathy 175
myoclonic seizures, described 173

## N

naltrexone 358
narcolepsy, focal seizures 173
NARHA *see* North American Riding
  for the Handicapped Association,
  Inc.
Nathanson, David 287
National Aphasia Association,
  contact information 575

National Autistic Society,
publications
attention deficit hyperactivity
disorder 193n
auditory integration training 326n
communication concerns 304n
daily life therapy 376n
diets 332n
facilitated communication 317n
gender factor, autism 23n
Higashi 376n
Son-Rise program 364n
vitamins 332n
National Dissemination Center for
Children with Disabilities
(NICHCY)
contact information 571
transition planning publication 491n
National Fragile X Foundation,
contact information 574
National Guideline Clearinghouse
(NGC), autism diagnosis
publication 226n
National Institute of Child Health
and Human Development (NICHD)
contact information 572
publications
autism overview 3n
glossary 557n
heredity, autism 77n
National Institute of Mental
Health (NIMH)
contact information 572
publications
adult living arrangements 538n
autism research 110n
autism spectrum disorders 213n
autism treatment 271n
medications 356n
National Institute of Neurological
Disorders and Stroke (NINDS),
publications
Angelman syndrome 153n
Asperger syndrome 51n
autism 46n
epilepsy 171n
Landau-Kleffner syndrome 155n
Tourette syndrome 163n
tuberous sclerosis 134n

National Institute on Deafness and
Other Communication Disorders
(NIDCD)
auditory processing disorder
publication 187n
Information Clearinghouse, contact
information 572
National Institutes of Health (NIH),
autism research publications 113n,
116n
National Institutes of Health
Autism Research Network,
website address 572
National Organization for Rare
Disorders (NORD), contact
information 572, 576
neocortical epilepsy, described 175
NEPSY *see* Developmental
Neuropsychological Assessment
neuroimaging studies, Tourette
syndrome 169–70
neuroleptic medications, Tourette
syndrome 166–67
neurologists, autism treatment
267–68
neurons
autism studies 121–23
epilepsy 171, 177
neuropathology, Tourette syndrome
170
neuropsychologists, autism
treatment 268
neurotransmitters
autism studies 48, 110–12, 123
chromosome 17 85
defined 560
Tourette syndrome 165
"New Research Suggests Oxytocin's
Potential for Treatment of Two
Core Autism Symptom Domains"
(ACNP) 360n
New York Families for Autistic
Children, contact information 572
NICHCY *see* National Dissemination
Center for Children with
Disabilities
NICHD *see* National Institute of
Child Health and Human
Development

nicotine receptors, autism studies 123–26

"Nicotine Receptors May Play Role in Development of Autism" (Archart-Treidhel) 123n

NIDCD *see* National Institute on Deafness and Other Communication Disorders

NIH *see* National Institutes of Health

NIMH *see* National Institute of Mental Health

NINDS *see* National Institute of Neurological Disorders and Stroke

NLD Ontario, website address 576

NLD on the Web!, website address 576

nonverbal communication skills, described 28–32

nonverbal learning disabilities (NVLD) described 34
diagnostic criteria 37–39

nonverbal learning disorder, information resources 576

NORD *see* National Organization for Rare Disorders

North American Riding for the Handicapped Association, Inc. (NARHA), contact information 575

NVLD *see* nonverbal learning disabilities

**O**

O.A.S.I.S., website address 574

obsessions, described 560

obsessive-compulsive disorder (OCD)
defined 560
Tourette syndrome 165, 168

occupational therapists
autism 12, 230
autism treatment 269
described 380
Rett syndrome 64

occupational therapy
Angelman syndrome 153, 155
Asperger syndrome 56
autism 250, 379–81
defined 560
information resource 576

"Occupational Therapy's Role with Autism" (American Occupational Therapy Association) 379n

OCD *see* obsessive-compulsive disorder

oculomotor exercises, described 325

olanzapine 289, 357

Olden, Kenneth 106

"Older Fathers More Likely to Have Autistic Children" (ScoutNews, LLC) 127n

"One-on-One Playdates" (Parrish) 429n

Online Asperger Syndrome Information and Support (O.A.S.I.S.), website address 574

Organization for Autism Research, contact information 572

oxytocin 360–62

**P**

pancreatic exocrine disease, diagnosis 561

"Parent, Pregnancy, and Birth Factors Found Possible Associations with the Risk of Autism" (CDC) 127n

parental training, Asperger syndrome 56

Parent Interview for Autism 229

Parents' Evaluations of Developmental Status 226

"Parent Skill Building Series: Eating Difficulties" (Ward) 422n

"Parent Skill Building Series: Sleeping Difficulties" (Ward) 420n

"Parent Skill Building Series: Toilet Training Difficulties" (Ward) 418n

Parent Stress Index (PSI) 245

parietal cortex, autism studies 114–15

paroxetine 167

Parrish, Marsha 429n

partial seizures *see* focal seizures

PBS *see* positive behavioral interventions and support

PDD *see* pervasive developmental disorders

PDDAS *see* Pervasive Developmental Disorder Assessment Scale

PDD-NOS *see* pervasive developmental disorder not otherwise specified

PDDST *see* Pervasive Developmental Disorders Screening Test

Peabody Picture Vocabulary Test - Revised (PPVT-III) 241–42

PECS *see* picture exchange communication system

pediatricians, autism treatment 267, 270

PEP *see* Psycho Educational Profile

PEP-R *see* Psychoeducational Profile - Revised

Perry, Elaine 124–25

pervasive, described 34

Pervasive Developmental Disorder Assessment Scale (PDDAS) 235

pervasive developmental disorder not otherwise specified (PDD-NOS)
    described 4, 34
    diagnostic criteria 36
    overview 70–71

"Pervasive Developmental Disorder - Not Otherwise Specified (PDD-NOS)" (Yale Developmental Disabilities Clinic) 70n

pervasive developmental disorders (PDD)
    defined 33–34, 560
    overview 3–18

Pervasive Developmental Disorders Screening Test (PDDST) 229, 233

PET *see* positron emission tomography

Peterson, Bradley 20–22

petit mal seizures, described 173

phakomas, tuberous sclerosis 136

physical therapists
    autism 12, 230
    autism treatment 269
    Rett syndrome 64

physical therapy
    Angelman syndrome 153, 155
    Asperger syndrome 56
    autism 250–51

"Picture Exchange Communication System" (Illinois Autism/PDD Training and Technical Assistance Project) 314n

picture exchange communication system (PECS)
    described 282–93
    overview 314–16
    tuberous sclerosis 144–45

pimozide 166

Pitocin (oxytocin) 361

pivotal response training (PRT), described 11, 283

"Planning for Successful Transitions across Grade Levels" (Pratt) 487n

play dates, overview 429–32

PLS-4 *see* Preschool Language Scale Fourth Edition

poliosis, tuberous sclerosis 137

positive behavioral interventions and support (PBS), described 11

positron emission tomography (PET)
    autism studies 110
    epilepsy 176
    savant syndrome 208

postsecondary education, disabilities 524–29

power of attorney, estate planning 552

PPVT-III *see* Peabody Picture Vocabulary Test - Revised

Prader-Willi syndrome
    chromosome 15 82
    defined 560
    information resource 576
    overview 157–60

Prader-Willi Syndrome Association
    contact information 576
    Prader-Willi publication 157n

pragmatic language, described 30

pragmatics, described 39

Pratt, Cathy 487n

Pratt, Michelle 436–37

prednisone 176

prefrontal cortex, autism studies 114–15

pregnancy
    autism 127–28
    fragile X syndrome 147

pre-intentional communication, described 305
premonitory urge, described 164
prenatal testing, fragile X syndrome 147
Preschool Language Scale Fourth Edition (PLS-4) 240
prevalence, defined 560
privacy concerns, internet health websites 566
prodigious savants, described 205–6
Professional Development in Autism Center, contact information 572
progressive epilepsy, described 175
proteins, defined 561
Prozac (fluoxetine) 289, 356
PRT *see* pivotal response training
PSI *see* Parent Stress Index
psychiatrists, autism treatment 268
Psycho Educational Profile (PEP) 282
Psychoeducational Profile - Revised (PEP-R) 240
psychologists, autism treatment 268
psychotherapy, Tourette syndrome 167
puberty, coping strategies 441–46
"Puberty and Sexuality" (IHC) 441n
"Putting Together Your Child's Treatment Team" (First Signs, Inc.; Waltz) 267n

# Q

QABF *see* Questions about Behavioral Function
Questions about Behavioral Function (QABF) 245
"Questions and Answers on Prader-Willi Syndrome" (Prader-Willi Syndrome Association) 157n
quetiapine 289

# R

Rady Children's Hospital and Health Center, dental care publication 424n
rapamycin 138–39

rasmussen encephalitis 175, 179
RDI *see* relationship development intervention
R-DPDQ *see* Revised Denver Pre-Screening Developmental Questionnaire
receptive verbal language, described 28
"Red Flags and Rules of Thumb for Evaluating Treatments" (AUTCOM) 271n
Reelin gene 84
regression
  autism 89
  autistic behavior 7
  Rett syndrome 58, 62
Rehabilitation Act (1973) 524
Reichenberg, Abraham 129–30
relationship development intervention (RDI) 285
repetitive behaviors
  autism 4, 78
  autism spectrum disorders 216–17
replicate, defined 561
research
  Asperger syndrome 57
  auditory processing disorder 189–90
  autism 50–51, 79–85
  Rett syndrome 64–65
  self-injurious behavior 411–12
  Tourette syndrome 169–70
"Researchers Gain Insight into Why Brain Areas Fail to Work Together in Autism" (NIH) 113n
Rett syndrome
  autism 4
  defined 34, 561
  diagnostic criteria 36
  information resources 576–77
  overview 58–68
"Rett Syndrome" (NICHD) 557n
Rett Syndrome Research Foundation (RSRF), contact information 577
Revised Denver Pre-Screening Developmental Questionnaire (R-DPDQ) 226
Rimland, Bernard 327
Risperdal (risperidone) 289, 357, 359, 410–11

risperidone 289, 357, 359, 410–11
Ritalin (methylphenidate) 198–99,
    289, 357
rituals
    described 560
routines
    autism 4, 78
    autism spectrum disorders 295
RSRF *see* Rett Syndrome Research
    Foundation
rubella, autism 96

**S**

safety considerations, homes 405–8
Sandman, Curt 411
savant syndrome
    information resource 577
    overview 205–9
SBAI *see* Social Behavior Assessment
    Inventory
SBIS-IV *see* Stanford-Binet
    Intelligence Scale, Fourth Edition
Scales of Independent Behavior -
    Revised 230
Schendel, Diana 128
schools
    autistic children 12–13
    individualized education programs
        449–71
    structured teaching 475–86
    TEACCH method 144, 282, 474–75
    transitional planning 487–89
    *see also* education
school transitions, overview 487–89
Schopler, Eric 475
Schroeder, Stephen 409n, 410–12
Schumann, Cynthia Mills 121–23
"Scientists Report Strong Evidence of
    Immune and Protein Alterations in
    Blood Samples of Children with
    Autism, Raising Hope for an Early
    Diagnostic Blood Test" (University
    of California) 103n
scoliosis, Rett syndrome 61, 62
ScoutNews, LLC, publications
    autism statistics 20n
    parental factors, autism 127n

SCQ *see* Social Communication
    Questionnaire
Screening Tool for Autism in
    Two-Year-Olds 229
secretin
    defined 561
    described 14–15
    overview 345–47
seizure disorders, autistic spectrum
    disorders 15
seizures
    Angelman syndrome 153
    autism spectrum disorders 217–18
    childhood disintegrative
        disorder 69
    defined 561
    epilepsy 171–74
    Landau-Kleffner syndrome 156
    medications 357
    Rett syndrome 61, 65
    treatment 50
    tuberous sclerosis 137, 138, 142
"Seizures and Epilepsy: Hope
    Through Research" (NINDS) 171n
selective serotonin reuptake
    inhibitors (SSRI)
    autism 288–89, 356–57
    defined 561
    described 14
    fragile X syndrome 150
    Tourette syndrome 167
self-injurious behavior
    medications 13
    overview 409–13
    tuberous sclerosis 137
"Self-Injurious Behavior" (Simpson)
    409n
semantic language, described 28
semantic-pragmatic language
    disorder (SPLD)
    described 34
    diagnostic criteria 39–41
semantics, described 39
sensory integration
    described 285–86
    overview 324–25
"Sensory Integration and Motor
    Therapies" (Autism Society
    Canada) 324n

sensory problems, autism spectrum disorders 217, 294–95, 296
Seroquel (quetiapine) 289
serotonin
  autism studies 48, 85
  autism treatment 338
  chromosome 17 83, 85
  defined 561
sertraline 167, 356
sexuality, coping strategies 441–46
shagreen patches, tuberous sclerosis 137
Shih, Andy 122
"Should You Explain the Diagnosis to the Child?" (Attwood) 260n
siblings
  autism diagnosis 226–27
  autism statistics 6
  coping strategies 397–404
  counseling 49
  information resources 577
  MMR vaccine 96
  stress sources 394
Sibling Support Project, contact information 577
Side Effects and Symptom Questionnaire 246
sign language, described 312
signs
  Asperger syndrome 51–52, 53
  autism 46–47
  autism spectrum disorders 213–19
  Rett syndrome 60–61
simple motor tics, described 164
Simpson, Joy 409n
Singer, Alison 20–22
single photon emission computed tomography (SPECT)
  autism studies 110
  epilepsy 177
  savant syndrome 208
skill-development homes, adult living arrangements 539
skills set, communication 28–32
skin abnormalities, tuberous sclerosis 137
skin tags, tuberous sclerosis 137
sleeping difficulties, autistic children 420–22

Social Behavior Assessment Inventory (SBAI) 242
Social Communication Questionnaire (SCQ) 235
social interactions
  Angelman syndrome 154
  autism 4, 78
  autism spectrum disorders 214–15
  communication skills 29–30
  Tourette syndrome 168
  Williams syndrome 162
Social Responsiveness Scale (SRS) 243
social skills
  hyperlexia 41
  nonverbal learning disabilities 38
  workplace 544–45
Social Skills Rating Scale (SSRS) 242
social skills training, Asperger syndrome 56
social stories
  described 284–85
  overview 300–302
"Social Stories" (Illinois Autism/PDD Training and Technical Assistance Project) 300n
social workers, autism treatment 268
Son-Rise program
  information resources 577
  overview 364–75
"The Son-Rise Program" (National Autistic Society) 364n
Southwest Autism Research and Resource Center, contact information 573
spatial orientation skills, nonverbal learning disabilities 37–38
special education services, described 12–13
special services teams, education 13
SPECT *see* single photon emission computed tomography
spectrum disorders, described 4
speech-language therapists
  auditory processing disorder 189
  autism 230
  described 11–12
  Rett syndrome 64

speech-language therapy
   Asperger syndrome 56
   autism 250
speech therapists, autism treatment
   269
speech therapy, Landau-Kleffner
   syndrome 155
SRS *see* Social Responsiveness Scale
SSRI *see* selective serotonin reuptake
   inhibitors
SSRS *see* Social Skills Rating Scale
Stanford-Binet Intelligence Scale,
   Fourth Edition (SBIS-IV) 238
statistics
   Angelman syndrome 154
   autism 6, 20–22, 95, 99–100, 222
   gender factor, autism 23
   Prader-Willi syndrome 157
   tuberous sclerosis 134, 141
status epilepticus 179, 182–83
*Stedman's Electronic Medical
   Dictionary* (Lippincott Williams
   and Wilkins) 557n
Stephens, Laurie 294n
stereotyped behaviors, defined 561
Stokes, Susan 475n
stress management
   family issues 392–96
   workplace 543
Stroop Test 244
structured teaching, overview
   475–86
"Structured Teaching: Strategies for
   Supporting Students with Autism"
   (Stokes) 475n
"Students with Disabilities Preparing
   for Postsecondary Education: Know
   Your Rights and Responsibilities"
   (DOE) 524n
"Studying Hyperlexia May Unlock
   How Brains Read" (Vedantam)
   202n
"Study Provides Evidence That
   Autism Affects Functioning of
   Entire Brain" (NIH) 116n
substance abuse, Tourette syndrome
   168
subungual fibromas, tuberous
   sclerosis 137

sudden unexplained death,
   epilepsy 183
"Summary of Applied Behavior
   Analysis" (Autism Outreach, Inc.)
   297n
supplements, autism treatment
   332–44
surgical procedures
   epilepsy 179–80
   Landau-Kleffner syndrome
      155–56
susceptibility, defined 561
swinging, described 325
Symbolic Play Scale 243
symbolic play skills, described 31

**T**

"Table of All Screening Tools and
   Rating Scales: Pervasive
   Developmental Disorder and
   Autism Spectrum" (Massachusetts
   General Hospital) 232n
TACA *see* Talk About Curing Autism
"Taking a Child with Autism to the
   Grocery Store" (Harchik) 434n
Talk About Curing Autism (TACA),
   contact information 573
tardive dyskinesia, Tourette
   syndrome 167
TEACCH *see* treatment and
   education of autistic and related
   communication handicapped
   children
Tegretol (carbamazepine) 357
temporal lobe epilepsy (TLE)
   described 175
   treatment 180
temporal lobes, tuberous
   sclerosis 141–42
Test of Language Development
   Primary and Intermediate - Third
   Edition (TOLD-3) 241
Test of Pragmatic Language
   (TOPL) 242
Test of Problem Solving, Elementary
   and Adolescent - Revised (TOPS-R)
   243

tests
  auditory processing disorder 189
  autism 107–8, 223, 226–51
  brain studies 114
  epilepsy 177
  fragile X syndrome 147
  hearing 227
  Prader-Willi syndrome 157–58
  Tourette syndrome 166
  tuberous sclerosis 143
theory of mind
  described 29
  pragmatic language 30
therapists, autism treatment 268–69
therapy
  Asperger syndrome 56
  autism 11–12, 49–50, 257–59
  Rett syndrome 64
  Tourette syndrome 167
thimerosal 21, 22
thioridazine 357
tics, Tourette syndrome 163–69
time management, workplace 542
"Tips from Parents of Children with
  ASDs" (Autism Society Canada)
  405n
TLE *see* temporal lobe epilepsy
TMS *see* transcranial magnetic
  stimulation
toilet training, autistic children
  418–19
TOLD-3 *see* Test of Language
  Development Primary and
  Intermediate - Third Edition
tonic-clonic seizures, described 174
tonic seizures, described 173
Topamax (topiramate) 357
"Topic: Secondary Transition"
  (DOE) 491n
topiramate 357
TOPL *see* Test of Pragmatic
  Language
TOPS-R *see* Test of Problem
  Solving, Elementary and
  Adolescent - Revised
Tourette, Georges Gilles de la 163
Tourette syndrome
  defined 561
  overview 163–70

"Tourette Syndrome Fact Sheet"
  (NINDS) 163n
Tower of Hanoi 244
Tower of London test 114
transcranial magnetic stimulation
  (TMS), epilepsy 181
transitional planning
  overview 491–522
  schools 460, 487–89
  structured teaching 482
"Transition Planning: A Team
  Effort" (NICHCY) 491n
travel concerns
  attention deficit hyperactivity
    disorder 196–97
  coping strategies 438–40
  safety considerations 407
"Treatment" (Autism Society of
  America) 275n
treatment and education of autistic
  and related communication
  handicapped children (TEACCH)
  described 282
  overview 474–86
  tuberous sclerosis 144
Treffert, Darold A. 205n
tricyclics, described 14
TSC (tuberous sclerosis complex)
  *see* tuberous sclerosis
tuberin 135
tuberous sclerosis
  autism 7
  autism spectrum disorders 218
  autistic spectrum disorders 15
  defined 561–62
  information resources 578
  overview 134–45
Tuberous Sclerosis Alliance
  contact information 577
  tuberous sclerosis publication 134n
tuberous sclerosis complex (TSC)
  *see* tuberous sclerosis
"Tuberous Sclerosis Complex and
  Autism Spectrum Disorders"
  (Tuberous Sclerosis Alliance) 134n
"Tuberous Sclerosis Fact Sheet"
  (NINDS) 134n
tumors, tuberous sclerosis 135–37,
  141–42

twins
  autism 223
  fraternal, defined 559
  identical, defined 559
twins studies, autism 79

## U

"UC Davis M.I.N.D. Institute Finds
  that Brain Regions Involving
  Memory and Emotion are Larger in
  Children with Autism" (University
  of California) 119n
"UC Davis M.I.N.D. Institute
  Researchers Find Fewer Neurons in
  the Amygdala of Males with Autism"
  (University of California) 121n
ungual fibromas, tuberous sclerosis
  137
University of California, publications
  autism research 119n, 121n
  immune system 103n
University of Florida, autism
  diagnosis publication 248n
University of Michigan, fragile X
  syndrome publication 146n
unspoken communication skills,
  described 28–32
unwritten rules, knowledge 30–31
US Department of Education (DOE),
  publications
  individualized education
    programs 449n
  postsecondary education
    planning 524n
  transition planning 491n
"The Use of Diet and Vitamins in the
  Treatment of Autism" (National
  Autistic Society) 332n
US Food and Drug Administration
  (FDA), Risperdal publication 359n

## V

vaccines, autism 5–6, 21, 22, 76,
  89–97, 104
vagus nerve stimulator 180–81

Valium (diazepam) 289, 358
valproic acid 357
Van de Water, Judy 103, 105–6
Vedantam, Shankar 202n
verbal adhesion 207
verbal behavior 299
verbal skills, gender factor 24
Vineland Adaptive Behavior
  Scales 230, 239
visualization, autism studies
  115–16
visual orientation skills, nonverbal
  learning disabilities 37–38
vitamin supplements
  autism treatment 290–91, 332–34,
    337
  epilepsy 182
VMI-4 *see* Beery-Buktenica
  Developmental Test of Visual-Motor
  Integration - 4th Edition
vocal tics, described 164–65
vocational rehabilitation agencies
  498–99
voice output communication aids,
  described 313

## W

Wada test 179
Wakefield, Andrew 21, 348–49
Waltz, Mitzi 254n, 257n, 267n
Ward, Kimberley 418n, 420n, 422n
Wechsler Intelligence Scale for
  Children (WISC) 33, 237–38
Wechsler Preschool and Primary
  Scales of Intelligence - Third
  Edition (WPPSI-III) 237–38
weighted vest, described 325
Wellbutrin 289
"What Are Your Treatment Options?"
  (Autism Society of America) 275n
"What Causes Autism?" (Autism
  Society of America) 75n
"What Is Williams Syndrome?"
  (Williams Syndrome Association)
  160n
White, Sandra 397n
Whitehouse, Peter 124

"Why Do More Boys than Girls
Develop Autism?" (National
Autistic Society) 23n
Wilbarger Protocol 325
Williams syndrome
information resource 578
overview 160–63
"Williams Syndrome" (Edelson) 160n
Williams Syndrome Association,
Williams syndrome publication
160n
Williams Syndrome Foundation,
contact information 577
wills, estate planning 549–52
Wing, Lorna 52
WISC *see* Wechsler Intelligence Scale
for Children
Wisconsin Card Sorting Test 244
Wisconsin Medical Society, contact
information 577
Wolf, Lori I. 549n
workplace
Asperger syndrome 540–47
autism 263
WPPSI-III *see* Wechsler Preschool
and Primary Scales of Intelligence -
Third Edition
Wright, Pamela Darr 449n
Wright, Peter W. D. 449n

**X**

Xanax 289
X chromosome
fragile X syndrome 83, 146
Rett syndrome 83, 561
X-chromosome inactivation, defined
562

**Y**

Yale Child Study Center, contact
information 573
Yale Developmental Disabilities
Clinic, publications
childhood disintegrative disorder
68n
pervasive developmental disorder
not otherwise specified 70n
yeast-free diet 336–37

**Z**

Zarcone, Jennifer 410
ziprasidone 357
Zoloft (sertraline) 356
Zyprexa (olanzapine) 289, 357

# Health Reference Series
## COMPLETE CATALOG
List price $87 per volume. **School and library price $78 per volume.**

## Adolescent Health Sourcebook, 2nd Edition

*Basic Consumer Health Information about the Physical, Mental, and Emotional Growth and Development of Adolescents, Including Medical Care, Nutritional and Physical Activity Requirements, Puberty, Sexual Activity, Acne, Tanning, Body Piercing, Common Physical Illnesses and Disorders, Eating Disorders, Attention Deficit Hyperactivity Disorder, Depression, Bullying, Hazing, and Adolescent Injuries Related to Sports, Driving, and Work*

*Along with Substance Abuse Information about Nicotine, Alcohol, and Drug Use, a Glossary, and Directory of Additional Resources*

Edited by Joyce Brennfleck Shannon. 683 pages. 2006. 978-0-7808-0943-7.

"It is written in clear, nontechnical language aimed at general readers. . . . Recommended for public libraries, community colleges, and other agencies serving health care consumers."
— *American Reference Books Annual, 2003*

"Recommended for school and public libraries. Parents and professionals dealing with teens will appreciate the easy-to-follow format and the clearly written text. This could become a 'must have' for every high school teacher." — *E-Streams, Jan '03*

"A good starting point for information related to common medical, mental, and emotional concerns of adolescents." — *School Library Journal, Nov '02*

"This book provides accurate information in an easy to access format. It addresses topics that parents and caregivers might not be aware of and provides practical, useable information."
— *Doody's Health Sciences Book Review Journal, Sep-Oct '02*

"Recommended reference source."
— *Booklist, American Library Association, Sep '02*

## AIDS Sourcebook, 3rd Edition

*Basic Consumer Health Information about Acquired Immune Deficiency Syndrome (AIDS) and Human Immunodeficiency Virus (HIV) Infection, Including Facts about Transmission, Prevention, Diagnosis, Treatment, Opportunistic Infections, and Other Complications, with a Section for Women and Children, Including Details about Associated Gynecological Concerns, Pregnancy, and Pediatric Care*

*Along with Updated Statistical Information, Reports on Current Research Initiatives, a Glossary, and Directories of Internet, Hotline, and Other Resources*

Edited by Dawn D. Matthews. 664 pages. 2003. 978-0-7808-0631-3.

"The 3rd edition of the *AIDS Sourcebook*, part of Omnigraphics' *Health Reference Series*, is a welcome update. . . . This resource is highly recommended for academic and public libraries."
— *American Reference Books Annual, 2004*

"Excellent sourcebook. This continues to be a highly recommended book. There is no other book that provides as much information as this book provides."
— *AIDS Book Review Journal, Dec-Jan '00*

"Recommended reference source."
— *Booklist, American Library Association, Dec '99*

## Alcoholism Sourcebook, 2nd Edition

*Basic Consumer Health Information about Alcohol Use, Abuse, and Dependence, Featuring Facts about the Physical, Mental, and Social Health Effects of Alcohol Addiction, Including Alcoholic Liver Disease, Pancreatic Disease, Cardiovascular Disease, Neurological Disorders, and the Effects of Drinking during Pregnancy*

*Along with Information about Alcohol Treatment, Medications, and Recovery Programs, in Addition to Tips for Reducing the Prevalence of Underage Drinking, Statistics about Alcohol Use, a Glossary of Related Terms, and Directories of Resources for More Help and Information*

Edited by Amy L. Sutton. 653 pages. 2006. 978-0-7808-0942-0.

"This title is one of the few reference works on alcoholism for general readers. For some readers this will be a welcome complement to the many self-help books on the market. Recommended for collections serving general readers and consumer health collections."
— *E-Streams, Mar '01*

"This book is an excellent choice for public and academic libraries."
— *American Reference Books Annual, 2001*

"Recommended reference source."
— *Booklist, American Library Association, Dec '00*

"Presents a wealth of information on alcohol use and abuse and its effects on the body and mind, treatment, and prevention." — *SciTech Book News, Dec '00*

"Important new health guide which packs in the latest consumer information about the problems of alcoholism." — *Reviewer's Bookwatch, Nov '00*

***SEE ALSO*** *Drug Abuse Sourcebook*

# Allergies Sourcebook, 3rd Edition

*Basic Consumer Health Information about Allergic Disorders, Such as Anaphylaxis, Hives, Eczema, Rhinitis, Sinusitis, and Conjunctivitis, and Their Triggers, Including Pollen, Mold, Dust Mites, Animal Dander, Insects, Chemicals, Food, Food Additives, and Medications;*

*Along with Advice about the Diagnosis and Treatment of Allergy Symptoms, a Glossary of Related Terms, a Directory of Resources for Help and Information, and Suggestions for Additional Reading*

Edited by Amy L. Sutton. 598 pages. 2007. 978-0-7808-0950-5.

"This book brings a great deal of useful material together. . . . This is an excellent addition to public and consumer health library collections."
— *American Reference Books Annual, 2003*

"This second edition would be useful to laypersons with little or advanced knowledge of the subject matter. This book would also serve as a resource for nursing and other health care professions students. It would be useful in public, academic, and hospital libraries with consumer health collections." — *E-Streams, Jul '02*

■

# Alternative Medicine Sourcebook

*SEE Complementary & Alternative Medicine Sourcebook*

■

# Alzheimer's Disease Sourcebook, 3rd Edition

*Basic Consumer Health Information about Alzheimer's Disease, Other Dementias, and Related Disorders, Including Multi-Infarct Dementia, AIDS Dementia Complex, Dementia with Lewy Bodies, Huntington's Disease, Wernicke-Korsakoff Syndrome (Alcohol-Related Dementia), Delirium, and Confusional States*

*Along with Information for People Newly Diagnosed with Alzheimer's Disease and Caregivers, Reports Detailing Current Research Efforts in Prevention, Diagnosis, and Treatment, Facts about Long-Term Care Issues, and Listings of Sources for Additional Information*

Edited by Karen Bellenir. 645 pages. 2003. 978-0-7808-0666-5.

"This very informative and valuable tool will be a great addition to any library serving consumers, students and health care workers."
— *American Reference Books Annual, 2004*

"This is a valuable resource for people affected by dementias such as Alzheimer's. It is easy to navigate and includes important information and resources."
— *Doody's Review Service, Feb '04*

"Recommended reference source."
— *Booklist, American Library Association, Oct '99*

***SEE ALSO*** *Brain Disorders Sourcebook*

# Arthritis Sourcebook, 2nd Edition

*Basic Consumer Health Information about Osteoarthritis, Rheumatoid Arthritis, Other Rheumatic Disorders, Infectious Forms of Arthritis, and Diseases with Symptoms Linked to Arthritis, Featuring Facts about Diagnosis, Pain Management, and Surgical Therapies*

*Along with Coping Strategies, Research Updates, a Glossary, and Resources for Additional Help and Information*

Edited by Amy L. Sutton. 593 pages. 2004. 978-0-7808-0667-2.

"This easy-to-read volume is recommended for consumer health collections within public or academic libraries." — *E-Streams, May '05*

"As expected, this updated edition continues the excellent reputation of this series in providing sound, usable health information. . . . Highly recommended."
— *American Reference Books Annual, 2005*

"Excellent reference." — *The Bookwatch, Jan '05*

■

# Asthma Sourcebook, 2nd Edition

*Basic Consumer Health Information about the Causes, Symptoms, Diagnosis, and Treatment of Asthma in Infants, Children, Teenagers, and Adults, Including Facts about Different Types of Asthma, Common Co-Occurring Conditions, Asthma Management Plans, Triggers, Medications, and Medication Delivery Devices*

*Along with Asthma Statistics, Research Updates, a Glossary, a Directory of Asthma-Related Resources, and More*

Edited by Karen Bellenir. 609 pages. 2006. 978-0-7808-0866-9.

"A worthwhile reference acquisition for public libraries and academic medical libraries whose readers desire a quick introduction to the wide range of asthma information." — *Choice, Association of College & Research Libraries, Jun '01*

"Recommended reference source."
— *Booklist, American Library Association, Feb '01*

"Highly recommended." — *The Bookwatch, Jan '01*

"There is much good information for patients and their families who deal with asthma daily."
— *American Medical Writers Association Journal, Winter '01*

"This informative text is recommended for consumer health collections in public, secondary school, and community college libraries and the libraries of universities with a large undergraduate population."
— *American Reference Books Annual, 2001*

■

# Attention Deficit Disorder Sourcebook

*Basic Consumer Health Information about Attention Deficit/Hyperactivity Disorder in Children and Adults,*

*Including Facts about Causes, Symptoms, Diagnostic Criteria, and Treatment Options Such as Medications, Behavior Therapy, Coaching, and Homeopathy*

*Along with Reports on Current Research Initiatives, Legal Issues, and Government Regulations, and Featuring a Glossary of Related Terms, Internet Resources, and a List of Additional Reading Material*

Edited by Dawn D. Matthews. 470 pages. 2002. 978-0-7808-0624-5.

**"Recommended reference source."**
—*Booklist, American Library Association, Jan '03*

**"This book is recommended for all school libraries and the reference or consumer health sections of public libraries."** —*American Reference Books Annual, 2003*

■

# Back & Neck Sourcebook, 2nd Edition

*Basic Consumer Health Information about Spinal Pain, Spinal Cord Injuries, and Related Disorders, Such as Degenerative Disk Disease, Osteoarthritis, Scoliosis, Sciatica, Spina Bifida, and Spinal Stenosis, and Featuring Facts about Maintaining Spinal Health, Self-Care, Pain Management, Rehabilitative Care, Chiropractic Care, Spinal Surgeries, and Complementary Therapies*

*Along with Suggestions for Preventing Back and Neck Pain, a Glossary of Related Terms, and a Directory of Resources*

Edited by Amy L. Sutton. 633 pages. 2004. 978-0-7808-0738-9.

**"Recommended . . . an easy to use, comprehensive medical reference book."** —*E-Streams, Sep '05*

**"The strength of this work is its basic, easy-to-read format. Recommended."** —*Reference and User Services Quarterly, American Library Association, Winter '97*

■

# Blood & Circulatory Disorders Sourcebook, 2nd Edition

*Basic Consumer Health Information about the Blood and Circulatory System and Related Disorders, Such as Anemia and Other Hemoglobin Diseases, Cancer of the Blood and Associated Bone Marrow Disorders, Clotting and Bleeding Problems, and Conditions That Affect the Veins, Blood Vessels, and Arteries, Including Facts about the Donation and Transplantation of Bone Marrow, Stem Cells, and Blood and Tips for Keeping the Blood and Circulatory System Healthy*

*Along with a Glossary of Related Terms and Resources for Additional Help and Information*

Edited by Amy L. Sutton. 659 pages. 2005. 978-0-7808-0746-4.

**"Highly recommended pick for basic consumer health reference holdings at all levels."** —*The Bookwatch, Aug '05*

**"Recommended reference source."**
—*Booklist, American Library Association, Feb '99*

**"An important reference sourcebook written in simple language for everyday, non-technical users. "**
—*Reviewer's Bookwatch, Jan '99*

■

# Brain Disorders Sourcebook, 2nd Edition

*Basic Consumer Health Information about Acquired and Traumatic Brain Injuries, Infections of the Brain, Epilepsy and Seizure Disorders, Cerebral Palsy, and Degenerative Neurological Disorders, Including Amyotrophic Lateral Sclerosis (ALS), Dementias, Multiple Sclerosis, and More*

*Along with Information on the Brain's Structure and Function, Treatment and Rehabilitation Options, Reports on Current Research Initiatives, a Glossary of Terms Related to Brain Disorders and Injuries, and a Directory of Sources for Further Help and Information*

Edited by Sandra J. Judd. 625 pages. 2005. 978-0-7808-0744-0.

**"Highly recommended pick for basic consumer health reference holdings at all levels."**
—*The Bookwatch, Aug '05*

**"Belongs on the shelves of any library with a consumer health collection."** —*E-Streams, Mar '00*

**"Recommended reference source."**
—*Booklist, American Library Association, Oct '99*

***SEE ALSO** Alzheimer's Disease Sourcebook*

■

# Breast Cancer Sourcebook, 2nd Edition

*Basic Consumer Health Information about Breast Cancer, Including Facts about Risk Factors, Prevention, Screening and Diagnostic Methods, Treatment Options, Complementary and Alternative Therapies, Post-Treatment Concerns, Clinical Trials, Special Risk Populations, and New Developments in Breast Cancer Research*

*Along with Breast Cancer Statistics, a Glossary of Related Terms, and a Directory of Resources for Additional Help and Information*

Edited by Sandra J. Judd. 595 pages. 2004. 978-0-7808-0668-9.

**"This book will be an excellent addition to public, community college, medical, and academic libraries."**
—*American Reference Books Annual, 2006*

**"It would be a useful reference book in a library or on loan to women in a support group."**
—*Cancer Forum, Mar '03*

**"Recommended reference source."**
—*Booklist, American Library Association, Jan '02*

**"This reference source is highly recommended. It is quite informative, comprehensive and detailed in na-**

ture, and yet it offers practical advice in easy-to-read language. It could be thought of as the 'bible' of breast cancer for the consumer." — *E-Streams, Jan '02*

"From the pros and cons of different screening methods and results to treatment options, *Breast Cancer Sourcebook* provides the latest information on the subject." — *Library Bookwatch, Dec '01*

"This thoroughgoing, very readable reference covers all aspects of breast health and cancer. . . . Readers will find much to consider here. Recommended for all public and patient health collections." — *Library Journal, Sep '01*

**SEE ALSO** *Cancer Sourcebook for Women, Women's Health Concerns Sourcebook*

---

# Breastfeeding Sourcebook

*Basic Consumer Health Information about the Benefits of Breastmilk, Preparing to Breastfeed, Breastfeeding as a Baby Grows, Nutrition, and More, Including Information on Special Situations and Concerns Such as Mastitis, Illness, Medications, Allergies, Multiple Births, Prematurity, Special Needs, and Adoption*

*Along with a Glossary and Resources for Additional Help and Information*

Edited by Jenni Lynn Colson. 388 pages. 2002. 978-0-7808-0332-9.

"Particularly useful is the information about professional lactation services and chapters on breastfeeding when returning to work. . . . *Breastfeeding Sourcebook* will be useful for public libraries, consumer health libraries, and technical schools offering nurse assistant training, especially in areas where Internet access is problematic." — *American Reference Books Annual, 2003*

**SEE ALSO** *Pregnancy & Birth Sourcebook*

---

# Burns Sourcebook

*Basic Consumer Health Information about Various Types of Burns and Scalds, Including Flame, Heat, Cold, Electrical, Chemical, and Sun Burns*

*Along with Information on Short-Term and Long-Term Treatments, Tissue Reconstruction, Plastic Surgery, Prevention Suggestions, and First Aid*

Edited by Allan R. Cook. 604 pages. 1999. 978-0-7808-0204-9.

"This is an exceptional addition to the series and is highly recommended for all consumer health collections, hospital libraries, and academic medical centers." — *E-Streams, Mar '00*

"This key reference guide is an invaluable addition to all health care and public libraries in confronting this ongoing health issue." — *American Reference Books Annual, 2000*

"Recommended reference source." — *Booklist, American Library Association, Dec '99*

**SEE ALSO** *Dermatological Disorders Sourcebook*

---

# Cancer Sourcebook, 5th Edition

*Basic Consumer Health Information about Major Forms and Stages of Cancer, Featuring Facts about Head and Neck Cancers, Lung Cancers, Gastrointestinal Cancers, Genitourinary Cancers, Lymphomas, Blood Cell Cancers, Endocrine Cancers, Skin Cancers, Bone Cancers, Metastatic Cancers, and More*

*Along with Facts about Cancer Treatments, Cancer Risks and Prevention, a Glossary of Related Terms, Statistical Data, and a Directory of Resources for Additional Information*

Edited by Karen Bellenir. 1,133 pages. 2007. 978-0-7808-0947-5.

"With cancer being the second leading cause of death for Americans, a prodigious work such as this one, which locates centrally so much cancer-related information, is clearly an asset to this nation's citizens and others." — *Journal of the National Medical Association, 2004*

"This title is recommended for health sciences and public libraries with consumer health collections." — *E-Streams, Feb '01*

". . . can be effectively used by cancer patients and their families who are looking for answers in a language they can understand. Public and hospital libraries should have it on their shelves." — *American Reference Books Annual, 2001*

"Recommended reference source." — *Booklist, American Library Association, Dec '00*

**SEE ALSO** *Breast Cancer Sourcebook, Cancer Sourcebook for Women, Pediatric Cancer Sourcebook, Prostate Cancer Sourcebook*

---

# Cancer Sourcebook for Women, 3rd Edition

*Basic Consumer Health Information about Leading Causes of Cancer in Women, Featuring Facts about Gynecologic Cancers and Related Concerns, Such as Breast Cancer, Cervical Cancer, Endometrial Cancer, Uterine Sarcoma, Vaginal Cancer, Vulvar Cancer, and Common Non-Cancerous Gynecologic Conditions, in Addition to Facts about Lung Cancer, Colorectal Cancer, and Thyroid Cancer in Women*

*Along with Information about Cancer Risk Factors, Screening and Prevention, Treatment Options, and Tips on Coping with Life after Cancer Treatment, a Glossary of Cancer Terms, and a Directory of Resources for Additional Help and Information*

Edited by Amy L. Sutton. 715 pages. 2006. 978-0-7808-0867-6.

"An excellent addition to collections in public, consumer health, and women's health libraries." — *American Reference Books Annual, 2003*

"Overall, the information is excellent, and complex topics are clearly explained. As a reference book for the consumer it is a valuable resource to assist them to make informed decisions about cancer and its treatments." — *Cancer Forum, Nov '02*

# Cancer Survivorship Sourcebook

*Basic Consumer Health Information about the Physical, Educational, Emotional, Social, and Financial Needs of Cancer Patients from Diagnosis, through Cancer Treatment, and Beyond, Including Facts about Researching Specific Types of Cancer and Learning about Clinical Trials and Treatment Options, and Featuring Tips for Coping with the Side Effects of Cancer Treatments and Adjusting to Life after Cancer Treatment Concludes*

*Along with Suggestions for Caregivers, Friends, and Family Members of Cancer Patients, a Glossary of Cancer Care Terms, and Directories of Related Resources*

Edited by Karen Bellenir. 6561 pages. 2007. 978-0-7808-0985-7.

# Cardiovascular Diseases & Disorders Sourcebook, 3rd Edition

*Basic Consumer Health Information about Heart and Vascular Diseases and Disorders, Such as Angina, Heart Attacks, Arrhythmias, Cardiomyopathy, Valve Disease, Atherosclerosis, and Aneurysms, with Information about Managing Cardiovascular Risk Factors and Maintaining Heart Health, Medications and Procedures Used to Treat Cardiovascular Disorders, and Concerns of Special Significance to Women*

*Along with Reports on Current Research Initiatives, a Glossary of Related Medical Terms, and a Directory of Sources for Further Help and Information*

Edited by Sandra J. Judd. 713 pages. 2005. 978-0-7808-0739-6.

# Caregiving Sourcebook

*Basic Consumer Health Information for Caregivers, Including a Profile of Caregivers, Caregiving Responsibilities and Concerns, Tips for Specific Conditions, Care Environments, and the Effects of Caregiving*

*Along with Facts about Legal Issues, Financial Information, and Future Planning, a Glossary, and a Listing of Additional Resources*

Edited by Joyce Brennfleck Shannon. 600 pages. 2001. 978-0-7808-0331-2.

# Child Abuse Sourcebook

*Basic Consumer Health Information about the Physical, Sexual, and Emotional Abuse of Children, with Additional Facts about Neglect, Munchausen Syndrome by Proxy (MSBP), Shaken Baby Syndrome, and Controversial Issues Related to Child Abuse, Such as Withholding Medical Care, Corporal Punishment, and Child Maltreatment in Youth Sports, and Featuring Facts about Child Protective Services, Foster Care, Adoption, Parenting Challenges, and Other Abuse Prevention Efforts*

*Along with a Glossary of Related Terms and Resources for Additional Help and Information*

Edited by Dawn D. Matthews. 620 pages. 2004. 978-0-7808-0705-1.

## Childhood Diseases & Disorders Sourcebook

*Basic Consumer Health Information about Medical Problems Often Encountered in Pre-Adolescent Children, Including Respiratory Tract Ailments, Ear Infections, Sore Throats, Disorders of the Skin and Scalp, Digestive and Genitourinary Diseases, Infectious Diseases, Inflammatory Disorders, Chronic Physical and Developmental Disorders, Allergies, and More*

*Along with Information about Diagnostic Tests, Common Childhood Surgeries, and Frequently Used Medications, with a Glossary of Important Terms and Resource Directory*

Edited by Chad T. Kimball. 662 pages. 2003. 978-0-7808-0458-6.

"This is an excellent book for new parents and should be included in all health care and public libraries."
—*American Reference Books Annual, 2004*

**SEE ALSO:** *Healthy Children Sourcebook*

■

## Colds, Flu & Other Common Ailments Sourcebook

*Basic Consumer Health Information about Common Ailments and Injuries, Including Colds, Coughs, the Flu, Sinus Problems, Headaches, Fever, Nausea and Vomiting, Menstrual Cramps, Diarrhea, Constipation, Hemorrhoids, Back Pain, Dandruff, Dry and Itchy Skin, Cuts, Scrapes, Sprains, Bruises, and More*

*Along with Information about Prevention, Self-Care, Choosing a Doctor, Over-the-Counter Medications, Folk Remedies, and Alternative Therapies, and Including a Glossary of Important Terms and a Directory of Resources for Further Help and Information*

Edited by Chad T. Kimball. 638 pages. 2001. 978-0-7808-0435-7.

"A good starting point for research on common illnesses. It will be a useful addition to public and consumer health library collections."
—*American Reference Books Annual, 2002*

"Will prove valuable to any library seeking to maintain a current, comprehensive reference collection of health resources. . . . Excellent reference."
—*The Bookwatch, Aug '01*

"Recommended reference source."
—*Booklist, American Library Association, Jul '01*

■

## Communication Disorders Sourcebook

*Basic Information about Deafness and Hearing Loss, Speech and Language Disorders, Voice Disorders, Balance and Vestibular Disorders, and Disorders of Smell, Taste, and Touch*

Edited by Linda M. Ross. 533 pages. 1996. 978-0-7808-0077-9.

"This is skillfully edited and is a welcome resource for the layperson. It should be found in every public and medical library." —*Booklist Health Sciences Supplement, American Library Association, Oct '97*

■

## Complementary & Alternative Medicine Sourcebook, 3rd Edition

*Basic Consumer Health Information about Complementary and Alternative Medical Therapies, Including Acupuncture, Ayurveda, Traditional Chinese Medicine, Herbal Medicine, Homeopathy, Naturopathy, Biofeedback, Hypnotherapy, Yoga, Art Therapy, Aromatherapy, Clinical Nutrition, Vitamin and Mineral Supplements, Chiropractic, Massage, Reflexology, Crystal Therapy, Therapeutic Touch, and More*

*Along with Facts about Alternative and Complementary Treatments for Specific Conditions Such as Cancer, Diabetes, Osteoarthritis, Chronic Pain, Menopause, Gastrointestinal Disorders, Headaches, and Mental Illness, a Glossary, and a Resource List for Additional Help and Information*

Edited by Sandra J. Judd. 657 pages. 2006. 978-0-7808-0864-5.

"Recommended for public, high school, and academic libraries that have consumer health collections. Hospital libraries that also serve the public will find this to be a useful resource." —*E-Streams, Feb '03*

"Recommended reference source."
—*Booklist, American Library Association, Jan '03*

"An important alternate health reference."
—*MBR Bookwatch, Oct '02*

"A great addition to the reference collection of every type of library." —*American Reference Books Annual, 2000*

■

## Congenital Disorders Sourcebook, 2nd Edition

*Basic Consumer Health Information about Nonhereditary Birth Defects and Disorders Related to Prematurity, Gestational Injuries, Congenital Infections, and Birth Complications, Including Heart Defects, Hydrocephalus, Spina Bifida, Cleft Lip and Palate, Cerebral Palsy, and More*

*Along with Facts about the Prevention of Birth Defects, Fetal Surgery and Other Treatment Options, Research Initiatives, a Glossary of Related Terms, and Resources for Additional Information and Support*

Edited by Sandra J. Judd. 647 pages. 2006. 978-0-7808-0945-1.

"Recommended reference source."
—*Booklist, American Library Association, Oct '97*

**SEE ALSO** *Pregnancy & Birth Sourcebook*

■

## Contagious Diseases Sourcebook

*Basic Consumer Health Information about Infectious Diseases Spread by Person-to-Person Contact through*

Direct Touch, Airborne Transmission, Sexual Contact, or Contact with Blood or Other Body Fluids, Including Hepatitis, Herpes, Influenza, Lice, Measles, Mumps, Pinworm, Ringworm, Severe Acute Respiratory Syndrome (SARS), Streptococcal Infections, Tuberculosis, and Others

Along with Facts about Disease Transmission, Antimicrobial Resistance, and Vaccines, with a Glossary and Directories of Resources for More Information

Edited by Karen Bellenir. 643 pages. 2004. 978-0-7808-0736-5.

"This easy-to-read volume is recommended for consumer health collections within public or academic libraries." —E-Streams, May '05

"This informative book is highly recommended for public libraries, consumer health collections, and secondary schools and undergraduate libraries." —American Reference Books Annual, 2005

"Excellent reference." — The Bookwatch, Jan '05

■

# Death & Dying Sourcebook, 2nd Edition

Basic Consumer Health Information about End-of-Life Care and Related Perspectives and Ethical Issues, Including End-of-Life Symptoms and Treatments, Pain Management, Quality-of-Life Concerns, the Use of Life Support, Patients' Rights and Privacy Issues, Advance Directives, Physician-Assisted Suicide, Caregiving, Organ and Tissue Donation, Autopsies, Funeral Arrangements, and Grief

Along with Statistical Data, Information about the Leading Causes of Death, a Glossary, and Directories of Support Groups and Other Resources

Edited by Joyce Brennfleck Shannon. 653 pages. 2006. 978-0-7808-0871-3.

"Public libraries, medical libraries, and academic libraries will all find this sourcebook a useful addition to their collections." —American Reference Books Annual, 2001

"An extremely useful resource for those concerned with death and dying in the United States." —Respiratory Care, Nov '00

"Recommended reference source." —Booklist, American Library Association, Aug '00

"This book is a definite must for all those involved in end-of-life care." — Doody's Review Service, 2000

■

# Dental Care & Oral Health Sourcebook, 2nd Edition

Basic Consumer Health Information about Dental Care, Including Oral Hygiene, Dental Visits, Pain Management, Cavities, Crowns, Bridges, Dental Implants, and Fillings, and Other Oral Health Concerns, Such as Gum Disease, Bad Breath, Dry Mouth, Genetic and Developmental Abnormalities, Oral Cancers, Orthodontics, and Temporomandibular Disorders

Along with Updates on Current Research in Oral Health, a Glossary, a Directory of Dental and Oral Health Organizations, and Resources for People with Dental and Oral Health Disorders

Edited by Amy L. Sutton. 609 pages. 2003. 978-0-7808-0634-4.

"This book could serve as a turning point in the battle to educate consumers in issues concerning oral health." —American Reference Books Annual, 2004

"Unique source which will fill a gap in dental sources for patients and the lay public. A valuable reference tool even in a library with thousands of books on dentistry. Comprehensive, clear, inexpensive, and easy to read and use. It fills an enormous gap in the health care literature." — Reference & User Services Quarterly, American Library Association, Summer '98

"Recommended reference source." —Booklist, American Library Association, Dec '97

■

# Depression Sourcebook

Basic Consumer Health Information about Unipolar Depression, Bipolar Disorder, Postpartum Depression, Seasonal Affective Disorder, and Other Types of Depression in Children, Adolescents, Women, Men, the Elderly, and Other Selected Populations

Along with Facts about Causes, Risk Factors, Diagnostic Criteria, Treatment Options, Coping Strategies, Suicide Prevention, a Glossary, and a Directory of Sources for Additional Help and Information

Edited by Karen Bellenir. 602 pages. 2002. 978-0-7808-0611-5.

"Depression Sourcebook is of a very high standard. Its purpose, which is to serve as a reference source to the lay reader, is very well served." — Journal of the National Medical Association, 2004

"Invaluable reference for public and school library collections alike." — Library Bookwatch, Apr '03

"Recommended for purchase." —American Reference Books Annual, 2003

■

# Dermatological Disorders Sourcebook, 2nd Edition

Basic Consumer Health Information about Conditions and Disorders Affecting the Skin, Hair, and Nails, Such as Acne, Rosacea, Rashes, Dermatitis, Pigmentation Disorders, Birthmarks, Skin Cancer, Skin Injuries, Psoriasis, Scleroderma, and Hair Loss, Including Facts about Medications and Treatments for Dermatological Disorders and Tips for Maintaining Healthy Skin, Hair, and Nails

Along with Information about How Aging Affects the Skin, a Glossary of Related Terms, and a Directory of Resources for Additional Help and Information

Edited by Amy L. Sutton. 645 pages. 2005. 978-0-7808-0795-2.

## Diabetes Sourcebook, 3rd Edition

*Basic Consumer Health Information about Type 1 Diabetes (Insulin-Dependent or Juvenile-Onset Diabetes), Type 2 Diabetes (Noninsulin-Dependent or Adult-Onset Diabetes), Gestational Diabetes, Impaired Glucose Tolerance (IGT), and Related Complications, Such as Amputation, Eye Disease, Gum Disease, Nerve Damage, and End-Stage Renal Disease, Including Facts about Insulin, Oral Diabetes Medications, Blood Sugar Testing, and the Role of Exercise and Nutrition in the Control of Diabetes*

*Along with a Glossary and Resources for Further Help and Information*

Edited by Dawn D. Matthews. 622 pages. 2003. 978-0-7808-0629-0.

## Diet & Nutrition Sourcebook, 3rd Edition

*Basic Consumer Health Information about Dietary Guidelines and the Food Guidance System, Recommended Daily Nutrient Intakes, Serving Proportions, Weight Control, Vitamins and Supplements, Nutrition Issues for Different Life Stages and Lifestyles, and the Needs of People with Specific Medical Concerns, Including Cancer, Celiac Disease, Diabetes, Eating Disorders, Food Allergies, and Cardiovascular Disease*

*Along with Facts about Federal Nutrition Support Programs, a Glossary of Nutrition and Dietary Terms, and Directories of Additional Resources for More Information about Nutrition*

Edited by Joyce Brennfleck Shannon. 633 pages. 2006. 978-0-7808-0800-3.

*SEE ALSO Digestive Diseases & Disorders Sourcebook, Eating Disorders Sourcebook, Gastrointestinal Diseases & Disorders Sourcebook, Vegetarian Sourcebook*

## Digestive Diseases & Disorders Sourcebook

*Basic Consumer Health Information about Diseases and Disorders that Impact the Upper and Lower Digestive System, Including Celiac Disease, Constipation, Crohn's Disease, Cyclic Vomiting Syndrome, Diarrhea, Diverticulosis and Diverticulitis, Gallstones, Heartburn, Hemorrhoids, Hernias, Indigestion (Dyspepsia), Irritable Bowel Syndrome, Lactose Intolerance, Ulcers, and More*

*Along with Information about Medications and Other Treatments, Tips for Maintaining a Healthy Digestive Tract, a Glossary, and Directory of Digestive Diseases Organizations*

Edited by Karen Bellenir. 335 pages. 2000. 978-0-7808-0327-5.

*SEE ALSO Eating Disorders Sourcebook, Gastrointestinal Diseases & Disorders Sourcebook*

## Disabilities Sourcebook

*Basic Consumer Health Information about Physical and Psychiatric Disabilities, Including Descriptions of Major Causes of Disability, Assistive and Adaptive Aids, Workplace Issues, and Accessibility Concerns*

*Along with Information about the Americans with Disabilities Act, a Glossary, and Resources for Additional Help and Information*

Edited by Dawn D. Matthews. 616 pages. 2000. 978-0-7808-0389-3.

"A much needed addition to the Omnigraphics *Health Reference Series*. A current reference work to provide people with disabilities, their families, caregivers or those who work with them, a broad range of information in one volume, has not been available until now. . . . It is recommended for all public and academic library reference collections." —*E-Streams, May '01*

"An excellent source book in easy-to-read format covering many current topics; highly recommended for all libraries." —*Choice, Association of College & Research Libraries, Jan '01*

"Recommended reference source." —*Booklist, American Library Association, Jul '00*

■

## Domestic Violence Sourcebook, 2nd Edition

*Basic Consumer Health Information about the Causes and Consequences of Abusive Relationships, Including Physical Violence, Sexual Assault, Battery, Stalking, and Emotional Abuse, and Facts about the Effects of Violence on Women, Men, Young Adults, and the Elderly, with Reports about Domestic Violence in Selected Populations, and Featuring Facts about Medical Care, Victim Assistance and Protection, Prevention Strategies, Mental Health Services, and Legal Issues*

*Along with a Glossary of Related Terms and Resources for Additional Help and Information*

Edited by Dawn D. Matthews. 628 pages. 2004. 978-0-7808-0669-6.

"Educators, clergy, medical professionals, police, and victims and their families will benefit from this realistic and easy-to-understand resource." —*American Reference Books Annual, 2005*

"Recommended for all collections supporting consumer health information. It should also be considered for any collection needing general, readable information on domestic violence." —*E-Streams, Jan '05*

"This sourcebook complements other books in its field, providing a one-stop resource . . . Recommended." —*Choice, Association of College & Research Libraries, Jan '05*

"Interested lay persons should find the book extremely beneficial. . . . A copy of *Domestic Violence and Child Abuse Sourcebook* should be in every public library in the United States." —*Social Science & Medicine, No. 56, 2003*

"This is important information. The Web has many resources but this sourcebook fills an important societal need. I am not aware of any other resources of this type." —*Doody's Review Service, Sep '01*

"Recommended reference source." —*Booklist, American Library Association, Apr '01*

"Important pick for college-level health reference libraries." —*The Bookwatch, Mar '01*

"Because this problem is so widespread and because this book includes a lot of issues within one volume, this work is recommended for all public libraries." —*American Reference Books Annual, 2001*

SEE ALSO *Child Abuse Sourcebook*

■

## Drug Abuse Sourcebook, 2nd Edition

*Basic Consumer Health Information about Illicit Substances of Abuse and the Misuse of Prescription and Over-the-Counter Medications, Including Depressants, Hallucinogens, Inhalants, Marijuana, Stimulants, and Anabolic Steroids*

*Along with Facts about Related Health Risks, Treatment Programs, Prevention Programs, a Glossary of Abuse and Addiction Terms, a Glossary of Drug-Related Street Terms, and a Directory of Resources for More Information*

Edited by Catherine Ginther. 607 pages. 2004. 978-0-7808-0740-2.

"Commendable for organizing useful, normally scattered government and association-produced data into a logical sequence." —*American Reference Books Annual, 2006*

"This easy-to-read volume is recommended for consumer health collections within public or academic libraries." —*E-Streams, Sep '05*

"An excellent library reference." —*The Bookwatch, May '05*

"Containing a wealth of information, this book will be useful to the college student just beginning to explore the topic of substance abuse. This resource belongs in libraries that serve a lower-division undergraduate or community college clientele as well as the general public." —*Choice, Association of College & Research Libraries, Jun '01*

"Recommended reference source." —*Booklist, American Library Association, Feb '01*

SEE ALSO *Alcoholism Sourcebook*

■

## Ear, Nose & Throat Disorders Sourcebook, 2nd Edition

*Basic Consumer Health Information about Disorders of the Ears, Hearing Loss, Vestibular Disorders, Nasal and Sinus Problems, Throat and Vocal Cord Disorders, and Otolaryngologic Cancers, Including Facts about Ear Infections and Injuries, Genetic and Congenital Deafness, Sensorineural Hearing Disorders, Tinnitus, Vertigo, Ménière Disease, Rhinitis, Sinusitis, Snoring, Sore Throats, Hoarseness, and More*

*Along with Reports on Current Research Initiatives, a Glossary of Related Medical Terms, and a Directory of Sources for Further Help and Information*

Edited by Sandra J. Judd. 659 pages. 2006. 978-0-7808-0872-0.

"Overall, this sourcebook is helpful for the consumer seeking information on ENT issues. It is recommended for public libraries."
— *American Reference Books Annual, 1999*

"Recommended reference source."
— *Booklist, American Library Association, Dec '98*

■

# Eating Disorders Sourcebook, 2nd Edition

*Basic Consumer Health Information about Anorexia Nervosa, Bulimia Nervosa, Binge Eating, Compulsive Exercise, Female Athlete Triad, and Other Eating Disorders, Including Facts about Body Image and Other Cultural and Age-Related Risk Factors, Prevention Efforts, Adverse Health Effects, Treatment Options, and the Recovery Process*

*Along with Guidelines for Healthy Weight Control, a Glossary, and Directories of Additional Resources*

Edited by Joyce Brennfleck Shannon. 585 pages. 2007. 978-0-7808-0948-2.

"Recommended for health science libraries that are open to the public, as well as hospital libraries. This book is a good resource for the consumer who is concerned about eating disorders." — *E-Streams, Mar '02*

"This volume is another convenient collection of excerpted articles. Recommended for school and public library patrons; lower-division undergraduates; and two-year technical program students."
— *Choice, Association of College & Research Libraries, Jan '02*

"Recommended reference source."
— *Booklist, American Library Association, Oct '01*

**SEE ALSO** *Diet & Nutrition Sourcebook, Digestive Diseases & Disorders Sourcebook, Gastrointestinal Diseases & Disorders Sourcebook*

■

# Emergency Medical Services Sourcebook

*Basic Consumer Health Information about Preventing, Preparing for, and Managing Emergency Situations, When and Who to Call for Help, What to Expect in the Emergency Room, the Emergency Medical Team, Patient Issues, and Current Topics in Emergency Medicine*

*Along with Statistical Data, a Glossary, and Sources of Additional Help and Information*

Edited by Jenni Lynn Colson. 494 pages. 2002. 978-0-7808-0420-3.

"Handy and convenient for home, public, school, and college libraries. Recommended."
— *Choice, Association of College & Research Libraries, Apr '03*

"This reference can provide the consumer with answers to most questions about emergency care in the United States, or it will direct them to a resource where the answer can be found."
— *American Reference Books Annual, 2003*

"Recommended reference source."
— *Booklist, American Library Association, Feb '03*

■

# Endocrine & Metabolic Disorders Sourcebook

*Basic Information for the Layperson about Pancreatic and Insulin-Related Disorders Such as Pancreatitis, Diabetes, and Hypoglycemia; Adrenal Gland Disorders Such as Cushing's Syndrome, Addison's Disease, and Congenital Adrenal Hyperplasia; Pituitary Gland Disorders Such as Growth Hormone Deficiency, Acromegaly, and Pituitary Tumors; Thyroid Disorders Such as Hypothyroidism, Graves' Disease, Hashimoto's Disease, and Goiter; Hyperparathyroidism; and Other Diseases and Syndromes of Hormone Imbalance or Metabolic Dysfunction*

*Along with Reports on Current Research Initiatives*

Edited by Linda M. Shin. 574 pages. 1998. 978-0-7808-0207-0.

"Omnigraphics has produced another needed resource for health information consumers."
— *American Reference Books Annual, 2000*

"Recommended reference source."
— *Booklist, American Library Association, Dec '98*

■

# Environmental Health Sourcebook, 2nd Edition

*Basic Consumer Health Information about the Environment and Its Effect on Human Health, Including the Effects of Air Pollution, Water Pollution, Hazardous Chemicals, Food Hazards, Radiation Hazards, Biological Agents, Household Hazards, Such as Radon, Asbestos, Carbon Monoxide, and Mold, and Information about Associated Diseases and Disorders, Including Cancer, Allergies, Respiratory Problems, and Skin Disorders*

*Along with Information about Environmental Concerns for Specific Populations, a Glossary of Related Terms, and Resources for Further Help and Information*

Edited by Dawn D. Matthews. 673 pages. 2003. 978-0-7808-0632-0.

"This recently updated edition continues the level of quality and the reputation of the numerous other volumes in Omnigraphics' *Health Reference Series*."
— *American Reference Books Annual, 2004*

"An excellent updated edition."
— *The Bookwatch, Oct '03*

"Recommended reference source."
— *Booklist, American Library Association, Sep '98*

"This book will be a useful addition to anyone's library." — *Choice Health Sciences Supplement, Association of College & Research Libraries, May '98*

". . . a good survey of numerous environmentally induced physical disorders . . . a useful addition to anyone's library."
— *Doody's Health Sciences Book Reviews, Jan '98*

# Ethnic Diseases Sourcebook

*Basic Consumer Health Information for Ethnic and Racial Minority Groups in the United States, Including General Health Indicators and Behaviors, Ethnic Diseases, Genetic Testing, the Impact of Chronic Diseases, Women's Health, Mental Health Issues, and Preventive Health Care Services*

*Along with a Glossary and a Listing of Additional Resources*

Edited by Joyce Brennfleck Shannon. 664 pages. 2001. 978-0-7808-0336-7.

"Recommended for health sciences libraries where public health programs are a priority."
— *E-Streams, Jan '02*

"Not many books have been written on this topic to date, and the *Ethnic Diseases Sourcebook* is a strong addition to the list. It will be an important introductory resource for health consumers, students, health care personnel, and social scientists. It is recommended for public, academic, and large hospital libraries."
— *American Reference Books Annual, 2002*

"Recommended reference source."
— *Booklist, American Library Association, Oct '01*

"Will prove valuable to any library seeking to maintain a current, comprehensive reference collection of health resources.... An excellent source of health information about genetic disorders which affect particular ethnic and racial minorities in the U.S."
— *The Bookwatch, Aug '01*

---

# Eye Care Sourcebook,
# 2nd Edition

*Basic Consumer Health Information about Eye Care and Eye Disorders, Including Facts about the Diagnosis, Prevention, and Treatment of Common Refractive Problems Such as Myopia, Hyperopia, Astigmatism, and Presbyopia, and Eye Diseases, Including Glaucoma, Cataract, Age-Related Macular Degeneration, and Diabetic Retinopathy*

*Along with a Section on Vision Correction and Refractive Surgeries, Including LASIK and LASEK, a Glossary, and Directories of Resources for Additional Help and Information*

Edited by Amy L. Sutton. 543 pages. 2003. 978-0-7808-0635-1.

". . . a solid reference tool for eye care and a valuable addition to a collection."
— *American Reference Books Annual, 2004*

---

# Family Planning Sourcebook

*Basic Consumer Health Information about Planning for Pregnancy and Contraception, Including Traditional Methods, Barrier Methods, Hormonal Methods, Permanent Methods, Future Methods, Emergency Contraception, and Birth Control Choices for Women at Each Stage of Life*

*Along with Statistics, a Glossary, and Sources of Additional Information*

Edited by Amy Marcaccio Keyzer. 520 pages. 2001. 978-0-7808-0379-4.

"Recommended for public, health, and undergraduate libraries as part of the circulating collection."
— *E-Streams, Mar '02*

"Information is presented in an unbiased, readable manner, and the sourcebook will certainly be a necessary addition to those public and high school libraries where Internet access is restricted or otherwise problematic." — *American Reference Books Annual, 2002*

"Recommended reference source."
— *Booklist, American Library Association, Oct '01*

"Will prove valuable to any library seeking to maintain a current, comprehensive reference collection of health resources. . . . Excellent reference."
— *The Bookwatch, Aug '01*

*SEE ALSO Pregnancy & Birth Sourcebook*

---

# Fitness & Exercise Sourcebook,
# 3rd Edition

*Basic Consumer Health Information about the Physical and Mental Benefits of Fitness, Including Cardiorespiratory Endurance, Muscular Strength, Muscular Endurance, and Flexibility, with Facts about Sports Nutrition and Exercise-Related Injuries and Tips about Physical Activity and Exercises for People of All Ages and for People with Health Concerns*

*Along with Advice on Selecting and Using Exercise Equipment, Maintaining Exercise Motivation, a Glossary of Related Terms, and a Directory of Resources for More Help and Information*

Edited by Amy L. Sutton. 663 pages. 2007. 978-0-7808-0946-8.

"This work is recommended for all general reference collections."
— *American Reference Books Annual, 2002*

"Highly recommended for public, consumer, and school grades fourth through college." — *E-Streams, Nov '01*

"Recommended reference source."
— *Booklist, American Library Association, Oct '01*

"The information appears quite comprehensive and is considered reliable. . . . This second edition is a welcomed addition to the series."
— *Doody's Review Service, Sep '01*

---

# Food Safety Sourcebook

*Basic Consumer Health Information about the Safe Handling of Meat, Poultry, Seafood, Eggs, Fruit Juices, and Other Food Items, and Facts about Pesticides, Drinking Water, Food Safety Overseas, and the Onset, Duration, and Symptoms of Foodborne Illnesses, Including Types of Pathogenic Bacteria, Parasitic Protozoa, Worms, Viruses, and Natural Toxins*

Along with the Role of the Consumer, the Food Handler, and the Government in Food Safety; a Glossary, and Resources for Additional Help and Information

Edited by Dawn D. Matthews. 339 pages. 1999. 978-0-7808-0326-8.

"This book is recommended for public libraries and universities with home economic and food science programs."
— E-Streams, Nov '00

"Recommended reference source."
— Booklist, American Library Association, May '00

"This book takes the complex issues of food safety and foodborne pathogens and presents them in an easily understood manner. [It does] an excellent job of covering a large and often confusing topic."
— American Reference Books Annual, 2000

## Forensic Medicine Sourcebook

Basic Consumer Information for the Layperson about Forensic Medicine, Including Crime Scene Investigation, Evidence Collection and Analysis, Expert Testimony, Computer-Aided Criminal Identification, Digital Imaging in the Courtroom, DNA Profiling, Accident Reconstruction, Autopsies, Ballistics, Drugs and Explosives Detection, Latent Fingerprints, Product Tampering, and Questioned Document Examination

Along with Statistical Data, a Glossary of Forensics Terminology, and Listings of Sources for Further Help and Information

Edited by Annemarie S. Muth. 574 pages. 1999. 978-0-7808-0232-2.

"Given the expected widespread interest in its content and its easy to read style, this book is recommended for most public and all college and university libraries."
— E-Streams, Feb '01

"Recommended for public libraries."
— Reference & User Services Quarterly, American Library Association, Spring 2000

"Recommended reference source."
— Booklist, American Library Association, Feb '00

"A wealth of information, useful statistics, references are up-to-date and extremely complete. This wonderful collection of data will help students who are interested in a career in any type of forensic field. It is a great resource for attorneys who need information about types of expert witnesses needed in a particular case. It also offers useful information for fiction and nonfiction writers whose work involves a crime. A fascinating compilation. All levels."
— Choice, Association of College & Research Libraries, Jan '00

"There are several items that make this book attractive to consumers who are seeking certain forensic data. . . . This is a useful current source for those seeking general forensic medical answers."
— American Reference Books Annual, 2000

## Gastrointestinal Diseases & Disorders Sourcebook, 2nd Edition

Basic Consumer Health Information about the Upper and Lower Gastrointestinal (GI) Tract, Including the Esophagus, Stomach, Intestines, Rectum, Liver, and Pancreas, with Facts about Gastroesophageal Reflux Disease, Gastritis, Hernias, Ulcers, Celiac Disease, Diverticulitis, Irritable Bowel Syndrome, Hemorrhoids, Gastrointestinal Cancers, and Other Diseases and Disorders Related to the Digestive Process

Along with Information about Commonly Used Diagnostic and Surgical Procedures, Statistics, Reports on Current Research Initiatives and Clinical Trials, a Glossary, and Resources for Additional Help and Information

Edited by Sandra J. Judd. 681 pages. 2006. 978-0-7808-0798-3.

". . . very readable form. The successful editorial work that brought this material together into a useful and understandable reference makes accessible to all readers information that can help them more effectively understand and obtain help for digestive tract problems."
— Choice, Association of College & Research Libraries, Feb '97

SEE ALSO Diet & Nutrition Sourcebook, Digestive Diseases & Disorders Sourcebook, Eating Disorders Sourcebook

## Genetic Disorders Sourcebook, 3rd Edition

Basic Consumer Health Information about Hereditary Diseases and Disorders, Including Facts about the Human Genome, Genetic Inheritance Patterns, Disorders Associated with Specific Genes, Such as Sickle Cell Disease, Hemophilia, and Cystic Fibrosis, Chromosome Disorders, Such as Down Syndrome, Fragile X Syndrome, and Turner Syndrome, and Complex Diseases and Disorders Resulting from the Interaction of Environmental and Genetic Factors, Such as Allergies, Cancer, and Obesity

Along with Facts about Genetic Testing, Suggestions for Parents of Children with Special Needs, Reports on Current Research Initiatives, a Glossary of Genetic Terminology, and Resources for Additional Help and Information

Edited by Karen Bellenir. 777 pages. 2004. 978-0-7808-0742-6.

"This text is recommended for any library with an interest in providing consumer health resources."
— E-Streams, Aug '05

"This is a valuable resource for anyone wishing to have an understandable description of any of the topics or disorders included. The editor succeeds in making complex genetic issues understandable."
— Doody's Book Review Service, May '05

"A good acquisition for public libraries."
— American Reference Books Annual, 2005

616

---

# Head Trauma Sourcebook

*Basic Information for the Layperson about Open-Head and Closed-Head Injuries, Treatment Advances, Recovery, and Rehabilitation*

*Along with Reports on Current Research Initiatives*

Edited by Karen Bellenir. 414 pages. 1997. 978-0-7808-0208-7.

# Headache Sourcebook

*Basic Consumer Health Information about Migraine, Tension, Cluster, Rebound and Other Types of Headaches, with Facts about the Cause and Prevention of Headaches, the Effects of Stress and the Environment, Headaches during Pregnancy and Menopause, and Childhood Headaches*

*Along with a Glossary and Other Resources for Additional Help and Information*

Edited by Dawn D. Matthews. 362 pages. 2002. 978-0-7808-0337-4.

---

# Healthy Aging Sourcebook

*Basic Consumer Health Information about Maintaining Health through the Aging Process, Including Advice on Nutrition, Exercise, and Sleep, Help in Making Decisions about Midlife Issues and Retirement, and Guidance Concerning Practical and Informed Choices in Health Consumerism*

*Along with Data Concerning the Theories of Aging, Different Experiences in Aging by Minority Groups, and Facts about Aging Now and Aging in the Future; and Featuring a Glossary, a Guide to Consumer Help, Additional Suggested Reading, and Practical Resource Directory*

Edited by Jenifer Swanson. 536 pages. 1999. 978-0-7808-0390-9.

*SEE ALSO Physical & Mental Issues in Aging Sourcebook*

---

# Healthy Children Sourcebook

*Basic Consumer Health Information about the Physical and Mental Development of Children between the Ages of 3 and 12, Including Routine Health Care, Preventative Health Services, Safety and First Aid,*

*Healthy Sleep, Dental Care, Nutrition, and Fitness, and Featuring Parenting Tips on Such Topics as Bedwetting, Choosing Day Care, Monitoring TV and Other Media, and Establishing a Foundation for Substance Abuse Prevention*

*Along with a Glossary of Commonly Used Pediatric Terms and Resources for Additional Help and Information.*

Edited by Chad T. Kimball. 647 pages. 2003. 978-0-7808-0247-6.

*SEE ALSO Childhood Diseases & Disorders Sourcebook*

---

# Healthy Heart Sourcebook for Women

*Basic Consumer Health Information about Cardiac Issues Specific to Women, Including Facts about Major Risk Factors and Prevention, Treatment and Control Strategies, and Important Dietary Issues*

*Along with a Special Section Regarding the Pros and Cons of Hormone Replacement Therapy and Its Impact on Heart Health, and Additional Help, Including Recipes, a Glossary, and a Directory of Resources*

Edited by Dawn D. Matthews. 336 pages. 2000. 978-0-7808-0329-9.

*SEE ALSO Cardiovascular Diseases & Disorders Sourcebook, Women's Health Concerns Sourcebook*

---

# Hepatitis Sourcebook

*Basic Consumer Health Information about Hepatitis A, Hepatitis B, Hepatitis C, and Other Forms of Hepatitis, Including Autoimmune Hepatitis, Alcoholic Hepatitis, Nonalcoholic Steatohepatitis, and Toxic Hepatitis, with*

Facts about Risk Factors, Screening Methods, Diagnostic Tests, and Treatment Options

Along with Information on Liver Health, Tips for People Living with Chronic Hepatitis, Reports on Current Research Initiatives, a Glossary of Terms Related to Hepatitis, and a Directory of Sources for Further Help and Information

Edited by Sandra J. Judd. 597 pages. 2005. 978-0-7808-0749-5.

"Highly recommended."
— American Reference Books Annual, 2006

∎

# Household Safety Sourcebook

Basic Consumer Health Information about Household Safety, Including Information about Poisons, Chemicals, Fire, and Water Hazards in the Home

Along with Advice about the Safe Use of Home Maintenance Equipment, Choosing Toys and Nursery Furniture, Holiday and Recreation Safety, a Glossary, and Resources for Further Help and Information

Edited by Dawn D. Matthews. 606 pages. 2002. 978-0-7808-0338-1.

"This work will be useful in public libraries with large consumer health and wellness departments."
— American Reference Books Annual, 2003

"As a sourcebook on household safety this book meets its mark. It is encyclopedic in scope and covers a wide range of safety issues that are commonly seen in the home."
— E-Streams, Jul '02

∎

# Hypertension Sourcebook

Basic Consumer Health Information about the Causes, Diagnosis, and Treatment of High Blood Pressure, with Facts about Consequences, Complications, and Co-Occurring Disorders, Such as Coronary Heart Disease, Diabetes, Stroke, Kidney Disease, and Hypertensive Retinopathy, and Issues in Blood Pressure Control, Including Dietary Choices, Stress Management, and Medications

Along with Reports on Current Research Initiatives and Clinical Trials, a Glossary, and Resources for Additional Help and Information

Edited by Dawn D. Matthews and Karen Bellenir. 613 pages. 2004. 978-0-7808-0674-0.

"Academic, public, and medical libraries will want to add the Hypertension Sourcebook to their collections."
— E-Streams, Aug '05

"The strength of this source is the wide range of information given about hypertension."
— American Reference Books Annual, 2005

∎

# Immune System Disorders Sourcebook, 2nd Edition

Basic Consumer Health Information about Disorders of the Immune System, Including Immune System Function and Response, Diagnosis of Immune Disorders, Information about Inherited Immune Disease, Acquired Immune Disease, and Autoimmune Diseases, Including Primary Immune Deficiency, Acquired Immunodeficiency Syndrome (AIDS), Lupus, Multiple Sclerosis, Type 1 Diabetes, Rheumatoid Arthritis, and Graves' Disease

Along with Treatments, Tips for Coping with Immune Disorders, a Glossary, and a Directory of Additional Resources.

Edited by Joyce Brennfleck Shannon. 671 pages. 2005. 978-0-7808-0748-8.

"Highly recommended for academic and public libraries." — American Reference Books Annual, 2006

"The updated second edition is a 'must' for any consumer health library seeking a solid resource covering the treatments, symptoms, and options for immune disorder sufferers. . . . An excellent guide."
— MBR Bookwatch, Jan '06

∎

# Infant & Toddler Health Sourcebook

Basic Consumer Health Information about the Physical and Mental Development of Newborns, Infants, and Toddlers, Including Neonatal Concerns, Nutrition Recommendations, Immunization Schedules, Common Pediatric Disorders, Assessments and Milestones, Safety Tips, and Advice for Parents and Other Caregivers

Along with a Glossary of Terms and Resource Listings for Additional Help

Edited by Jenifer Swanson. 585 pages. 2000. 978-0-7808-0246-9.

"As a reference for the general public, this would be useful in any library." — E-Streams, May '01

"Recommended reference source."
— Booklist, American Library Association, Feb '01

"This is a good source for general use."
— American Reference Books Annual, 2001

∎

# Infectious Diseases Sourcebook

Basic Consumer Health Information about Non-Contagious Bacterial, Viral, Prion, Fungal, and Parasitic Diseases Spread by Food and Water, Insects and Animals, or Environmental Contact, Including Botulism, E. Coli, Encephalitis, Legionnaires' Disease, Lyme Disease, Malaria, Plague, Rabies, Salmonella, Tetanus, and Others, and Facts about Newly Emerging Diseases, Such as Hantavirus, Mad Cow Disease, Monkeypox, and West Nile Virus

Along with Information about Preventing Disease Transmission, the Threat of Bioterrorism, and Current Research Initiatives, with a Glossary and Directory of Resources for More Information

Edited by Karen Bellenir. 634 pages. 2004. 978-0-7808-0675-7.

"This reference continues the excellent tradition of the *Health Reference Series* in consolidating a wealth of information on a selected topic into a format that is easy to use and accessible to the general public."
— *American Reference Books Annual, 2005*

"Recommended for public and academic libraries."
— *E-Streams, Jan '05*

■

# Injury & Trauma Sourcebook

*Basic Consumer Health Information about the Impact of Injury, the Diagnosis and Treatment of Common and Traumatic Injuries, Emergency Care, and Specific Injuries Related to Home, Community, Workplace, Transportation, and Recreation*

*Along with Guidelines for Injury Prevention, a Glossary, and a Directory of Additional Resources*

Edited by Joyce Brennfleck Shannon. 696 pages. 2002. 978-0-7808-0421-0.

"This publication is the most comprehensive work of its kind about injury and trauma."
— *American Reference Books Annual, 2003*

"This sourcebook provides concise, easily readable, basic health information about injuries. . . . This book is well organized and an easy to use reference resource suitable for hospital, health sciences and public libraries with consumer health collections."
— *E-Streams, Nov '02*

"Practitioners should be aware of guides such as this in order to facilitate their use by patients and their families."
— *Doody's Health Sciences Book Review Journal, Sep-Oct '02*

"Recommended reference source."
— *Booklist, American Library Association, Sep '02*

"Highly recommended for academic and medical reference collections."
— *Library Bookwatch, Sep '02*

■

# Kidney & Urinary Tract Diseases & Disorders Sourcebook

SEE *Urinary Tract & Kidney Diseases & Disorders Sourcebook*

■

# Learning Disabilities Sourcebook, 2nd Edition

*Basic Consumer Health Information about Learning Disabilities, Including Dyslexia, Developmental Speech and Language Disabilities, Non-Verbal Learning Disorders, Developmental Arithmetic Disorder, Developmental Writing Disorder, and Other Conditions That Impede Learning Such as Attention Deficit/Hyperactivity Disorder, Brain Injury, Hearing Impairment, Klinefelter Syndrome, Dyspraxia, and Tourette's Syndrome*

*Along with Facts about Educational Issues and Assistive Technology, Coping Strategies, a Glossary of Related Terms, and Resources for Further Help and Information*

Edited by Dawn D. Matthews. 621 pages. 2003. 978-0-7808-0626-9.

"The second edition of Learning Disabilities Sourcebook far surpasses the earlier edition in that it is more focused on information that will be useful as a consumer health resource."
— *American Reference Books Annual, 2004*

"Teachers as well as consumers will find this an essential guide to understanding various syndromes and their latest treatments. [An] invaluable reference for public and school library collections alike."
— *Library Bookwatch, Apr '03*

Named "Outstanding Reference Book of 1999."
— *New York Public Library, Feb '00*

"An excellent candidate for inclusion in a public library reference section. It's a great source of information. Teachers will also find the book useful. Definitely worth reading."
— *Journal of Adolescent & Adult Literacy, Feb 2000*

"Readable . . . provides a solid base of information regarding successful techniques used with individuals who have learning disabilities, as well as practical suggestions for educators and family members. Clear language, concise descriptions, and pertinent information for contacting multiple resources add to the strength of this book as a useful tool."
— *Choice, Association of College & Research Libraries, Feb '99*

"Recommended reference source."
— *Booklist, American Library Association, Sep '98*

"A useful resource for libraries and for those who don't have the time to identify and locate the individual publications."
— *Disability Resources Monthly, Sep '98*

■

# Leukemia Sourcebook

*Basic Consumer Health Information about Adult and Childhood Leukemias, Including Acute Lymphocytic Leukemia (ALL), Chronic Lymphocytic Leukemia (CLL), Acute Myelogenous Leukemia (AML), Chronic Myelogenous Leukemia (CML), and Hairy Cell Leukemia, and Treatments Such as Chemotherapy, Radiation Therapy, Peripheral Blood Stem Cell and Marrow Transplantation, and Immunotherapy*

*Along with Tips for Life During and After Treatment, a Glossary, and Directories of Additional Resources*

Edited by Joyce Brennfleck Shannon. 587 pages. 2003. 978-0-7808-0627-6.

"Unlike other medical books for the layperson, . . . the language does not talk down to the reader. . . . This volume is highly recommended for all libraries."
— *American Reference Books Annual, 2004*

". . . a fine title which ranges from diagnosis to alternative treatments, staging, and tips for life during and after diagnosis."
— *The Bookwatch, Dec '03*

619

# Liver Disorders Sourcebook

*Basic Consumer Health Information about the Liver and How It Works; Liver Diseases, Including Cancer, Cirrhosis, Hepatitis, and Toxic and Drug Related Diseases; Tips for Maintaining a Healthy Liver; Laboratory Tests, Radiology Tests, and Facts about Liver Transplantation*

*Along with a Section on Support Groups, a Glossary, and Resource Listings*

Edited by Joyce Brennfleck Shannon. 591 pages. 2000. 978-0-7808-0383-1.

"A valuable resource."
*—American Reference Books Annual, 2001*

"This title is recommended for health sciences and public libraries with consumer health collections."
*— E-Streams, Oct '00*

"Recommended reference source."
*—Booklist, American Library Association, Jun '00*

■

# Lung Disorders Sourcebook

*Basic Consumer Health Information about Emphysema, Pneumonia, Tuberculosis, Asthma, Cystic Fibrosis, and Other Lung Disorders, Including Facts about Diagnostic Procedures, Treatment Strategies, Disease Prevention Efforts, and Such Risk Factors as Smoking, Air Pollution, and Exposure to Asbestos, Radon, and Other Agents*

*Along with a Glossary and Resources for Additional Help and Information*

Edited by Dawn D. Matthews. 678 pages. 2002. 978-0-7808-0339-8.

"This title is a great addition for public and school libraries because it provides concise health information on the lungs."
*— American Reference Books Annual, 2003*

"Highly recommended for academic and medical reference collections." *— Library Bookwatch, Sep '02*

**SEE ALSO** *Respiratory Diseases & Disorders Sourcebook*

■

# Medical Tests Sourcebook, 2nd Edition

*Basic Consumer Health Information about Medical Tests, Including Age-Specific Health Tests, Important Health Screenings and Exams, Home-Use Tests, Blood and Specimen Tests, Electrical Tests, Scope Tests, Genetic Testing, and Imaging Tests, Such as X-Rays, Ultrasound, Computed Tomography, Magnetic Resonance Imaging, Angiography, and Nuclear Medicine*

*Along with a Glossary and Directory of Additional Resources*

Edited by Joyce Brennfleck Shannon. 654 pages. 2004. 978-0-7808-0670-2.

"Recommended for hospital and health sciences libraries with consumer health collections."
*—E-Streams, Mar '00*

"This is an overall excellent reference with a wealth of general knowledge that may aid those who are reluctant to get vital tests performed."
*—Today's Librarian, Jan '00*

"A valuable reference guide."
*—American Reference Books Annual, 2000*

■

# Men's Health Concerns Sourcebook, 2nd Edition

*Basic Consumer Health Information about the Medical and Mental Concerns of Men, Including Theories about the Shorter Male Lifespan, the Leading Causes of Death and Disability, Physical Concerns of Special Significance to Men, Reproductive and Sexual Concerns, Sexually Transmitted Diseases, Men's Mental and Emotional Health, and Lifestyle Choices That Affect Wellness, Such as Nutrition, Fitness, and Substance Use*

*Along with a Glossary of Related Terms and a Directory of Organizational Resources in Men's Health*

Edited by Robert Aquinas McNally. 644 pages. 2004. 978-0-7808-0671-9.

"A very accessible reference for non-specialist general readers and consumers." *— The Bookwatch, Jun '04*

"This comprehensive resource and the series are highly recommended."
*—American Reference Books Annual, 2000*

"Recommended reference source."
*—Booklist, American Library Association, Dec '98*

■

# Mental Health Disorders Sourcebook, 3rd Edition

*Basic Consumer Health Information about Mental and Emotional Health and Mental Illness, Including Facts about Depression, Bipolar Disorder, and Other Mood Disorders, Phobias, Post-Traumatic Stress Disorder (PTSD), Obsessive-Compulsive Disorder, and Other Anxiety Disorders, Impulse Control Disorders, Eating Disorders, Personality Disorders, and Psychotic Disorders, Including Schizophrenia and Dissociative Disorders*

*Along with Statistical Information, a Special Section Concerning Mental Health Issues in Children and Adolescents, a Glossary, and Directories of Resources for Additional Help and Information*

Edited by Karen Bellenir. 661 pages. 2005. 978-0-7808-0747-1.

"Recommended for public libraries and academic libraries with an undergraduate program in psychology."
*—American Reference Books Annual, 2006*

"Recommended reference source."
*—Booklist, American Library Association, Jun '00*

# Mental Retardation Sourcebook

*Basic Consumer Health Information about Mental Retardation and Its Causes, Including Down Syndrome, Fetal Alcohol Syndrome, Fragile X Syndrome, Genetic Conditions, Injury, and Environmental Sources*

*Along with Preventive Strategies, Parenting Issues, Educational Implications, Health Care Needs, Employment and Economic Matters, Legal Issues, a Glossary, and a Resource Listing for Additional Help and Information*

Edited by Joyce Brennfleck Shannon. 642 pages. 2000. 978-0-7808-0377-0.

"Public libraries will find the book useful for reference and as a beginning research point for students, parents, and caregivers."
— *American Reference Books Annual, 2001*

"The strength of this work is that it compiles many basic fact sheets and addresses for further information in one volume. It is intended and suitable for the general public. This sourcebook is relevant to any collection providing health information to the general public."
— *E-Streams, Nov '00*

"From preventing retardation to parenting and family challenges, this covers health, social and legal issues and will prove an invaluable overview."
— *Reviewer's Bookwatch, Jul '00*

# Movement Disorders Sourcebook

*Basic Consumer Health Information about Neurological Movement Disorders, Including Essential Tremor, Parkinson's Disease, Dystonia, Cerebral Palsy, Huntington's Disease, Myasthenia Gravis, Multiple Sclerosis, and Other Early-Onset and Adult-Onset Movement Disorders, Their Symptoms and Causes, Diagnostic Tests, and Treatments*

*Along with Mobility and Assistive Technology Information, a Glossary, and a Directory of Additional Resources*

Edited by Joyce Brennfleck Shannon. 655 pages. 2003. 978-0-7808-0628-3.

". . . a good resource for consumers and recommended for public, community college and undergraduate libraries." — *American Reference Books Annual, 2004*

# Muscular Dystrophy Sourcebook

*Basic Consumer Health Information about Congenital, Childhood-Onset, and Adult-Onset Forms of Muscular Dystrophy, Such as Duchenne, Becker, Emery-Dreifuss, Distal, Limb-Girdle, Facioscapulohumeral (FSHD), Myotonic, and Ophthalmoplegic Muscular Dystrophies, Including Facts about Diagnostic Tests, Medical and Physical Therapies, Management of Co-Occurring Conditions, and Parenting Guidelines*

*Along with Practical Tips for Home Care, a Glossary, and Directories of Additional Resources*

Edited by Joyce Brennfleck Shannon. 577 pages. 2004. 978-0-7808-0676-4.

"This book is highly recommended for public and academic libraries as well as health care offices that support the information needs of patients and their families."
— *E-Streams, Apr '05*

"Excellent reference." — *The Bookwatch, Jan '05*

# Obesity Sourcebook

*Basic Consumer Health Information about Diseases and Other Problems Associated with Obesity, and Including Facts about Risk Factors, Prevention Issues, and Management Approaches*

*Along with Statistical and Demographic Data, Information about Special Populations, Research Updates, a Glossary, and Source Listings for Further Help and Information*

Edited by Wilma Caldwell and Chad T. Kimball. 376 pages. 2001. 978-0-7808-0333-6.

"The book synthesizes the reliable medical literature on obesity into one easy-to-read and useful resource for the general public."
— *American Reference Books Annual, 2002*

"This is a very useful resource book for the lay public."
— *Doody's Review Service, Nov '01*

"Well suited for the health reference collection of a public library or an academic health science library that serves the general population." — *E-Streams, Sep '01*

"Recommended reference source."
— *Booklist, American Library Association, Apr '01*

"Recommended pick both for specialty health library collections and any general consumer health reference collection." — *The Bookwatch, Apr '01*

# Oral Health Sourcebook

*SEE Dental Care & Oral Health Sourcebook*

# Osteoporosis Sourcebook

*Basic Consumer Health Information about Primary and Secondary Osteoporosis and Juvenile Osteoporosis and Related Conditions, Including Fibrous Dysplasia, Gaucher Disease, Hyperthyroidism, Hypophosphatasia, Myeloma, Osteopetrosis, Osteogenesis Imperfecta, and Paget's Disease*

*Along with Information about Risk Factors, Treatments, Traditional and Non-Traditional Pain Management, a Glossary of Related Terms, and a Directory of Resources*

Edited by Allan R. Cook. 584 pages. 2001. 978-0-7808-0239-1.

"This would be a book to be kept in a staff or patient library. The targeted audience is the layperson, but the therapist who needs a quick bit of information on a particular topic will also find the book useful."
— *Physical Therapy, Jan '02*

"This resource is recommended as a great reference source for public, health, and academic libraries, and is another triumph for the editors of Omnigraphics."
— *American Reference Books Annual, 2002*

"Recommended for all public libraries and general health collections, especially those supporting patient education or consumer health programs."
— *E-Streams, Nov '01*

"Will prove valuable to any library seeking to maintain a current, comprehensive reference collection of health resources. . . . From prevention to treatment and associated conditions, this provides an excellent survey."
— *The Bookwatch, Aug '01*

"Recommended reference source."
— *Booklist, American Library Association, Jul '01*

**SEE ALSO** *Healthy Aging Sourcebook, Physical & Mental Issues in Aging Sourcebook, Women's Health Concerns Sourcebook*

# Pain Sourcebook, 2nd Edition

*Basic Consumer Health Information about Specific Forms of Acute and Chronic Pain, Including Muscle and Skeletal Pain, Nerve Pain, Cancer Pain, and Disorders Characterized by Pain, Such as Fibromyalgia, Shingles, Angina, Arthritis, and Headaches*

*Along with Information about Pain Medications and Management Techniques, Complementary and Alternative Pain Relief Options, Tips for People Living with Chronic Pain, a Glossary, and a Directory of Sources for Further Information*

Edited by Karen Bellenir. 670 pages. 2002. 978-0-7808-0612-2.

"A source of valuable information. . . . This book offers help to nonmedical people who need information about pain and pain management. It is also an excellent reference for those who participate in patient education."
— *Doody's Review Service, Sep '02*

"Highly recommended for academic and medical reference collections." — *Library Bookwatch, Sep '02*

"The text is readable, easily understood, and well indexed. This excellent volume belongs in all patient education libraries, consumer health sections of public libraries, and many personal collections."
— *American Reference Books Annual, 1999*

"The information is basic in terms of scholarship and is appropriate for general readers. Written in journalistic style . . . intended for non-professionals. Quite thorough in its coverage of different pain conditions and summarizes the latest clinical information regarding pain treatment." — *Choice, Association of College and Research Libraries, Jun '98*

"Recommended reference source."
— *Booklist, American Library Association, Mar '98*

# Pediatric Cancer Sourcebook

*Basic Consumer Health Information about Leukemias, Brain Tumors, Sarcomas, Lymphomas, and Other Cancers in Infants, Children, and Adolescents, Including Descriptions of Cancers, Treatments, and Coping Strategies*

*Along with Suggestions for Parents, Caregivers, and Concerned Relatives, a Glossary of Cancer Terms, and Resource Listings*

Edited by Edward J. Prucha. 587 pages. 1999. 978-0-7808-0245-2.

"An excellent source of information. Recommended for public, hospital, and health science libraries with consumer health collections." — *E-Streams, Jun '00*

"Recommended reference source."
— *Booklist, American Library Association, Feb '00*

"A valuable addition to all libraries specializing in health services and many public libraries."
— *American Reference Books Annual, 2000*

**SEE ALSO** *Childhood Diseases & Disorders Sourcebook, Healthy Children Sourcebook*

# Physical & Mental Issues in Aging Sourcebook

*Basic Consumer Health Information on Physical and Mental Disorders Associated with the Aging Process, Including Concerns about Cardiovascular Disease, Pulmonary Disease, Oral Health, Digestive Disorders, Musculoskeletal and Skin Disorders, Metabolic Changes, Sexual and Reproductive Issues, and Changes in Vision, Hearing, and Other Senses*

*Along with Data about Longevity and Causes of Death, Information on Acute and Chronic Pain, Descriptions of Mental Concerns, a Glossary of Terms, and Resource Listings for Additional Help*

Edited by Jenifer Swanson. 660 pages. 1999. 978-0-7808-0233-9.

"This is a treasure of health information for the layperson." — *Choice Health Sciences Supplement, Association of College & Research Libraries, May '00*

"Recommended for public libraries."
— *American Reference Books Annual, 2000*

"Recommended reference source."
— *Booklist, American Library Association, Oct '99*

**SEE ALSO** *Healthy Aging Sourcebook*

# Podiatry Sourcebook, 2nd Edition

*Basic Consumer Health Information about Disorders, Diseases, Deformities, and Injuries that Affect the Foot and Ankle, Including Sprains, Corns, Calluses, Bunions, Plantar Warts, Plantar Fasciitis, Neuromas, Clubfoot, Flat Feet, Achilles Tendonitis, and Much More*

*Along with Information about Selecting a Foot Care Specialist, Foot Fitness, Shoes and Socks, Diagnostic Tests and Corrective Procedures, Financial Assistance for Corrective Devices, a Glossary of Related Terms, and a Directory of Resources for Additional Help and Information*

Edited by Ivy L. Alexander. 543 pages. 2007. 978-0-7808-0944-4.

**"Recommended reference source."**
— *Booklist, American Library Association, Feb '02*

**"There is a lot of information presented here on a topic that is usually only covered sparingly in most larger comprehensive medical encyclopedias."**
— *American Reference Books Annual, 2002*

# Pregnancy & Birth Sourcebook, 2nd Edition

*Basic Consumer Health Information about Conception and Pregnancy, Including Facts about Fertility, Infertility, Pregnancy Symptoms and Complications, Fetal Growth and Development, Labor, Delivery, and the Postpartum Period, as Well as Information about Maintaining Health and Wellness during Pregnancy and Caring for a Newborn*

*Along with Information about Public Health Assistance for Low-Income Pregnant Women, a Glossary, and Directories of Agencies and Organizations Providing Help and Support*

Edited by Amy L. Sutton. 626 pages. 2004. 978-0-7808-0672-6.

**"Will appeal to public and school reference collections strong in medicine and women's health. . . . Deserves a spot on any medical reference shelf."**
— *The Bookwatch, Jul '04*

**"A well-organized handbook. Recommended."**
— *Choice, Association of College & Research Libraries, Apr '98*

**"Recommended reference source."**
— *Booklist, American Library Association, Mar '98*

**"Recommended for public libraries."**
— *American Reference Books Annual, 1998*

*SEE ALSO Breastfeeding Sourcebook, Congenital Disorders Sourcebook, Family Planning Sourcebook*

# Prostate & Urological Disorders Sourcebook

*Basic Consumer Health Information about Urogenital and Sexual Disorders in Men, Including Prostate and Other Andrological Cancers, Prostatitis, Benign Prostatic Hyperplasia, Testicular and Penile Trauma, Cryptorchidism, Peyronie Disease, Erectile Dysfunction, and Male Factor Infertility, and Facts about Commonly Used Tests and Procedures, Such as Prostatectomy, Vasectomy, Vasectomy Reversal, Penile Implants, and Semen Analysis*

*Along with a Glossary of Andrological Terms and a Directory of Resources for Additional Information*

Edited by Karen Bellenir. 631 pages. 2005. 978-0-7808-0797-6.

# Prostate Cancer Sourcebook

*Basic Consumer Health Information about Prostate Cancer, Including Information about the Associated Risk Factors, Detection, Diagnosis, and Treatment of Prostate Cancer*

*Along with Information on Non-Malignant Prostate Conditions, and Featuring a Section Listing Support and Treatment Centers and a Glossary of Related Terms*

Edited by Dawn D. Matthews. 358 pages. 2001. 978-0-7808-0324-4.

**"Recommended reference source."**
— *Booklist, American Library Association, Jan '02*

**"A valuable resource for health care consumers seeking information on the subject. . . . All text is written in a clear, easy-to-understand language that avoids technical jargon. Any library that collects consumer health resources would strengthen their collection with the addition of the *Prostate Cancer Sourcebook*."**
— *American Reference Books Annual, 2002*

*SEE ALSO Men's Health Concerns Sourcebook*

# Reconstructive & Cosmetic Surgery Sourcebook

*Basic Consumer Health Information on Cosmetic and Reconstructive Plastic Surgery, Including Statistical Information about Different Surgical Procedures, Things to Consider Prior to Surgery, Plastic Surgery Techniques and Tools, Emotional and Psychological Considerations, and Procedure-Specific Information*

*Along with a Glossary of Terms and a Listing of Resources for Additional Help and Information*

Edited by M. Lisa Weatherford. 374 pages. 2001. 978-0-7808-0214-8.

**"An excellent reference that addresses cosmetic and medically necessary reconstructive surgeries. . . . The style of the prose is calm and reassuring, discussing the many positive outcomes now available due to advances in surgical techniques."**
— *American Reference Books Annual, 2002*

**"Recommended for health science libraries that are open to the public, as well as hospital libraries that are open to the patients. This book is a good resource for the consumer interested in plastic surgery."**
— *E-Streams, Dec '01*

**"Recommended reference source."**
— *Booklist, American Library Association, Jul '01*

# Rehabilitation Sourcebook

*Basic Consumer Health Information about Rehabilitation for People Recovering from Heart Surgery, Spinal Cord Injury, Stroke, Orthopedic Impairments, Amputation, Pulmonary Impairments, Traumatic Injury, and More, Including Physical Therapy, Occupational Therapy, Speech/Language Therapy, Massage Therapy, Dance Therapy, Art Therapy, and Recreational Therapy*

Along with Information on Assistive and Adaptive Devices, a Glossary, and Resources for Additional Help and Information

Edited by Dawn D. Matthews. 531 pages. 1999. 978-0-7808-0236-0.

"This is an excellent resource for public library reference and health collections."
—American Reference Books Annual, 2001

"Recommended reference source."
—Booklist, American Library Association, May '00

■

# Respiratory Diseases & Disorders Sourcebook

Basic Information about Respiratory Diseases and Disorders, Including Asthma, Cystic Fibrosis, Pneumonia, the Common Cold, Influenza, and Others, Featuring Facts about the Respiratory System, Statistical and Demographic Data, Treatments, Self-Help Management Suggestions, and Current Research Initiatives

Edited by Allan R. Cook and Peter D. Dresser. 771 pages. 1995. 978-0-7808-0037-3.

"Designed for the layperson and for patients and their families coping with respiratory illness. . . . an extensive array of information on diagnosis, treatment, management, and prevention of respiratory illnesses for the general reader."　—Choice, Association of College & Research Libraries, Jun '96

"A highly recommended text for all collections. It is a comforting reminder of the power of knowledge that good books carry between their covers."
—Academic Library Book Review, Spring '96

"A comprehensive collection of authoritative information presented in a nontechnical, humanitarian style for patients, families, and caregivers."
—Association of Operating Room Nurses, Sep/Oct '95

SEE ALSO Lung Disorders Sourcebook

■

# Sexually Transmitted Diseases Sourcebook, 3rd Edition

Basic Consumer Health Information about Chlamydial Infections, Gonorrhea, Hepatitis, Herpes, HIV/AIDS, Human Papillomavirus, Pubic Lice, Scabies, Syphilis, Trichomoniasis, Vaginal Infections, and Other Sexually Transmitted Diseases, Including Facts about Risk Factors, Symptoms, Diagnosis, Treatment, and the Prevention of Sexually Transmitted Infections

Along with Updates on Current Research Initiatives, a Glossary of Related Terms, and Resources for Additional Help and Information

Edited by Amy L. Sutton. 629 pages. 2006. 978-0-7808-0824-9.

"Recommended for consumer health collections in public libraries, and secondary school and community college libraries."
—American Reference Books Annual, 2002

"Every school and public library should have a copy of this comprehensive and user-friendly reference book."
—Choice, Association of College & Research Libraries, Sep '01

"This is a highly recommended book. This is an especially important book for all school and public libraries."
—AIDS Book Review Journal, Jul-Aug '01

"Recommended reference source."
—Booklist, American Library Association, Apr '01

■

# Sleep Disorders Sourcebook, 2nd Edition

Basic Consumer Health Information about Sleep and Sleep Disorders, Including Insomnia, Sleep Apnea, Restless Legs Syndrome, Narcolepsy, Parasomnias, and Other Health Problems That Affect Sleep, Plus Facts about Diagnostic Procedures, Treatment Strategies, Sleep Medications, and Tips for Improving Sleep Quality

Along with a Glossary of Related Terms and Resources for Additional Help and Information

Edited by Amy L. Sutton. 567 pages. 2005. 978-0-7808-0743-3.

"This book will be useful for just about everybody, especially the 40 million Americans with sleep disorders."
—American Reference Books Annual, 2006

"Recommended for public libraries and libraries supporting health care professionals." —E-Streams, Sep '05

". . . key medical library acquisition."
—The Bookwatch, Jun '05

■

# Smoking Concerns Sourcebook

Basic Consumer Health Information about Nicotine Addiction and Smoking Cessation, Featuring Facts about the Health Effects of Tobacco Use, Including Lung and Other Cancers, Heart Disease, Stroke, and Respiratory Disorders, Such as Emphysema and Chronic Bronchitis

Along with Information about Smoking Prevention Programs, Suggestions for Achieving and Maintaining a Smoke-Free Lifestyle, Statistics about Tobacco Use, Reports on Current Research Initiatives, a Glossary of Related Terms, and Directories of Resources for Additional Help and Information

Edited by Karen Bellenir. 621 pages. 2004. 978-0-7808-0323-7.

"Provides everything needed for the student or general reader seeking practical details on the effects of tobacco use."　—The Bookwatch, Mar '05

"Public libraries and consumer health care libraries will find this work useful."
—American Reference Books Annual, 2005

## Sports Injuries Sourcebook, 3rd Edition

*Basic Consumer Health Information about Sprains and Strains, Fractures, Growth Plate Injuries, Overtraining Injuries, and Injuries to the Head, Face, Shoulders, Elbows, Hands, Spinal Column, Knees, Ankles, and Feet, and with Facts about Heat-Related Illness, Steroids and Sport Supplements, Protective Equipment, Diagnostic Procedures, Treatment Options, and Rehabilitation*

*Along with a Glossary of Related Terms and a Directory of Resources for Additional Help and Information*

Edited by Sandra J. Judd. 651 pages. 2007. 978-0-7808-0949-9.

**"This is an excellent reference for consumers and it is recommended for public, community college, and undergraduate libraries."**
— *American Reference Books Annual, 2003*

**"Recommended reference source."**
— *Booklist, American Library Association, Feb '03*

■

## Stress-Related Disorders Sourcebook

*Basic Consumer Health Information about Stress and Stress-Related Disorders, Including Stress Origins and Signals, Environmental Stress at Work and Home, Mental and Emotional Stress Associated with Depression, Post-Traumatic Stress Disorder, Panic Disorder, Suicide, and the Physical Effects of Stress on the Cardiovascular, Immune, and Nervous Systems*

*Along with Stress Management Techniques, a Glossary, and a Listing of Additional Resources*

Edited by Joyce Brennfleck Shannon. 610 pages. 2002. 978-0-7808-0560-6.

**"Well written for a general readership, the *Stress-Related Disorders Sourcebook* is a useful addition to the health reference literature."**
— *American Reference Books Annual, 2003*

**"I am impressed by the amount of information. It offers a thorough overview of the causes and consequences of stress for the layperson. . . . A well-done and thorough reference guide for professionals and nonprofessionals alike."** — *Doody's Review Service, Dec '02*

■

## Stroke Sourcebook

*Basic Consumer Health Information about Stroke, Including Ischemic, Hemorrhagic, Transient Ischemic Attack (TIA), and Pediatric Stroke, Stroke Triggers and Risks, Diagnostic Tests, Treatments, and Rehabilitation Information*

*Along with Stroke Prevention Guidelines, Legal and Financial Information, a Glossary, and a Directory of Additional Resources*

Edited by Joyce Brennfleck Shannon. 606 pages. 2003. 978-0-7808-0630-6.

**"This volume is highly recommended and should be in every medical, hospital, and public library."**
— *American Reference Books Annual, 2004*

**"Highly recommended for the amount and variety of topics and information covered."** — *Choice, Nov '03*

■

## Surgery Sourcebook

*Basic Consumer Health Information about Inpatient and Outpatient Surgeries, Including Cardiac, Vascular, Orthopedic, Ocular, Reconstructive, Cosmetic, Gynecologic, and Ear, Nose, and Throat Procedures and More*

*Along with Information about Operating Room Policies and Instruments, Laser Surgery Techniques, Hospital Errors, Statistical Data, a Glossary, and Listings of Sources for Further Help and Information*

Edited by Annemarie S. Muth and Karen Bellenir. 596 pages. 2002. 978-0-7808-0380-0.

**"Large public libraries and medical libraries would benefit from this material in their reference collections."**
— *American Reference Books Annual, 2004*

**"Invaluable reference for public and school library collections alike."** — *Library Bookwatch, Apr '03*

■

## Thyroid Disorders Sourcebook

*Basic Consumer Health Information about Disorders of the Thyroid and Parathyroid Glands, Including Hypothyroidism, Hyperthyroidism, Graves Disease, Hashimoto Thyroiditis, Thyroid Cancer, and Parathyroid Disorders, Featuring Facts about Symptoms, Risk Factors, Tests, and Treatments*

*Along with Information about the Effects of Thyroid Imbalance on Other Body Systems, Environmental Factors That Affect the Thyroid Gland, a Glossary, and a Directory of Additional Resources*

Edited by Joyce Brennfleck Shannon. 599 pages. 2005. 978-0-7808-0745-7.

**"Recommended for consumer health collections."**
— *American Reference Books Annual, 2006*

**"Highly recommended pick for basic consumer health reference holdings at all levels."**
— *The Bookwatch, Aug '05*

■

## Transplantation Sourcebook

*Basic Consumer Health Information about Organ and Tissue Transplantation, Including Physical and Financial Preparations, Procedures and Issues Relating to Specific Solid Organ and Tissue Transplants, Rehabilitation, Pediatric Transplant Information, the Future of Transplantation, and Organ and Tissue Donation*

*Along with a Glossary and Listings of Additional Resources*

Edited by Joyce Brennfleck Shannon. 628 pages. 2002. 978-0-7808-0322-0.

"Along with these advances [in transplantation technology] have come a number of daunting questions for potential transplant patients, their families, and their health care providers. This reference text is the best single tool to address many of these questions. . . . It will be a much-needed addition to the reference collections in health care, academic, and large public libraries."
— *American Reference Books Annual, 2003*

"Recommended for libraries with an interest in offering consumer health information." — *E-Streams, Jul '02*

"This is a unique and valuable resource for patients facing transplantation and their families."
— *Doody's Review Service, Jun '02*

■

## Traveler's Health Sourcebook

*Basic Consumer Health Information for Travelers, Including Physical and Medical Preparations, Transportation Health and Safety, Essential Information about Food and Water, Sun Exposure, Insect and Snake Bites, Camping and Wilderness Medicine, and Travel with Physical or Medical Disabilities*

*Along with International Travel Tips, Vaccination Recommendations, Geographical Health Issues, Disease Risks, a Glossary, and a Listing of Additional Resources*

Edited by Joyce Brennfleck Shannon. 613 pages. 2000. 978-0-7808-0384-8.

"Recommended reference source."
— *Booklist, American Library Association, Feb '01*

"This book is recommended for any public library, any travel collection, and especially any collection for the physically disabled."
— *American Reference Books Annual, 2001*

SEE ALSO *Worldwide Health Sourcebook*

■

## Urinary Tract & Kidney Diseases & Disorders Sourcebook, 2nd Edition

*Basic Consumer Health Information about the Urinary System, Including the Bladder, Urethra, Ureters, and Kidneys, with Facts about Urinary Tract Infections, Incontinence, Congenital Disorders, Kidney Stones, Cancers of the Urinary Tract and Kidneys, Kidney Failure, Dialysis, and Kidney Transplantation*

*Along with Statistical and Demographic Information, Reports on Current Research in Kidney and Urologic Health, a Summary of Commonly Used Diagnostic Tests, a Glossary of Related Terms, and a Directory of Resources for Additional Help and Information*

Edited by Ivy L. Alexander. 649 pages. 2005. 978-0-7808-0750-1.

"A good choice for a consumer health information library or for a medical library needing information to refer to their patients."
— *American Reference Books Annual, 2006*

## Vegetarian Sourcebook

*Basic Consumer Health Information about Vegetarian Diets, Lifestyle, and Philosophy, Including Definitions of Vegetarianism and Veganism, Tips about Adopting Vegetarianism, Creating a Vegetarian Pantry, and Meeting Nutritional Needs of Vegetarians, with Facts Regarding Vegetarianism's Effect on Pregnant and Lactating Women, Children, Athletes, and Senior Citizens*

*Along with a Glossary of Commonly Used Vegetarian Terms and Resources for Additional Help and Information*

Edited by Chad T. Kimball. 360 pages. 2002. 978-0-7808-0439-5.

"Organizes into one concise volume the answers to the most common questions concerning vegetarian diets and lifestyles. This title is recommended for public and secondary school libraries." — *E-Streams, Apr '03*

"Invaluable reference for public and school library collections alike." — *Library Bookwatch, Apr '03*

"The articles in this volume are easy to read and come from authoritative sources. The book does not necessarily support the vegetarian diet but instead provides the pros and cons of this important decision. The Vegetarian Sourcebook is recommended for public libraries and consumer health libraries."
— *American Reference Books Annual, 2003*

SEE ALSO *Diet & Nutrition Sourcebook*

■

## Women's Health Concerns Sourcebook, 2nd Edition

*Basic Consumer Health Information about the Medical and Mental Concerns of Women, Including Maintaining Health and Wellness, Gynecological Concerns, Breast Health, Sexuality and Reproductive Issues, Menopause, Cancer in Women, Leading Causes of Death and Disability among Women, Physical Concerns of Special Significance to Women, and Women's Mental and Emotional Health*

*Along with a Glossary of Related Terms and Directories of Resources for Additional Help and Information*

Edited by Amy L. Sutton. 746 pages. 2004. 978-0-7808-0673-3.

"This is a useful reference book, which makes the reader knowledgeable about several issues that concern women's health. It is recommended for public libraries and home library collections." — *E-Streams, May '05*

"A useful addition to public and consumer health library collections."
— *American Reference Books Annual, 2005*

"A highly recommended title."
— *The Bookwatch, May '04*

"Handy compilation. There is an impressive range of diseases, devices, disorders, procedures, and other physical and emotional issues covered . . . well organized, illustrated, and indexed." — *Choice, Association of College & Research Libraries, Jan '98*

SEE ALSO *Breast Cancer Sourcebook, Cancer Sourcebook for Women, Healthy Heart Sourcebook for Women, Osteoporosis Sourcebook*

# Workplace Health & Safety Sourcebook

*Basic Consumer Health Information about Workplace Health and Safety, Including the Effect of Workplace Hazards on the Lungs, Skin, Heart, Ears, Eyes, Brain, Reproductive Organs, Musculoskeletal System, and Other Organs and Body Parts*

*Along with Information about Occupational Cancer, Personal Protective Equipment, Toxic and Hazardous Chemicals, Child Labor, Stress, and Workplace Violence*

Edited by Chad T. Kimball. 626 pages. 2000. 978-0-7808-0231-5.

"As a reference for the general public, this would be useful in any library." — *E-Streams, Jun '01*

"Provides helpful information for primary care physicians and other caregivers interested in occupational medicine. . . . General readers; professionals." — *Choice, Association of College & Research Libraries, May '01*

"Recommended reference source." — *Booklist, American Library Association, Feb '01*

"Highly recommended." — *The Bookwatch, Jan '01*

# Worldwide Health Sourcebook

*Basic Information about Global Health Issues, Including Malnutrition, Reproductive Health, Disease Dispersion and Prevention, Emerging Diseases, Risky Health Behaviors, and the Leading Causes of Death*

*Along with Global Health Concerns for Children, Women, and the Elderly, Mental Health Issues, Research and Technology Advancements, and Economic, Environmental, and Political Health Implications, a Glossary, and a Resource Listing for Additional Help and Information*

Edited by Joyce Brennfleck Shannon. 614 pages. 2001. 978-0-7808-0330-5.

"Named an Outstanding Academic Title." — *Choice, Association of College & Research Libraries, Jan '02*

"Yet another handy but also unique compilation in the extensive *Health Reference Series,* this is a useful work because many of the international publications reprinted or excerpted are not readily available. Highly recommended." — *Choice, Association of College & Research Libraries, Nov '01*

"Recommended reference source." — *Booklist, American Library Association, Oct '01*

SEE ALSO *Traveler's Health Sourcebook*

627

# Teen Health Series
## Helping Young Adults Understand, Manage, and Avoid Serious Illness

List price $65 per volume. **School and library price $58 per volume.**

## Alcohol Information for Teens
### Health Tips about Alcohol and Alcoholism

*Including Facts about Underage Drinking, Preventing Teen Alcohol Use, Alcohol's Effects on the Brain and the Body, Alcohol Abuse Treatment, Help for Children of Alcoholics, and More*

Edited by Joyce Brennfleck Shannon. 370 pages. 2005. 978-0-7808-0741-9.

**"Boxed facts and tips add visual interest to the well-researched and clearly written text."**
— *Curriculum Connection, Apr '06*

## Allergy Information for Teens
### Health Tips about Allergic Reactions Such as Anaphylaxis, Respiratory Problems, and Rashes

*Including Facts about Identifying and Managing Allergies to Food, Pollen, Mold, Animals, Chemicals, Drugs, and Other Substances*

Edited by Karen Bellenir. 410 pages. 2006. 978-0-7808-0799-0.

## Asthma Information for Teens
### Health Tips about Managing Asthma and Related Concerns

*Including Facts about Asthma Causes, Triggers, Symptoms, Diagnosis, and Treatment*

Edited by Karen Bellenir. 386 pages. 2005. 978-0-7808-0770-9.

**"Highly recommended for medical libraries, public school libraries, and public libraries."**
— *American Reference Books Annual, 2006*

**"It is so clearly written and well organized that even hesitant readers will be able to find the facts they need, whether for reports or personal information. . . . A succinct but complete resource."**
— *School Library Journal, Sep '05*

## Body Information for Teens
### Health Tips about Maintaining Well-Being for a Lifetime

*Including Facts about the Development and Functioning of the Body's Systems, Organs, and Structures and the Health Impact of Lifestyle Choices*

Edited by Sandra Augustyn Lawton. 458 pages. 2007. 978-0-7808-0443-2.

## Cancer Information for Teens
### Health Tips about Cancer Awareness, Prevention, Diagnosis, and Treatment

*Including Facts about Frequently Occurring Cancers, Cancer Risk Factors, and Coping Strategies for Teens Fighting Cancer or Dealing with Cancer in Friends or Family Members*

Edited by Wilma R. Caldwell. 428 pages. 2004. 978-0-7808-0678-8.

**"Recommended for school libraries, or consumer libraries that see a lot of use by teens."**
— *E-Streams, May '05*

**"A valuable educational tool."**
— *American Reference Books Annual, 2005*

**"Young adults and their parents alike will find this new addition to the *Teen Health Series* an important reference to cancer in teens."**
— *Children's Bookwatch, Feb '05*

## Complementary and Alternative Medicine Information for Teens
### Health Tips about Non-Traditional and Non-Western Medical Practices

*Including Information about Acupuncture, Chiropractic Medicine, Dietary and Herbal Supplements, Hypnosis, Massage Therapy, Prayer and Spirituality, Reflexology, Yoga, and More*

Edited by Sandra Augustyn Lawton. 405 pages. 2006. 978-0-7808-0966-6.

## Diabetes Information for Teens
### Health Tips about Managing Diabetes and Preventing Related Complications

*Including Information about Insulin, Glucose Control, Healthy Eating, Physical Activity, and Learning to Live with Diabetes*

Edited by Sandra Augustyn Lawton. 410 pages. 2006. 978-0-7808-0811-9.

# Diet Information for Teens, 2nd Edition

### Health Tips about Diet and Nutrition

*Including Facts about Dietary Guidelines, Food Groups, Nutrients, Healthy Meals, Snacks, Weight Control, Medical Concerns Related to Diet, and More*

Edited by Karen Bellenir. 432 pages. 2006. 978-0-7808-0820-1.

"Full of helpful insights and facts throughout the book. ... An excellent resource to be placed in public libraries or even in personal collections."
— *American Reference Books Annual, 2002*

"Recommended for middle and high school libraries and media centers as well as academic libraries that educate future teachers of teenagers. It is also a suitable addition to health science libraries that serve patrons who are interested in teen health promotion and education." — *E-Streams, Oct '01*

"This comprehensive book would be beneficial to collections that need information about nutrition, dietary guidelines, meal planning, and weight control. ... This reference is so easy to use that its purchase is recommended." — *The Book Report, Sep-Oct '01*

"This book is written in an easy to understand format describing issues that many teens face every day, and then provides thoughtful explanations so that teens can make informed decisions. This is an interesting book that provides important facts and information for today's teens." — *Doody's Health Sciences Book Review Journal, Jul-Aug '01*

"A comprehensive compendium of diet and nutrition. The information is presented in a straightforward, plain-spoken manner. This title will be useful to those working on reports on a variety of topics, as well as to general readers concerned about their dietary health." — *School Library Journal, Jun '01*

# Drug Information for Teens, 2nd Edition

### Health Tips about the Physical and Mental Effects of Substance Abuse

*Including Information about Marijuana, Inhalants, Club Drugs, Stimulants, Hallucinogens, Opiates, Prescription and Over-the-Counter Drugs, Herbal Products, Tobacco, Alcohol, and More*

Edited by Sandra Augustyn Lawton. 468 pages. 2006. 978-0-7808-0862-1.

"A clearly written resource for general readers and researchers alike." — *School Library Journal*

"This book is well-balanced. ... a must for public and school libraries."
— *VOYA: Voice of Youth Advocates, Dec '03*

"The chapters are quick to make a connection to their teenage reading audience. The prose is straightforward and the book lends itself to spot reading. It should be useful both for practical information and for research, and it is suitable for public and school libraries."
— *American Reference Books Annual, 2003*

"Recommended reference source."
— *Booklist, American Library Association, Feb '03*

"This is an excellent resource for teens and their parents. Education about drugs and substances is key to discouraging teen drug abuse and this book provides this much needed information in a way that is interesting and factual." — *Doody's Review Service, Dec '02*

# Eating Disorders Information for Teens

### Health Tips about Anorexia, Bulimia, Binge Eating, and Other Eating Disorders

*Including Information on the Causes, Prevention, and Treatment of Eating Disorders, and Such Other Issues as Maintaining Healthy Eating and Exercise Habits*

Edited by Sandra Augustyn Lawton. 337 pages. 2005. 978-0-7808-0783-9.

"An excellent resource for teens and those who work with them."
— *VOYA: Voice of Youth Advocates, Apr '06*

"A welcome addition to high school and undergraduate libraries." — *American Reference Books Annual, 2006*

"This book covers the topic in a lucid manner but delves deeper into every aspect of an eating disorder. A solid addition for any nonfiction or reference collection." — *School Library Journal, Dec '05*

# Fitness Information for Teens

### Health Tips about Exercise, Physical Well-Being, and Health Maintenance

*Including Facts about Aerobic and Anaerobic Conditioning, Stretching, Body Shape and Body Image, Sports Training, Nutrition, and Activities for Non-Athletes*

Edited by Karen Bellenir. 425 pages. 2004. 978-0-7808-0679-5.

"Another excellent offering from Omnigraphics in their *Teen Health Series*. ... This book will be a great addition to any public, junior high, senior high, or secondary school library."
— *American Reference Books Annual, 2005*

# Learning Disabilities Information for Teens

### Health Tips about Academic Skills Disorders and Other Disabilities That Affect Learning

*Including Information about Common Signs of Learning Disabilities, School Issues, Learning to Live with a Learning Disability, and Other Related Issues*

Edited by Sandra Augustyn Lawton. 337 pages. 2005. 978-0-7808-0796-9.

"This book provides a wealth of information for any reader interested in the signs, causes, and consequences

of learning disabilities, as well as related legal rights and educational interventions. . . . Public and academic libraries should want this title for both students and general readers."
— *American Reference Books Annual, 2006*

# Mental Health Information for Teens, 2nd Edition

*Health Tips about Mental Wellness and Mental Illness*

*Including Facts about Mental and Emotional Health, Depression and Other Mood Disorders, Anxiety Disorders, Behavior Disorders, Self-Injury, Psychosis, Schizophrenia, and More*

Edited by Karen Bellenir. 400 pages. 2006. 978-0-7808-0863-8.

"In both language and approach, this user-friendly entry in the *Teen Health Series* is on target for teens needing information on mental health concerns."
— *Booklist, American Library Association, Jan '02*

"Readers will find the material accessible and informative, with the shaded notes, facts, and embedded glossary insets adding appropriately to the already interesting and succinct presentation."
— *School Library Journal, Jan '02*

"This title is highly recommended for any library that serves adolescents and parents/caregivers of adolescents."
— *E-Streams, Jan '02*

"Recommended for high school libraries and young adult collections in public libraries. Both health professionals and teenagers will find this book useful."
— *American Reference Books Annual, 2002*

"This is a nice book written to enlighten the society, primarily teenagers, about common teen mental health issues. It is highly recommended to teachers and parents as well as adolescents."
— *Doody's Review Service, Dec '01*

# Sexual Health Information for Teens

*Health Tips about Sexual Development, Human Reproduction, and Sexually Transmitted Diseases*

*Including Facts about Puberty, Reproductive Health, Chlamydia, Human Papillomavirus, Pelvic Inflammatory Disease, Herpes, AIDS, Contraception, Pregnancy, and More*

Edited by Deborah A. Stanley. 391 pages. 2003. 978-0-7808-0445-6.

"This work should be included in all high school libraries and many larger public libraries. . . . highly recommended."
— *American Reference Books Annual, 2004*

"*Sexual Health* approaches its subject with appropriate seriousness and offers easily accessible advice and information."
— *School Library Journal, Feb '04*

# Skin Health Information for Teens

*Health Tips about Dermatological Concerns and Skin Cancer Risks*

*Including Facts about Acne, Warts, Hives, and Other Conditions and Lifestyle Choices, Such as Tanning, Tattooing, and Piercing, That Affect the Skin, Nails, Scalp, and Hair*

Edited by Robert Aquinas McNally. 429 pages. 2003. 978-0-7808-0446-3.

"This volume, as with others in the series, will be a useful addition to school and public library collections."
— *American Reference Books Annual, 2004*

"There is no doubt that this reference tool is valuable."
— *VOYA: Voice of Youth Advocates, Feb '04*

"This volume serves as a one-stop source and should be a necessity for any health collection."
— *Library Media Connection*

# Sports Injuries Information for Teens

*Health Tips about Sports Injuries and Injury Protection*

*Including Facts about Specific Injuries, Emergency Treatment, Rehabilitation, Sports Safety, Competition Stress, Fitness, Sports Nutrition, Steroid Risks, and More*

Edited by Joyce Brennfleck Shannon. 405 pages. 2003. 978-0-7808-0447-0.

"This work will be useful in the young adult collections of public libraries as well as high school libraries."
— *American Reference Books Annual, 2004*

# Suicide Information for Teens

*Health Tips about Suicide Causes and Prevention*

*Including Facts about Depression, Risk Factors, Getting Help, Survivor Support, and More*

Edited by Joyce Brennfleck Shannon. 368 pages. 2005. 978-0-7808-0737-2.

# Tobacco Information for Teens

*Health Tips about the Hazards of Using Cigarettes, Smokeless Tobacco, and Other Nicotine Products*

*Including Facts about Nicotine Addiction, Immediate and Long-Term Health Effects of Tobacco Use, Related Cancers, Smoking Cessation, Tobacco Use Prevention, and Tobacco Use Statistics*

Edited by Karen Bellenir. 440 pages. 2007. 978-0-7808-0976-5.

# Health Reference Series

Adolescent Health Sourcebook,
2nd Edition

AIDS Sourcebook, 3rd Edition

Alcoholism Sourcebook, 2nd Edition

Allergies Sourcebook, 3rd Edition

Alzheimer's Disease Sourcebook,
3rd Edition

Arthritis Sourcebook, 2nd Edition

Asthma Sourcebook, 2nd Edition

Attention Deficit Disorder Sourcebook

Back & Neck Sourcebook, 2nd Edition

Blood & Circulatory Disorders
Sourcebook, 2nd Edition

Brain Disorders Sourcebook, 2nd Edition

Breast Cancer Sourcebook, 2nd Edition

Breastfeeding Sourcebook

Burns Sourcebook

Cancer Sourcebook, 5th Edition

Cancer Sourcebook for Women,
3rd Edition

Cancer Survivorship Sourcebook

Cardiovascular Diseases & Disorders
Sourcebook, 3rd Edition

Caregiving Sourcebook

Child Abuse Sourcebook

Childhood Diseases & Disorders
Sourcebook

Colds, Flu & Other Common Ailments
Sourcebook

Communication Disorders Sourcebook

Complementary & Alternative Medicine
Sourcebook, 3rd Edition

Congenital Disorders Sourcebook,
2nd Edition

Contagious Diseases Sourcebook

Cosmetic & Reconstructive Surgery
Sourcebook, 2nd

Death & Dying Sourcebook, 2nd Edition

Dental Care & Oral Health Sourcebook,
2nd Edition

Depression Sourcebook

Dermatological Disorders Sourcebook,
2nd Edition

Diabetes Sourcebook, 3rd Edition

Diet & Nutrition Sourcebook,
3rd Edition

Digestive Diseases & Disorder
Sourcebook

Disabilities Sourcebook

Domestic Violence Sourcebook,
2nd Edition

Drug Abuse Sourcebook, 2nd Edition

Ear, Nose & Throat Disorders
Sourcebook, 2nd Edition

Eating Disorders Sourcebook, 2nd Edition

Emergency Medical Services Sourcebook

Endocrine & Metabolic Disorders
Sourcebook, 2nd Edition

EnvironmentalHealth Sourcebook,
2nd Edition

Ethnic Diseases Sourcebook

Eye Care Sourcebook, 2nd Edition

Family Planning Sourcebook

Fitness & Exercise Sourcebook,
3rd Edition

Food Safety Sourcebook

Forensic Medicine Sourcebook

Gastrointestinal Diseases & Disorders
Sourcebook, 2nd Edition

Genetic Disorders Sourcebook,
3rd Edition

Head Trauma Sourcebook

Headache Sourcebook

Health Insurance Sourcebook

Healthy Aging Sourcebook

Healthy Children Sourcebook

Healthy Heart Sourcebook for Women

Hepatitis Sourcebook

Household Safety Sourcebook

Hypertension Sourcebook

Immune System Disorders Sourcebook,
2nd Edition

Infant & Toddler Health Sourcebook

Infectious Diseases Sourcebook